2ND EDITION

Nurse-Midwifery
Handbook

A Practical Guide to
Prenatal and Postpartum Care

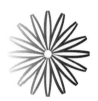

2 ND EDITION

Nurse-Midwifery Handbook

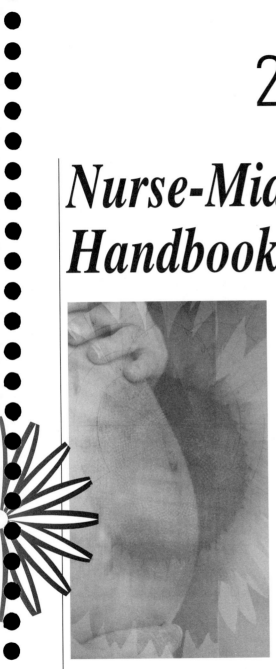

A Practical Guide to Prenatal and Postpartum Care

Linda Wheeler, CNM, EdD
Oregon Health and Science University
Portland, Oregon

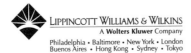

LIPPINCOTT WILLIAMS & WILKINS
A **Wolters Kluwer** Company

Philadelphia · Baltimore · New York · London
Buenos Aires · Hong Kong · Sydney · Tokyo

Acquisitions Editor: Jennifer E. Brogan
Assistant Editor: Susan Barta Rainey
Senior Project Editor: Erika Kors
Senior Production Manager: Helen Ewan
Managing Editor/Production: Barbara Ryalls
Art Director: Carolyn O'Brien
Design: BJ Crim
Manufacturing Manager: William Alberti
Compositor: Lippincott Williams & Wilkins
Printer: Vicks Litho

Edition 2

9 8 7 6 5 4 3 2 1

Library of Congress Cataloging-in-Publication Data
Wheeler, Linda A.
   Nurse-midwifery handbook: a practical guide to prenatal and postpartum care / Linda Wheeler.—2nd ed.
      p. cm.
   Includes bibliographical references and index.
   ISBN 0-7817-2929-7 (alk. paper)
      1. Midwifery—Handbooks, manuals, etc. 2. Prenatal care—Handbooks, manuals, etc. 3. Postnatal care—Handbooks, manuals, etc. I. Title.
   RG950.W48 2002
   618.2—dc21   2001050540

Care has been taken to confirm the accuracy of the information presented and to describe generally accepted practices. However, the authors, editors, and publisher are not responsible for errors or omissions or for any consequences from application of the information in this book and make no warranty, express or implied, with respect to the content of the publication.

The authors, editors, and publisher have exerted every effort to ensure that drug selection and dosage set forth in this text are in accordance with the current recommendations and practice at the time of publication. However, in view of ongoing research, changes in government regulations, and the constant flow of information relating to drug therapy and drug reactions, the reader is urged to check the package insert for each drug for any change in indications and dosage and for added warnings and precautions. This is particularly important when the recommended agent is a new or infrequently employed drug.

Some drugs and medical devices presented in this publication have Food and Drug Administration (FDA) clearance for limited use in restricted research settings. It is the responsibility of the health care provider to ascertain the FDA status of each drug or device planned for use in his or her clinical practice.

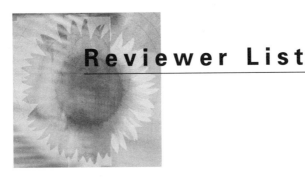

Reviewer List

Nancy Alley, MS, PhD, RN-C
Professor/Associate Dean
College of Nursing
East Tennessee State University
Johnson City, Tennessee

Diana Dowdy, RN, MN, CNM, RDMS
Certified Nurse-Midwife/Registered Sonographer (OB-GYN)
Clinic for Women
Huntsville, Alabama

Linda Glenn, CNM, PMHNP, MN, MPH
Instructor
Oregon Health and Science University
Portland, Oregon

Sally Hersh, CNM, MSN
Instructor
Oregon Health and Science University
Portland, Oregon

Susan Rice, PhD
Samford University
Ida V. Moffett School of Nursing
Birmingham, Alabama

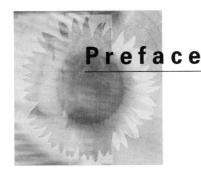

Preface

In my journey as teacher and clinician I remain in awe of the process of birth and the importance of respecting a woman's desire for the way it should be conducted. Yet, although midwifery care acknowledges that a baby's birth can be a life-changing event for women, midwives know that pregnancy and birth occur not as isolated incidents, but within the context of a woman's life. Accordingly, the kind of care a woman receives prenatally and postpartally is of the utmost importance. Not only must that care consist of an awareness of the physical problems a pregnant woman and her baby may face, but midwifery care must also address the meaning of the pregnancy to the woman on social, emotional, and spiritual levels.

The second edition of Nurse-Midwifery Handbook: A Practical Guide To Prenatal And Postpartum Care continues to be a guide for novice practitioners of midwifery. It combines recent factual information on which to base care with suggestions for providing holistic care and for addressing difficult issues. Readers will find some changes in this edition. The four parts into which the first edition was divided (preconception care, the initial prenatal visit, the return visit, and postpartum care) have been subdivided into chapters for quicker reference. Useful facts have been put in boxes and tables so that the information is easy to obtain. Findings from more than 200 new references have been incorporated. To avoid repetition, substantial information on many topics can be found in the initial prenatal visit chapter. A topic is addressed again in other chapters either to stress its importance or to address its application at a different time or in a different context.

The appendices contain information for both practitioners and patients. Feel free to copy the patient-related information to give to patients. Better yet, revise it to suit your client population or reflect the nuances of your own practice.

You may find it useful to laminate copies of the information contained in some of the boxes, tables, and figures. Laminated copies measuring approximately 4 × 6 inches fit nicely in a lab coat pocket and make guidelines and important facts readily available for repeated use. Try copying each topic onto paper of a different color so that each subject can be easily found from within your pocket. Among the topics often found to be useful when laminated are the "Healthy Pregnancy Questions," "How to Review an AP Chart," the "Food Guide Pyramid/Serving Sizes," and "Determining Body Mass Index." You might want to enlarge and then laminate (on 8×11 inch paper) the BMI Index and "Essential Information and Key Moments in Prenatal Care." Post them for easy reference in your clinic or office. Add laminated information from other areas of your practice and put them on a small key ring.

I find that use of patient history forms increases the amount of time I can spend with clients attending to psychosocial issues. Whether it is the Initial Prenatal Visit form, the Return Prenatal Visit form, or the Postpartum History form, I can quickly scan the information given by the client and highlight responses that should be discussed whereas, if I take the time to ask each question individually, I end up with similar information but minimal time to address it. Again, feel free to copy the history forms for use with your own clients, making revisions that reflect topics you wish to address using phrasing with which you are comfortable and that is understood by your clients.

In this digital age, I encourage all midwives to buy a PDA (personal digital assistant) to store information important to patient care. It is impossible to recall all of the facts, approaches, and management guidelines needed to provide the very best prenatal care—help is at hand with the PDA.

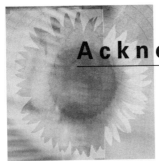

Acknowledgments

I wish to express my gratitude to Linda Glenn, CNM, PMHNP, MN, MPH, and Sally Hersh, CNM, MS, for serving as reviewers for this book. Their comments were invaluable. Any errors or omissions, however, are my own.

I also wish to express my gratitude to my midwifery sisters at Oregon Health and Science University. Their clinical skill and devotion to the families who have come to us for care make me proud to be one of them. The women I have worked with at OHSU for many years include:

* Linda Glenn, a graduate of the Nurse-Midwifery Program at the University of Mississippi and a special friend, who has the amazing ability to deliver the same exquisite care to families from every walk of life and in every setting. She is masterful at helping families understand all of their options, supporting their decisions, and championing their rights. Going "the extra mile" for patients, students, and friends is routine for Linda.

* Carol Howe, a graduate of the Yale University Nurse-Midwifery Program, who started both the OHSU Nurse-Midwifery Service and the Education Program. A quiet leader, Carol is unfailingly kind, flexible, and supportive. She is an accomplished teacher. Tough issues do not faze her. Her clear thinking and practical problem solving have earned her the respect of the OHSU School of Nursing faculty.

* Polly Malby, a graduate of the Nurse-Midwifery Program at the University of Mississippi, who is passionate about the wonders of birth and the strength of women. Also an artist and a dedicated teacher, Polly's creative approaches to helping students learn and her commitment to doing whatever it takes to help them succeed make her an incredible role model as both clinician and teacher.

* Linda Robrecht, a graduate of the Intercampus Graduate Studies Program of the University of California at San Francisco and the

University of California at San Diego, who is a brilliant teacher with an amazing ability to translate science into art. Her innovative teaching methods resonate with students, and her ability to analyze student strengths is enviable. Who else could make research exciting for midwifery students!

❖ Nancy Sullivan, a graduate of the Columbia University Nurse-Midwifery Program, who was born with a midwifery heart. Nancy is a gifted clinician who has the respect not only of her midwifery colleagues, but of nurses and physicians as well. While grounded in respect for birth as normal, Nancy has a practical side that has kept us financially solvent. Additionally, her computer skills have led to the establishment of an extraordinary database that allows us to analyze both practices and outcomes.

I also wish to acknowledge the following:

1. The nurses and residents at OHSU Hospital. Their support of midwifery practice at this institution has made working here a delight.
2. The OHSU Department of OB/GYN physician faculty who have consistently endorsed midwifery care with words and actions and have helped us deliver quality care to the families whose births we attend.
3. Renne Lann, RN, BS, clinic nurse for the OHSU CNMs, whose dedication to our patients is unsurpassed and whose skill, good humor, and willingness to try anything new make our prenatal clinic such an exciting place to be.
4. Marie Brown, CNM, PNP, PhD, and Virginia Capan, CNM, MN, MA, friends of many years who have influenced not only my professional life, but my personal life as well.

Contents

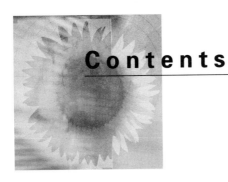

xiv   ❖ *Contents*

Chapter 6
Health Education at the
Initial Prenatal Visit   174

PART 4   The Postpartum
              Period   273

Chapter 10
Transition to
Parenthood   275

Chapter 11
Postpartum Complications   279

Chapter 15
Health Issues
for Women   346

PART 1 Preconception Counseling

Every pregnant woman desires a healthy outcome for both herself and her baby. In the United States, the chances for a successful pregnancy are overwhelmingly in the favor of most women. Part I of this book discusses the preconception visit, an opportunity for a woman or couple to consider the risks that pregnancy or birth might pose. To this end the visit consists of a medical history (personal and family) and an obstetric history, upon which a midwife might recommend laboratory testing and, at times, a referral to specialists.

Preconception counseling can help a woman and her family make a good decision about attempting pregnancy, and women whose pregnancies are considered high risk can receive information about the tests, procedures, and medicines likely to be recommended. Information obtained from the preconception interview may indicate a need for genetic counseling and possible testing that could help parents make a decision about becoming pregnant.

Chapter 1 discusses the historical information that should be obtained at a preconception visit. An additional advantage to a preconception interview with a nurse-midwife is the opportunity to discuss ways to have a healthier pregnancy, readiness for parenting, and options for childbirth. Chapter 2 addresses these topics.

Chapter 1

Health and Health-Related Information

Pregnancy outcome is influenced by many factors. Information needed to assess the risks of pregnancy for either the mother or her baby includes the mother's age, menstrual history, presence of certain organic diseases, previous reproductive history, health habits, use of medications, exposure to environmental toxins, and family medical problems. The medical history of the baby's father and his family as well as information about other pregnancies in which he was the father of the baby should also be obtained. Midwives, bringing a holistic approach to pregnancy and birth, will also seek information about the client's emotional well-being.

✳ Communication Skills

Good communication increases the chances for a productive interview. Asking questions in a way that invites the client to share parts of her life with you, parts that, at times, the client may be reluctant to disclose, is an art that develops with time and with practice. Studies show that most clinicians do a good job of establishing the reason for the client's visit. What worries the client and what the client thinks she needs are pieces of information elicited less frequently, even though the answers to these questions may be key to the client's willingness to respond to your questions and adhere to a plan of care.

✳ HELPFUL HINT

Ask colleagues how they phrase sensitive questions. Listen to interviews conducted by other health professionals to get ideas for approaches that will increase your skill.

Right from the start you want to convey interest, thoughtfulness, understanding, and concern for the client's comfort and privacy. Be aware of your personal appearance. In general, conservative clothing and hairstyle are more readily accepted in most settings. Tie back long hair so that it does not fall across the client's body or need to be repeatedly flipped back over your ears as you bend your head to chart or perform a physical examination. Commit to short fingernails. Note mannerisms you have that may be distracting. For example, frequent use of "okay," "uh," "basically," and even head nodding can be annoying. The way you ask questions, the words you use, your tone of voice, and expressions of interest can influence how much the client will tell you.

 HELPFUL HINT

Purchase old teacups at a garage sale and offer tea to the client and her family. Enjoy a cup yourself as you sit and talk.

 HELPFUL HINT

Arrange to videotape a history-taking session (with the client's permission, of course). Because most of us are unaware of personal mannerisms that can be distracting, the videotape can be enlightening!

Barriers to Good Communication

Be aware of obstacles to a productive interview. These might include the physical setting, time constraints imposed by the workplace, your own fears and resistance (feeling intrusive, embarrassed, helpless, or awkward; wanting to fix things), and reservations on the part of the client. Respect the client's decisions about what she will share. As the interview progresses, ask the client, "Is that something that worries you?" and "What would relieve your concern?" Respect cultural proscriptions by learning about the values and customs of the families that frequent your clinic or office. And be aware of the potential for violating "boundaries" with physical contact. For example, a hug can be frightening to a woman who has been sexually abused. In fact, women with a history of sexual abuse may not wish any unnecessary physical contact from the clinician. Also, keep in mind that as the health care provider, you are in a position of power. Always use that power in an ethical way.

No one interview approach works well with all women. This is particularly true when it comes to asking questions about sensitive subjects—social support, substance abuse, domestic violence, sexual abuse, emotional problems, mental illness. Yet, these topics are just as important as genetic, medical, and obstetric factors.

❖ Maternal Age

Pregnancy, labor, and birth are safest in most respects when a baby is born to a woman between the ages of 20 and 34. Both younger (aged 13–17) and older (aged 18 or 19) teenage mothers have an increased chance of delivering premature and growth restricted (IUGR) babies. Problems encountered by older women (age 35 or older at delivery, 34 years of age in some institutions) are often the result of chromosomal abnormalities or medical complications from chronic illness. Table 1-1 summarizes the risk of chromosomal abnormalities identified in the second trimester for infants born to women at various ages.

Women who will be 34 or 35 years of age or older at the birth of their babies should be offered genetic counseling. Counseling should include the range of options for diagnostic testing as well as the timing of tests and procedures. The lay public often knows of the increased risk of Down syndrome (trisomy 21) in babies of older women giving birth. In fact, Down syndrome accounts for only half of the risk of a chromosomal error in babies of this age group. "Counseling for advanced maternal age should correct this misperception and include a full discussion of the spectrum of chromosomal abnormalities and their phenotypes. This discussion should cover the trisomies 21, 18, and 13 as well as the sex aneuploidies of 47, XXX, and 46, XXY" (Scioscia, 1999).

In addition to the increased risk of giving birth to a baby with genetic/chromosomal abnormalities, older gravidas are more likely to have medical problems that contribute to a greater risk for spontaneous abortion, premature separation of the placenta, intrauterine growth restriction (IUGR), preeclampsia, macrosomia (abnormally large baby), and stillbirth. Preterm delivery increases because labor is induced more often for maternal medical problems and small-for-dates babies.

Fortunately, treatment is available for many chronic medical disorders, and the number of stillborn babies in this age group is low. When older women without chronic disease carry a chromosomally normal baby, clinicians should be optimistic about the outcome of pregnancy (Cunningham & Leveno, 1995). Classifying all older gravidas as high risk because of biologic aging is not appropriate.

❖ Menstrual History

The menstrual history is an important part of the preconception interview as it provides information about the likelihood of ovulation occurring. Normal menstrual cycles have a range of 18 to 40 days. In two thirds of women, menstruation occurs at 28-day intervals, plus or minus 3 days (American College of Obstetricians and Gynecologists [ACOG], 1989). "Uniformity of the men-

TABLE 1.1 Midtrimester Risk of Chromosomal Abnormalities

Maternal Age*	Risk for Down Syndrome	Total Risk for Chromosomal Abnormalities[†]
20	1:1667	1:526
21	1:1667	1:526
22	1:1429	1:500
23	1:1429	1:500
24	1:1250	1:476
25	1:1250	1:476
26	1:1176	1:476
27	1:1111	1:455
28	1:1053	1:435
29	1:1000	1:417
30	1:952	1:385
31	1:909	1:385
32	1:769	1:322
33	1:602	1:286
34	1:485	1:238
35	1:378	1:192
36	1:289	1:156
37	1:224	1:127
38	1:173	1:102
39	1:136	1:83
40	1:106	1:66
41	1:82	1:53
42	1:63	1:42
43	1:49	1:33
44	1:38	1:26
45	1:30	1:21
46	1:23	1:16
47	1:18	1:13
48	1:14	1:10
49	1:11	1:8

*Because sample size for some intervals is relatively small, 95% confidence limits are sometimes relatively large. Nonetheless, these figures are suitable for genetic counseling.

†47 XXX excluded for ages 20–32 (data not available) (Source: American College of Obstetricians and Gynecologists. *Antenatal diagnosis of genetic disorders*. Technical Bulletin No. 108. Washington, DC: ACOG © 1987. Reprinted with permission.)

strual interval, duration of flow, and amount of flow are strongly indicative of an ovulatory menstrual pattern. Of even greater importance is the presence of characteristic menstrual molimina (bloating sensation, mood changes, uterine cramping, and breast tenderness). In contrast, an unpredictable menstrual pattern is highly suggestive of an anovulatory or oligoovulatory disorder"

(ACOG, 1994, p. 1). Women whose menstrual cycles fall outside the range of normal should be asked about pubertal milestones, employment, diet, exercise habits, use of medications or drugs, environmental exposures, psychological stress, and any family history of amenorrhea or genetic anomalies as these can influence the cycle. Referral to a specialist may be indicated if the client with menstrual irregularities decides she wishes to become pregnant, particularly if she is older.

❈ Personal Medical History

Organic Disease

Certain medical conditions have the potential for affecting the mother or baby or both. A prospective mother needs to know if her own disease may worsen or interfere with her baby's well-being. Some of the more common, serious medical conditions in this category are seizure disorders, diabetes mellitus, hypertension, cancer, autoimmune disorders, heart disease, hematologic disorders, and HIV disease.

Seizure Disorders

While most women with seizure disorders find that pregnancy has no effect on their disease, one third find an increase in seizure activity. The latter are likely to be women with severe epilepsy (Wilhelm, Morris, & Hotham, 1990). Compared with nonepileptics, women with epilepsy have a twofold increased risk of giving birth to a child with malformations (Cunningham, Gant, Leveno, Gilstrap, Hauth, & Wenstrom, 2001) and a 2% to 3% risk of having a child with a seizure disorder. They are also at increased risk for preeclampsia and preterm labor.

The most important step toward a good pregnancy outcome for women who are epileptic is seizure control before pregnancy. Close follow-up during pregnancy is particularly important because changes in metabolism lower the levels of antiepileptic drugs during pregnancy. Medication dosage may need to be increased.

Activities known to trigger seizures should be avoided insofar as possible. Adequate sleep may be helpful. Babies of women who take phenytoin (Dilantin) for seizure control are at risk for fetal hydantoin syndrome and hemorrhagic disease of the newborn. Fetal hydantoin syndrome is characterized by IUGR, microcephaly, facial abnormalities, developmental delays, and mental retardation. The exact contribution of phenytoin to fetal abnormalities is unknown, as it is difficult to distinguish between the effects of disease and those of the medicine. Fetal hydantoin syndrome may even be a combination of each.

Women with epilepsy need 4 mg of folic acid daily rather than the 0.4 mg (400 μg) usually recommended to prevent neural tube defects. Consultation with a physician prior to conception should occur when a woman is epileptic.

Insulin-Dependent Diabetes Mellitus

Many years ago few women with diabetes were able to conceive. Those who did become pregnant experienced high rates of fetal loss. Stillbirth was common. The advent of insulin made motherhood possible for diabetic women, but the road to a healthy baby without maternal morbidity can be difficult, especially for women with poorly managed or difficult-to-control diabetes.

Women with insulin-dependent diabetes mellitus (IDDM) may develop severe hypertension, preeclampsia, ketoacidosis, excessive amniotic fluid, and even blindness and renal failure. The fetus is at increased risk for congenital abnormalities and may be unusually large (macrosomic) or small (IUGR). If the baby is macrosomic, vaginal delivery can be traumatic to both mother and baby. Difficulty delivering the baby's shoulders can lacerate maternal tissue and damage the baby's arm and clavicle. Postpartum hemorrhage is more likely to occur. Women with IDDM should be followed by an obstetrician or perinatologist when possible.

Hypertension

Most women with Stage 1 and 2 chronic hypertension (systolic blood pressure of 140–179 mm Hg or diastolic blood pressure of 90–109 mm Hg) are at low risk for cardiovascular complications during pregnancy, and most will have good maternal and neonatal outcomes if normal renal function is present. Serum creatinine is a marker of renal function, and levels above 1.4 mg/dL at conception increase the risk of fetal loss and progression of maternal renal disease. "Women with renal diseases that tend to progress should be encouraged to complete their childbearing while their renal function is well preserved" (National High Blood Pressure Education Program Working Group on High Blood Pressure in Pregnancy, 2000, p. 13).

Hypertension-related perinatal morbidity and mortality is usually due to superimposed preeclampsia, a complication that occurs in almost 25% of pregnancies in women with preexisting hypertension. "The incidence is even higher if the high blood pressure is associated with renal insufficiency, the presence of hypertension for at least 4 years, and a history of hypertension in a previous pregnancy. The incidence of placental abruption is markedly increased in the presence of superimposed preeclampsia" (National High Blood Pressure Education Program Working Group on High Blood Pressure in Pregnancy, 2000, p. 12). Fetal growth restriction also occurs with chronic hypertension. Ultrasound examinations for growth will be important during pregnancy, as may additional testing for fetal well-being.

Cancer

Although spontaneous abortion is increased in cancer survivors, the risk of cancer to their offspring is not increased unless a parent carries a cancer-susceptibility gene. A woman who has had cancer is likely to ask about her risk for a recurrence of the cancer as well as the child's risk for cancer. These women should be referred to a genetic counselor who can help an individual woman evaluate her risk. Congenital malformation rates after radiation and chemotherapy do not seem to be increased (Schneider, 1994b).

Autoimmune Disorders

In pathogenic situations the immune system turns against itself (autoimmune disorder), causing severe and debilitating illness. Antiphospholipid syndrome and systemic lupus erythematosus are two examples of these disorders. During pregnancy, autoantibodies can cause thrombosis and stroke, preeclampsia, IUGR, and fetal death. Birth is often preterm as labor is likely to be induced or a cesarean section performed because of maternal or fetal complications.

Antiphospholipid Syndrome

Antiphospholipid syndrome (APS) is an autoimmune disorder characterized by thrombosis (usually in a lower extremity as well as pulmonary embolus) and thrombocytopenia. The antiphospholipid antibodies, lupus anticoagulant, and anticardiolipin antibodies are present and, in pregnancy, are associated with repeated spontaneous abortion, second and third trimester fetal loss, preeclampsia, IUGR, and preterm birth.

Systemic Lupus Erythematosus

Systemic lupus erythematosus (SLE), a multisystem connective tissue disease of unknown etiology, can cause spontaneous abortion, IUGR, preterm rupture of membranes and delivery, congenital cardiac defects including heart block, and perinatal death. The effect of SLE on pregnant women is variable. Some women experience no new problems. Others experience an exacerbation of symptoms with hospitalization required. Complications during pregnancy include cerebral infarction, disease flares, and preeclampsia. During labor and birth, complications include uterine rupture, bilateral retinal detachment, retinopathy, stroke, and deep vein thrombosis (Chang & Ramsey-Goldman, 2001).

Preconception counseling for these women should include a discussion about complications, risks for pregnancy loss, and contraindications to pregnancy. Physician involvement is essential. Pregnancy should await a 6-month period of remission. Women who are taking cyclophosphamide or warfarin should not consider pregnancy until these drugs are discontinued. Before conception an evaluation of organ function (cardiac, lung, neurologic, renal, hematologic) and current disease activity should occur. Multiple laboratory tests should be performed. Prospective parents should be advised that pregnancy management is likely to include weekly clinic or office visits, early and frequent tests of fetal well-being, serial sonograms, and preterm induction of labor or planned cesarean birth (Silver & Branch, 1999).

Tuberculosis

Tuberculosis can be a serious and potentially debilitating disease. The concern for pregnant women with tuberculosis is not the effect that pregnancy has on the disease or vice versa; rather, the concern is for the potential effects on the fetus of the chemotherapeutic agents used for treatment. Fetal infection is rare.

Thyroid Disease

Fatigue and menstrual irregularities occur in both hypothyroidism and hyperthyroidism. Weight gain, cold intolerance, or both are characteristic of hypothyroidism, and weight loss, heat intolerance, or both are characteristic of hyperthyroidism. Testing for thyroid disease is appropriate when these symptoms are reported during the preconception interview.

Both hypothyroid and hyperthyroid disease can pose problems for women and their babies. Infertility may preclude pregnancy. Pregnant women with untreated thyroid disease have higher rates of low-birth-weight and stillborn babies. While hypothyroidism is rarely a problem in pregnancy as long as a woman who is hypothyroid continues to take thyroid medication (usually levothyroxine), without appropriate medicine the newborn may have congenital hypothyroidism and associated mental retardation. Thyroid replacement therapy for the baby must be initiated soon after birth. Women with hyperthyroidism are at increased risk for preeclampsia and heart failure. Their babies can have neonatal thyrotoxicosis and die in utero (ACOG, 1993).

Heart Disease

The preconception evaluation should identify persons with existing cardiac disease, considering cardiac disease contributes substantially to maternal death. Referral to a specialist is important as pregnancy is contraindicated in certain cardiac diseases. Maternal mortality varies from less than 1% with some conditions (corrected tetralogy of Fallot) to as high as 50% in others (pulmonary hypertension, complicated coarctation of the aorta, Marfan syndrome with aortic involvement). A decision about whether to attempt pregnancy when cardiac disease is present is best made by a perinatologist working in conjunction with a cardiac specialist.

Hematologic Disorders

Certain anemias have health implications for both mother and baby. For example, some of the thalassemias are associated with preterm labor, IUGR, and increased fetal loss. Babies may have severe anemia. Sickle cell trait increases the risk of urinary tract infection in pregnant women.

Women with hematologic problems need consultation with a perinatologist before making a final decision about whether to attempt pregnancy. Often the father of the baby should be tested to identify the nature and extent of the risk.

Sexually Transmitted Infections

Perinatal outcome can be influenced by various sexually transmitted diseases. Infections caused by *Chlamydia trachomatis* and *Neisseria gonorrhoeae* can cause pelvic inflammatory disease (PID), infertility, and ectopic pregnancy. Salpingitis, one of the sequelae of these infections, increases the risk for infertility and ectopic pregnancy by causing "agglutination of the absorbent folds of the tubal mucosa with narrowing of the lumen or formation of blind pockets. Reduced ciliation of the tubal mucosa because of infection also may contribute to tubal implantation of the zygote" (Cunningham et al., 2001, p. 884). A single instance of PID increases a woman's chances of having an ectopic pregnancy sevenfold (Oregon Health Division, 1995). Vaginal delivery of a baby born to a mother with gonorrhea can lead to blindness in the baby if untreated, and chlamydia can cause both conjunctivitis and pneumonia.

Infants born vaginally to women with a primary outbreak of the type-2 herpes virus have a 40% chance of developing neonatal herpes infections. The risk of neonatal infection with a recurrent lesion is probably 1% to 2% (Gibbs & Sweet, 1999). Still, genital herpes lesions or prodromal herpes symptoms are considered reasons for cesarean delivery. With the development of herpes type-specific serologic testing, identification of women who are negative for the type-2 virus is increasingly possible. Considering most women infected with the herpes virus are unaware of their infection, testing can identify women who should be counseled about avoiding intercourse during pregnancy with someone known to have the type-2 virus. Women who have never noted symptoms of a herpes infection but have a partner who admits to a type-2 infection should undergo type-specific serologic testing. If test results are negative, they should avoid intercourse during pregnancy. Condom use does not give sufficient protection against transmission of the virus.

The AIDS epidemic has not bypassed pregnant women. Women are 8 times more likely than men to contract HIV during intercourse. In nine cities, AIDS is the leading cause of death for women age 22 to 44 (Lee, 2000). Whether HIV disease is affected by pregnancy is not known. It is known, however, that the virus can be passed from the mother to her baby. While at one time it was thought that perinatal transmission might be as high as 50%, maternal treatment with zidovudine (ZDV) prenatally and during labor reduces the transmission rate from 25% to 6%. Scheduled cesarean birth plus prophylactic ZDV further reduces the risk to 2% (ACOG, 1999f).

Decisions about pregnancy in women who are HIV-positive are highly personal and complex. Prenatal care should be shared with specialist physicians and mental health counselors who have experience caring for HIV-positive pregnant women.

❖ Obstetric History

Information about previous pregnancies should be obtained to identify complications that may recur in a subsequent pregnancy. The information obtained often provides an entry for discussions about fears or anxieties about a new pregnancy, as well as an opportunity to discuss emotional responses to previous reproductive problems. Gather the following information:

- Dates of births (term and preterm), miscarriages, elective abortions, ectopic pregnancies, and midpregnancy losses to establish a context for the pregnancies. Three consecutive losses (or two losses in a women older than 35) should prompt referral to a perinatologist.
- Gestational age (in weeks) when the pregnancy ended to identify preterm birth and possible incompetent cervix, conditions likely to recur
- Type of delivery (spontaneous, cesarean, or vacuum/forceps assisted) to identify potentially recurring problems, to determine whether the client would like to attempt a vaginal birth after a cesarean birth should pregnancy occur, and to identify lingering emotional problems related to previous complications
- Length of labor to identify problems associated with a long labor as well as talk about the client's perceptions of the birth experience
- Birth weight to identify babies with low birth weight, intrauterine growth problems, and excessive size, problems with a high recurrence rate
- Sex of the child or children to discuss gender-related issues
- Complications during pregnancy, birth, or the year after the birth to identify problems likely to recur (such as severe preeclampsia and postpartum depression) and to provide an opportunity for the client to talk about her perception of the problems as well as their physical and emotional impact on her and her family
- Perception of previous pregnancy, labor, and birth experience to provide an opportunity for the client to talk about disappointments, present fears, desires for a future birth
- Current health of the child or children to identify problems likely to recur as well as provide an opportunity to talk about the emotional impact of a child who has died or a child with serious physical, mental, or behavioral problems

- Description of where children live to understand the current family constellation and to provide an opportunity for the client to talk about any children being with the other parent, in foster care, or relinquished for adoption

These topics are summarized in Box 1-1.

❋ Risks To Health

Smoking

Babies in utero experience decreased uteroplacental perfusion if their mothers smoke. Mothers who smoke more than half a pack of cigarettes per day give birth to babies likely to weigh less than they would have weighed if the mother had not smoked. In some cases, the effect on the baby is enough to significantly affect birth weight and jeopardize fetal health—11% of the incidences of low birth weight in singleton pregnancies in one study (Pollack, Lantz, & Frohna, 2000). Long-term effects on babies born into households where people smoke include an increased incidence of sudden infant death syndrome (SIDS), meningococcal disease, pneumonia, asthma, bronchitis, colds, and ear infections. Women who are smoking and contemplating pregnancy should stop smoking before conception.

Smokers must deal with both nicotine addiction and psychologic dependence on cigarettes. Whereas nicotine dependence can be eliminated within 2 weeks of complete cessation, psychologic dependence is a more significant force and continues until adequate countering behaviors are adopted (Doerr, 2000, p. 46).

Box 1.1

Data To Be Obtained for the Obstetric History

1. Dates of births (term and preterm), miscarriages, elective abortions, ectopic pregnancies, midpregnancy losses
2. Gestational age (in weeks) when the pregnancy ended
3. Type of delivery (spontaneous, cesarean, or vacuum/forceps assisted)
4. Length of labor(s)
5. Birth weight(s)
6. Sex of the child or children
7. Complications during pregnancy, birth, or the year after the birth
8. Perception of previous pregnancy, labor, and birth experiences
9. Current health of the child or children
10. Description of where child or children are living

The highest success rates for stopping smoking occur with nicotine replacement therapy or antidepressant medication and individual or group counseling. The mechanism by which drugs such as bupropion and nortriptyline work to aid smoking cessation is unknown. When the dosage is excessive (and occasionally with therapeutic doses), bupropion can cause severe anxiety, hypertension, and seizures, particularly in individuals with bulimia or anorexia nervosa (Benowitz, 1997).

However, even brief office intervention can be successful. A strong dose–response relationship between the intensity of tobacco dependence counseling and its effectiveness has been noted. Practical counseling that includes problem-solving help, social support from office or clinic personnel, and social support outside of the office or clinic is helpful.

Treating Tobacco Use and Dependence (U.S. Public Health Service, 2000) is an invaluable clinical guide containing information about the chronic nature of tobacco dependence, effective treatment strategies, and instructions on how to use the five first-line pharmacologic agents to treat tobacco dependence (Table 1-2). Problems and approaches in special populations, including pregnant women, are included. Every clinician should have a copy of this book.

There is no one, perfect, stop-smoking method. In most cities, the American Cancer Society and the American Lung Association maintain lists of resources that can help. A few states have developed "Quit Lines" to provide immediate encouragement, initiate planning for a "quit date," and at times, refer people to agencies that may be able to assist financially. Few people successfully quit on the first attempt. Each office or clinic should establish a mechanism for flagging the medical record of smokers and should make an assessment of client smoking status a part of every initial clinic or office visit. Individuals who have quit smoking should be identified as well because relapse rates are high. These smoking assessments should be documented. Clinician activities to help clients stop smoking are summarized in Box 1-2.

Alcohol

Pregnant women who drink at least one or more drinks per day have a twofold increase in spontaneous abortions (Harlap & Shiono, 1980), and for every two drinks consumed daily in late pregnancy, infant birth weight has been found to decrease by 160 g (Little, 1977). Women who drink while pregnant also risk having a baby with fetal alcohol syndrome (FAS), a syndrome of abnormal facial features, stunted growth, behavior problems, and varying degrees of intellectual handicap. FAS is the leading cause of congenital mental retardation. As FAS children get older, they are likely to have mental health problems (attention-deficit disorder, attention-deficit hyperactivity disorder, conduct disorder, alcohol and drug abuse, depression), as well as problems with mem-

TABLE 1.2 First-Line* Drugs to Aid in Smoking Cessation†

	Dosage	Comments
Bupropion SR (sustained release)	150 mg every morning for 3 days, then increase to b.i.d. for 7 to 12 wk after the quit date	Begin treatment 1 to 2 weeks before quitting. May use b.i.d. for up to 6 months for maintenance.
Nicotine Gum	2 mg for clients smoking <25 cigarettes/day; 4 mg for >25 cigarettes/day	Use for up to 24 weeks. Use no more than 24 pieces/day. Chew gum slowly until a peppery or minty taste is noted, and then "park" gum between cheek and gum for mucosal absorption. Chew and "park" gum for about 30 min.
Nicotine Inhaler	Each cartridge = 4 mg of nicotine over 80 inhalations; use 6 to 16 cartridges/day	Taper dosage during final 3 months of treatment.
Nicotine Nasal Spray	1–2 sprays to each nostril (1 dose) per hr; increase as needed; 8 to 40 doses per day	To avoid irritating effects, do not sniff, swallow, or inhale through nose when administering. Use for 3 to 6 mo. Each bottle contains 100 doses.
Nicotine Patch	Nicoderm CQ: 21 mg/24 h for 4 wk, then 14 mg for 2 wk, then 7 mg for 2 wk	The 16- and 24-h patches have same efficacy.
	Nicotrol: 15 mg/16 h for 8 wk	Consider using lower-dose patch in clients smoking <10 cigarettes/day.

*Safe, effective, and FDA approved
†Adapted from U.S. Public Health Service. (2000). *Treating tobacco use and dependence.* Washington, DC: U.S. Department of Health and Human Services.

Box 1.2

Clinician Activities to Help Clients Stop Smoking

1. Determine the reasons that the client smokes.
2. Determine the stage of readiness for quitting.
3. Identify the sources of support for quitting.
4. Identify the barriers against quitting (such as living with a smoker who is not interested in quitting).
5. Emphasize the benefits.
6. Help the client anticipate and deal with the absence of cigarettes in social situations after eating or drinking coffee.
7. Offer pharmacologic support and referral to groups offering quit-smoking programs.
8. Follow up within 2 weeks of the date the client agrees to quit and again within the next 2 weeks (most relapses occur within the first 3 months).
9. Reassure the client that she can still stop when a relapse occurs (Doerr, 2000).

---

ory, abstract thinking, judgment, and impulse control. They are easily distracted and hypersensitive to criticism, and they find it difficult to follow through with tasks. Psychosocial problems persist into adulthood.

The amount and duration of intrauterine exposure to alcohol required to produce FAS effects is unknown, although a dose-response relationship generally occurs. Greater exposure is associated with more serious effects (Streissguth, Sampson, & Barr, 1989). Individual differences in maternal metabolism of alcohol may account for the large number of babies whose mothers drink heavily in pregnancy but escape the syndrome. The number of drinks consumed, exposure during a period of organogenesis, and genetic sensitivity may also play a role.

While there is no agreed-on definition of alcoholism, the National Institute on Alcohol Abuse and Alcoholism defines the risk of alcohol-related problems as more than seven drinks per week for women (National Institute on Alcohol Abuse and Alcoholism, 1995). Another guideline is the number of drinks it takes before a woman feels high (8 oz of beer equals 5 oz of wine equals 1½ oz 80-proof alcohol). Because most women feel the effects of alcohol by the second drink, a woman who states that it takes three or more drinks before she feels the effect might be a problem drinker.

If you suspect that the client drinks too much, ask, "Do you think you have a drinking problem?" ("Drinking problem" may be better understood and accepted than "alcoholism.") If the client does not feel that a problem exists, yet you do, ask "What would it take for you to think you had a problem?" This question can identify beliefs that interfere with recognition of a personal problem with alcohol. For example, a woman who was 5 months pregnant and worked the evening shift drank 40 oz of beer each night when she arrived home from work. She felt she needed the beer to help her "wind down" enough to sleep and did not feel she had a drinking problem. When asked what it would take for her to feel she had a problem, she replied, "Drinking all day like my sister does."

Clinicians may fear offending clients by asking about alcohol use. Establishing a good relationship with the client and finding the right way to introduce the subject are key factors. At times, it may be helpful to approach this topic peripherally. For example, ask, "How has alcohol affected your life in the past?" to allow the client to talk about growing up in an alcoholic family and her own use, as well as the recent or current use by significant people in her life. You might also say, "Can you tell me a little bit about your experience with alcohol?"

Be sure to ask the client about her partner's consumption of alcohol. A high alcohol intake increases the likelihood of physical and emotional abuse and the use of illicit drugs. Box 1-3 lists questions that may be helpful in assessing a client's use of alcohol.

Illicit Drugs

The true extent of illicit drug use is unknown because the illegal status of these drugs makes users reluctant to discuss them, and they often deny use. Drug use in pregnancy can cause problems during pregnancy, at birth, and into childhood. Longitudinal studies tracking adults exposed to drugs in utero are not available.

As with alcohol, clinicians sometimes hesitate to ask women about drug use for fear of offending them. However, considering neither socioeconomic status nor race /ethnicity help predict which women will have a positive urine drug screen, all women should be asked about past and present use of drugs. Box 1-4 contains questions that can be helpful in identifying the extent of illicit drug use. Ask specifically about marijuana use, as some clients do not place it in the drug category. Most drug users use more than one drug, and almost all drink alcohol as well. Drug use should cease before conception.

In addition to determining whether the client is using drugs, ask about drug use by her partner. Heavy marijuana use can make the user emotionally unavailable to others. All drug use by both partners should cease before any attempt is made to conceive a child. Further discussion of the effect of drugs on the developing fetus can be found in Chapter 3.

Box 1.3

Questions to Ask About Alcohol Use

DIRECT APPROACH

1. How old were you when you first tasted something alcoholic? When did you start seriously drinking?
2. How often do you have a drink of beer, wine, a wine cooler, hard liquor, or anything containing alcohol?
3. When you drink, how often do you have one or two drinks, three or four drinks, or go on binges? You could also ask, "How much alcohol do you drink a week, a month, or a day?" Offer specific choices—a six-pack, a case? Or ask, "On a typical day when you drink, how many drinks do you have?"
4. What is the greatest number of drinks you have had at any one time in the past month?
5. How many drinks does it take to make you feel high?
6. Has anyone ever expressed concern to you about your drinking?
7. Has your drinking ever led to problems between you and your family?
8. Have you ever been in trouble with the law because of your drinking? Have you ever been arrested for driving under the influence of alcohol (DUI)? How many times?
9. Do others encourage you to drink?
10. How many close friends or family members drink a lot or have a drinking problem?

PERIPHERAL APPROACH

1. How has alcohol affected your life?

or

2. Could you tell me a little about your experience with alcohol?

❈ Prescription Medicine, Over-the-Counter Drugs, and Herbal Products

Most pregnant women are aware that certain medicines can be harmful to the growing baby. Many, however, do not know which medicines should be avoided. These are listed in Box 1-5. Fewer women are concerned about teratogenic effects of over-the-counter drugs and herbs. For example, many women do not know that vitamin A consumed in amounts greater than 10,000 IU per day has been found to contribute to cranial-neural crest defects when taken within the first 7 weeks of pregnancy (Rothman et al., 1995). In fact, ACOG does not advocate routine supplementation with vitamin A for women in the United States and recommends a maximum of 5,000 IU per day before pregnancy (ACOG, 1998d).

Box 1.4

Questions to Ask About the Use of Illicit and Recreational Drugs

1. Can you tell me how drugs have affected your life?
2. How old were you when you were first given a drug to try?
3. What drugs have you used?
4. Have you ever been a regular user? For how many months or years?
5. When was the last time you used . . .?
6. How much did you use?
7. Have you also used . . .?
8. How much of that did you use?
9. What about . . .?
10. Have you ever been in a drug treatment program? How many times?
11. Have you ever lost a job or been in trouble with the law because of drugs?
12. How did you use the drugs—smoke, snort, swallow, or inject them?
13. Have you ever shared needles for drugs?

The effectiveness and safety of most herbal products is unknown. In the United States, they are not regulated for either purity or potency. Both adulteration and contamination are possible. Even though the word "standardized" may appear on a product label, the FDA neither sets nor monitors manufacturing standards for herbal products.

"In a survey of adulterants in Chinese herbal products and the side effects occurring with their use, 2,000 cases were screened; 20.4% of the herbal prod-

---

Box 1.5

Medications Associated With Adverse Fetal Effects

ACE inhibitor	Phenytoin
Acetylsalicylic acid	Propylthiouracil, methimazole
Alcohol	Quinolones
Aminopterin methotrexate	Retinoic acid
Carbamazepine	Tetracycline
Daunorubicin	Trimethadione
Lithium	Valproic acid
Methyl mercury	Warfarin

From Dacus, J. V., Meyer, N. L., & Sibai, B. M. (1995). How preconception counseling improves pregnancy outcome. *Contemporary OB/GYN, 40*(6), 115.

ucts were adulterated. The maximum number of adulterants identified in a single herbal product was seven.

In an FDA analysis of 125 products containing ephedra alkaloids, the actual contents ranged from 0 to 110 mg/dose. Some ephedra products contained 6 to 20 additional ingredients. An analysis of 10 brands of ginseng products found a 20-fold variation in the ginsenoside content. Even the quantities stated on the label may not be helpful; for example, in two different brand-name products labeled as containing 648 mg of ginsenoside, there was a 10-fold difference in the actual amount in each product . . ."(Tatro, 1999, p. 35).

Another study of ephedra-containing products showed that of the 20 supplements studied, half had discrepancies of more than 20% in alkaloid content from the content claimed on the label, and one product demonstrated no ephedra alkaloids (Gurley, Gardner, & Hubbard, 2000).

❖ Environmental Exposures

Exposure to toxic elements in the environment can occur while at work, at home, or at play. Unfortunately, except for higher incidences of cancer, little is known about the effect of these substances on humans. While appropriate use of most chemicals is not known to be harmful to the unborn fetus, women should be encouraged to eliminate chemicals from their environment before pregnancy or observe appropriate precautions.

Ask women contemplating pregnancy about current and past exposure to biologic agents, radiation, metals, dust or fibers, fumes, pesticides, and chemicals. Ask also about sick building syndrome, a relatively new phenomenon in which vague symptoms cannot be traced to a single cause. The symptoms probably result from pollutants that are 2 to 5 times and occasionally 100 times more concentrated indoors than outdoors. Among the concerns are:

- Carbon monoxide sucked into a building when air-intake vents overhang loading docks and parking garages
- Volatile organic compounds (VOCs) from furniture, paint, carpet, and office equipment
- Molds and bacteria from heating, ventilation, and air conditioning (HVAC) systems
- Smoke from people puffing on cigarettes at building entrances, which is sucked back into the building when doors open
- Windows that won't open to allow fresh air to enter
- Possible carcinogens in carbonless copy paper
- Spray pesticides (Arndt, 2000)

Health care providers also need to know when their clients have lived in areas where exposure to radiation has occurred. Information specific to the site may be available to both the client and provider. Known exposure to harmful agents should be documented. Appendix A contains a sample exposure history form that can be used if toxic exposure is suspected.

❊ Psychosocial History

"Hard" data on the role of social and emotional factors on the outcome of pregnancy are difficult to find. Part of the problem is that many factors may be involved, and isolating one or two is impossible. Experienced and caring clinicians, nevertheless, *know* that poverty, inadequate housing, problems with relationships, a history of abuse, depression, poor self-esteem, low levels of education, high levels of stress, and meager systems of social support put pregnant women at risk. The preconception counseling visit can be used to identify stressors and sources of support.

History of Abuse

Questions about abuse are best asked when the clinician is alone with the client. If the client is accompanied by a partner, conclude the visit by saying, "I always like to spend a little time alone with each of the potential parents. Would you excuse us for just a few minutes?" When alone, ask the client if there is any information she would like to share in private. After she responds to your question, tell her that you would like to ask her a few personal questions, questions that are asked of everyone who comes for care. You can add, "You don't have to answer any question that you feel is intrusive or none of my business. We know that many women in this country have been physically, emotionally, or sexually hurt at some time in their lives. I am wondering if you have ever been in a relationship in which you were hurt—perhaps slapped or hit, yelled at, put down with words, made to do something you didn't want to do."

A client may or may not wish to admit to a previous or current abusive relationship. Incest is particularly difficult to acknowledge because of its profound negative connotations. If a woman reports having been abused, ask if she has ever talked about the abuse with anyone. Does she have someone with whom she talks now? Perhaps the most important realization is that "Simply asking about abuse—and then listening to a patient's story—can be as important as providing resources and physical care" (Titus, 1996, p. 1865).

Not all women with a history of abuse will want or need discussions on this topic. Human beings are amazingly resilient, and it is inappropriate to create a problem where one does not exist. Some women are not ready to acknowledge an abusive past but respond to continuing expressions of concern from the clinician. Women in abusive relationships who indicate an interest in becoming pregnant should be informed that physical abuse frequently increases during pregnancy.

Discussion of painful issues can be difficult for both clinician and client. Some practitioners hesitate to ask about abuse because they feel they are being intrusive, fear being overwhelmed by the stories, find the stories too painful, think it will take too much time, feel the information is irrelevant, or were taught they should not ask about things for which they can do nothing. Some have misperceptions about which women are abused. A personal history of abuse may arouse feelings of anxiety. In these instances, the clinician may find it helpful to work with a counselor or another supportive person until it is possible to be a helpful listener. In the interim, working with a colleague who can elicit the needed information and act in a therapeutic manner may be necessary.

Box 1-6 lists questions that can be appropriate to ask about physical and emotional abuse. This list of questions will not be suitable in all situations, nor will the approach and phrasing of the questions fit every clinician's style. Develop a personal list of questions or modify those suggested as you gain experience and as you listen to the way colleagues approach this subject.

Intimate Partner Violence

Key factors in helping women in abusive situations include respecting confidentiality, believing and validating the client's experiences, acknowledging the injustice done to her, helping her plan for future safety, promoting access to community services, and respecting her right to make decisions for herself. A woman in a relationship that is currently abusive should be asked if she is in immediate danger. Does she fear for her life? Is there a gun in the house? Are the children in jeopardy? Has she ever thought of leaving her partner because of the abuse? Development of an "action plan" may be appropriate for women who are thinking about leaving abusive situations. Box 1-7 lists items for the mother and her children that should be left in a safe place, perhaps with a neighbor or at work.

At times it is appropriate for the clinician to make the initial contact with a domestic violence shelter or other safe place. A list of names and phone numbers should be available in every clinic or office. Small cards with a list of shelters and emergency phone numbers should be placed in the women's rest rooms. Clinicians should be familiar with counselors, support groups, and organizations in the community with expertise in counseling women who have been abused.

Some women in abusive situations or with a history of abuse appreciate suggestions of books to read as well as a list of support groups. Lists of these should be available. When you find a book you like, call your local library to

Box 1.6

Questions to Ask About Physical or Emotional Abuse

GENERAL QUESTIONS

1. Have you ever been called names, put down, or unfairly accused?
2. Have you ever been pushed, shoved, slapped, hit, punched, or kicked; had something thrown at you; or were hurt in any way?

QUESTIONS ABOUT THE CURRENT PARTNER

1. Does your partner ever do anything that scares you?
2. Are you ever frightened by your partner's temper?
3. Do you ever "give in" because you are afraid of your partner's reaction?
4. Does your partner ever withhold affection as punishment?
5. Does your partner ever threaten to withhold money?
6. Does your partner ever threaten to have an affair?
7. Do you ever apologize to others for your partner's behavior?
8. Has your partner ever tried to stop you from seeing friends?
9. Do you feel isolated?
10. Is your partner jealous of your friends?
11. Do you need your partner's permission to do anything?
12. Has your partner ever threatened to hurt the children, relatives, or pets?
13. Are you afraid of what will happen next or that you can't survive alone?
14. Do you think your partner is capable of killing you?
15. Do you believe accusations of being stupid or worthless, or not doing things right?
16. How many times in the last year have you been involved in yelling or screaming fights?
17. How many times in the past year have you been hit or had something thrown at you?
18. Do you ever hit back?
19. Do you ever hit first?

Adapted from Slaughter, R., & Kanter, L. (1993). Women being alive. *Domestic violence: Is it happening to you?*

see if the book is one that circulates in the library system. If not, ask for the procedure for recommending new books.

If the client agrees to counseling, be sure that it is freely chosen. Avoid suggesting therapy and court mediation to couples because the immediate issue is *not* marital conflict and because court mediation operates on the assumption that two people are equal parties who can negotiate in good faith and arrive at a reasonably equitable solution. Such an assumption is erroneous

---

Box 1.7

Items Women in an Abusive Situation Should Leave in a Safe Place

A change of clothes
Cash for a taxi, change for phone calls, and a prepaid phone card
Car, house, and office keys
A list of emergency phone numbers
Important documents
    Rent receipts, lease agreement, deed to house
    Divorce papers
    Checkbook
    Bank statements
    Car title and vehicle registration
    Insurance papers
    Medical records
    Social security card
    Passport and/or immigration papers
    Medicaid certification
    Birth certificates for self and children
    Immunization records so that the children can enroll in school
Personal hygiene items
Photographs and other personal treasures
Medications
Credit card
Driver's license
A favorite blanket, stuffed animal, book, or small toy for each child

---

when applied to an abuser and reflects ignorance of the dynamics of battering (Fish, 1988).

Clinicians may find it difficult to understand why some women refuse to go to a domestic violence shelter. Unfortunately, life in a shelter is not easy. The rules may be difficult to abide by, the environment is often chaotic, and some shelters will not house male children over the age of 10. Some shelters require a commitment to leaving the relationship. Pets are rarely permitted, leaving women fearful for their pets' safety should they leave. Shelters are often nonexistent in rural communities. Perhaps even more important is that the woman may reasonably fear for the lives of herself and her children should she leave. Clinicians should not focus on the client leaving the situation when leaving is not the option that the client wishes to pursue. Living violence-free is a process rather than an event. The goal must be living free of violence rather than leaving.

HELPFUL HINT

Establish an office or clinic policy stating that all clients meet alone with the clinician at the initial visit. If a partner balks when the clinician addresses meeting alone with the client, invoke the clinic policy. Controlling partners who understand that all clients are treated in this manner may be less threatened and permit the one-to-one discussion.

Sexual Abuse

Information about past or present sexual abuse is also important to obtain. Memories of the abuse (flashbacks) can surface during a pelvic examination, in labor, at birth, and while breastfeeding. Let the client know that you are always ready to listen and can serve as a resource should questions or concerns surface. Respect the desires of the client who does not want to talk with you at this time. It is inappropriate to destroy defense mechanisms, including denial, that help a woman cope with her life. Responses to a disclosure of childhood sexual abuse can be found in Appendix B.

❋ Family History

The family history can identify risk for having a child with a birth defect or an inherited disorder that may appear later in life. The family history should include questions about race/ethnicity and medical and obstetrical problems. Should a risk factor be identified, a referral for genetic counseling may be indicated. A genetic consultation is probably not necessary when the family history includes only one case of a generally noninherited condition, such as cerebral palsy, or when the family history includes a single distant relative (great-aunts, great-uncles, cousins) with a multifactorial condition (cleft lip or palate, clubfoot, multiple sclerosis) other than neural tube defects or congenital heart disease. Box 1-8 summarizes indications for genetic counseling.

Racial and Ethnic Background

Racial/ethnic background can identify women from groups known to be at risk for certain genetic disorders. These include women at risk for hemoglobinopathies as well as women at risk for Tay-Sachs disease (TSD), Canavan disease (CD), and cystic fibrosis. Carrier testing should be offered to women in these groups.

Box 1.8

Conditions or Situations in Which Genetic Counseling Is Appropriate

CONDITIONS OR SITUATIONS IN EITHER PARENT OR HIS OR HER FAMILY

1. Possible carrier status for a genetic disease such as sickle cell (African heritage), Tay-Sachs disease (Ashkenazi Jewish and French Canadian heritage), thalassemias (from North, West, and Central Africa; Italy; Sicily; Greece; the Middle East; South and, Southeast Asia; Southern China; Pacific Islands)
2. Adult-onset disability of genetic origin
3. Behavioral disorders of genetic origin
4. Down syndrome or other chromosomal abnormality
5. A family history of a known genetic disorder
6. Mental retardation or developmental delay
7. Chronic neurologic or neuromuscular childhood disorders
8. Short stature for ethnic group
9. Infertility or sterility
10. Exposure to potentially mutagenic or teratogenic agents
11. Multiple family members with the same condition, even when it is not thought to be genetic

CONDITIONS OR SITUATIONS IN THE MOTHER

12. Has had three or more unexplained, consecutive, spontaneous first-trimester losses or two or more spontaneous first-trimester losses if she is over 35 years of age
13. Is age 35 or older
14. Has had a previous infant with a birth defect when no cytogenic study was performed (single anomalies, multiple defects, metabolic disorders)
15. Has had a neonatal death or an unexplained stillborn baby
16. Has had a baby die with a case of atypical SIDS (death before 1 month of age or after 12 months)
17. Has a risk because of consanguinity

CONDITIONS OR SITUATIONS IN THE FATHER

18. Has been the father in three consecutive first-trimester losses
19. Has a family history of genetic disease
20. Has been the father of a baby with a birth defect

Thalassemia, the most common genetic disease, occurs worldwide but most frequently in people from West and Central Africa, the Mediterranean basin (Italy, Sicily, Greece, North Africa), the Middle East, South and Southeast Asia, Southern China, and the Pacific Islands. Women of Southeast Asian descent are at increased risk for alpha thalassemia, and women of Mediterranean descent are at increased risk for beta thalassemia (ACOG, 2000b).

However, "the ever-widening ethnic and geographic distribution of human hemoglobinopathies has made the identification of individuals at increased risk by ethnic or racial origin less reliable" (ACOG, 2000b, p.1). Carriers of hemoglobinopathies are usually healthy except for microcytic anemia, while carriers of hemoglobin variants (such as hemoglobin S, E, and C) do not have microcytosis and need hemoglobin electrophoresis testing.

TSD, a fatal genetic disorder in children, is caused by the absence of the enzyme hexosaminidase A (Hex-A). Absence of Hex-A leads to progressive destruction of the central nervous system. No cure or treatment exists, and affected children usually die by the age of 5. Parents who are carriers of the inactive Tay-Sachs gene have a 25% chance in each pregnancy that their child will have the disease. For their unaffected children, there is a 2 in 3 chance that each child will be a carrier.

TSD, like other recessive diseases, occurs more frequently (but not exclusively) in a particular population—in this case, persons of eastern European (Ashkenazi) Jewish background. The chances that a person of Ashkenazi Jewish descent is a TSD carrier are 1 in 27. Other populations with a significantly higher chance of being TSD carriers are French Canadians living near the St. Lawrence River and Cajuns from the Cajun community of Louisiana. While TSD is found more often in certain populations, anyone in any population can be a carrier. In fact, most of the babies born today with TSD are born to couples not known to be at risk. Testing will identify 95% of Ashkenazi Jewish carriers and about 60% of non-Jewish carriers (National Tay-Sachs & Allied Diseases Association, no date). Carrier testing for TSD is extremely important for couples in high-risk populations who contemplate pregnancy.

CD is an incurable, progressive neurological disease causing mental retardation and motor disability. It is often fatal in childhood. CD is caused by a deficiency in the enzyme aspartocyclase and, like TSD, is inherited in an autosomal recessive pattern. Also like TSD, CD occurs in higher frequency in persons of Ashkenazi Jewish background. Approximately one person out of 30 to 40 persons in this group is a carrier. If both partners are of Ashkenazi Jewish descent or if a family history consistent with CD is present, carrier testing should be offered before pregnancy. If only one partner is of Ashkenazi Jewish background, that person should be offered carrier testing. Testing will identify 97% of Ashkenazi Jewish carriers (New England Regional Genetics Group, 1999). Screening for CD should be combined with screening for TSD because both diseases are found more commonly in the same ethnic group.

Family Medical History

As outlined above, questions about racial and ethnic background can elicit information about possible familial genetic problems and can indicate a need for certain tests. Women with thalassemia often have a normal hemoglobin and hematocrit but a low mean corpuscular volume (MCV) (<80 fL, but a MCV in the 60s is common). Hemoglobin electrophoresis is indicated when the MCV is low.

Identification of additional significant inherited disorders in first-degree (parents, siblings, children) and second-degree (grandparents, grandchildren, aunts and uncles, nieces, and nephews) relatives can be obtained by asking about the family medical history. Women with a family history of lupus, rheumatoid arthritis, rashes, and arthralgias may be referred to a perinatologist for a discussion of risk for diagnosis of an autoimmune disorder.

A family history of mental retardation is significant when two or more family members are affected and/or the retardation is associated with dysmorphic features. Fragile X syndrome is the most common heritable form of mental retardation, occurring in about 1 in 1200 males and 1 in 2500 females. Physical features commonly associated with fragile X include a long face, large ears, macrocephaly, and slightly shortened height in adulthood. Behavior may resemble autism and attention-deficit disorder. Retardation varies from mild to severe, although 20% of males with the mutation appear normal and have no intellectual impairment. Females have less mental retardation (about 30% are affected intellectually), and the physical features are more subtle (Hagerman, 1994). DNA testing is available for individuals at risk because of a family history of fragile X syndrome. Women with a family history of unexplained mental retardation, regardless of whether it is associated with fragile X syndrome, should be offered genetic evaluation to assess the risk of having an affected child.

Some psychiatric disorders—schizophrenia, depression, and bipolar disease, for example—have hereditary components. Considering emotional and psychiatric problems often are not officially diagnosed, you might ask the client if depression or unstable and unexpected behavior was present in any family member. A referral to a genetic counselor may be appropriate. When mental illness is present in a family, be sure to ask the client if she has fears about developing the illness herself and inquire about the effect the illness may have had on the client's life. Living with or in close association with someone with a mental disease can be difficult, and the client's life may have been unpredictable and chaotic.

Family Obstetrical History

Occasionally, the family obstetrical history will alert the midwife to potential problems. A small but significant increase in the incidence of preeclampsia occurs when a mother or sister has had severe preeclampsia. A family history of polycystic ovary syndrome carries a higher incidence of fertility problems. Reproductive loss in close family members is important, as a baby may be stillborn because of an unrecognized genetic disorder. A neonatal death may be caused by an inherited metabolic disorder. A baby who died early in life may have died from SIDS but also may have had a genetic disorder, particularly in the case of atypical SIDS (death before 1 month of age or after 12 months) or multiple deaths attributed to SIDS. Three or more miscarriages in a first-degree relative may indicate a chromosome translocation. In all of these instances, referral to a genetics counselor can clarify whether genetic testing might be helpful.

Diethylstilbestrol (DES), a drug used until the early 1970s to prevent miscarriage and other complications of pregnancy, increases a daughter's risk for cervicovaginal clear cell adenocarcinoma, reproductive tract anomalies, and premature births. DES daughters are probably at risk for ectopic pregnancy and infertility as well (National Institutes of Health, 1999). Ask women born before 1974 if their mothers may have used DES when pregnant with the client. DES daughters should be advised to seek care as soon as they suspect they are pregnant and a pregnancy test is positive. Appendix C contains guidelines for caring for DES-exposed women.

Substance Abuse in Family Members

Talking about family issues around alcohol and drug abuse can lead to important discussions about parenting and the possible hereditary component of substance abuse. Ask about past and present use of alcohol and/or drugs in close family members (parents, stepparents, parental partners, siblings). Not only does violence occur frequently in families with substance abuse problems, but also physical and emotional nurturing may have been lacking as parents struggled to support their habit, maintain a home, and find or keep a job. Multiple foster care placements involving repeated separation and loss may have occurred.

Asking questions about family substance abuse is difficult for some clinicians. When this is the case, you might try an indirect approach. "Tell me about your family's feelings about alcohol? How about drugs?" You can then continue with these questions:

- How much alcohol did your parents use when you were growing up?
- How often did they drink?
- What about drugs? How often did they smoke marijuana or use other drugs?
- Did your brothers and sisters use drugs or alcohol?

When it is evident that substance abuse occurred, ask the client, "How old were you when this was happening?" and "What was it like for you growing up in that environment?" The effect on the child can be dependent on the child's developmental stage at the time of the parental substance abuse. Rarely do individuals who grew up in families where substance abuse was common escape without some emotional sequela. Parents-to-be often appreciate acknowledgment of the difficulties these situations may have caused.

❋ The Baby's Father

Important information can be obtained by asking questions about the medical history of the father of the baby and his family. Ask particularly if the baby's father has had herpes. If yes, there is a good chance that the client also has had herpes, even though she may be asymptomatic. In such cases the mother should be taught symptoms of an outbreak. She should also be sero-tested for HSV-2 when this test is available.

In addition to racial and ethnic background, ask the father if his family has a history of mental retardation, developmental delay, a birth defect, unusual facial features, a genetic disorder, or a chromosome abnormality. Ask, as well, if he has been involved in any relationship in which three or more miscarriages have occurred. Order a karyotype of any man who was the father of three babies that were miscarried. A genetic consultation is probably not necessary if the baby's father was exposed to a teratogen.

Paternal age can also have an effect on pregnancy outcome. Although the risk for chromosomal anomalies does not appear to be increased, advancing age exponentially increases the risk for autosomal dominant diseases such as neurofibromatosis, achondroplasia, Apert syndrome, and Marfan syndrome. However, the exact risk is small (ACOG, 1997a).

The so-called "grandfather effect," in which older men transmit through carrier daughters to affected grandsons, may occur with X-linked disorders including hemophilia A and Duchenne muscular dystrophy (ACOG, 1997a). Genetic counseling may be welcomed by individuals as it is not possible at present to screen for all autosomally dominant and X-linked conditions that might occur. Chromosomal analysis is not helpful in these cases.

❋ Laboratory Testing

Information obtained from the history will determine what tests, if any, might be indicated before conception is attempted. Among the tests likely to be appropriate prior to conception are a CBC, rubella and varicella titers, and a Pap smear. Cultures for chlamydia and gonorrhea, serologic testing for herpes, and testing for thyroid-stimulating hormone (TSH) may also be advised.

Box 1.9

Women at Risk for the Hepatitis B Virus*

- Adolescents
- Women with multiple sexual partners
- Women who live with chronic carriers of the virus
- Women whose jobs could expose them to human blood or body fluids
- Women who use illicit drugs
- Women who travel internationally to endemic areas
- Women who were born in Asia, Africa, the Amazon basin in South America, the Pacific Islands, Eastern Europe, or the Middle East
- Women who are Native Americans or Alaskan natives
- Women who are monogamous but whose partners are at risk for hepatitis B infection

---

*From the National Coalition for Adult Immunization

Women in high-risk groups should consider tests for hemoglobinopathies, hepatitis (Box 1-9), tuberculosis (Box 1-10), and HIV (Box 1-11). Genetic testing may be indicated. It is helpful to have a list and approximate costs of common laboratory tests as well as tests that might be unique to a given pregnancy, such as amniocentesis or special blood work that would be indicated with an autoimmune disorder. Financial support from organizations or state programs is sometimes available.

Box 1.10

Women At Risk for Tuberculosis

Women who are
- Symptomatic
- HIV-positive
- A close contact of a person with pulmonary tuberculosis
- Alcoholics or IV drug users
- From a country with a high prevalence rate
- Residents of a correctional institution or a long-term care facility
- Health care workers
- Poor and medically underserved
- Homeless or in a shelter

Box 1.11

Women At Risk for HIV Infection

Women who have
- Had sex with more than two men in 1 year
- More than one partner now
- Had sex when they were high
- Injected drugs or medicine
- Had anal sex
- Traded sex for drugs, food, money, housing, or anything else
- Had a partner who:
    used recreational drugs
    has been in jail
    has been diagnosed as HIV-positive
    had a blood transfusion between 1975 and 1978 or had hemophilia
    had sex with a prostitute
    had sex with someone who used IV drugs
    had sex with another woman or both men and women
    had any warts, blisters, sores, discharge, or painful urination
    had anal sex

Box 1.12

Information To Be Obtained at a Preconception Interview and Commonly Requested Laboratory Tests

INFORMATION TO OBTAIN

1. Maternal age
2. Menstrual history
3. Personal medical history (including gynecologic information)
4. Obstetric history
5. Use of cigarettes
6. Substance abuse
7. Use of prescription drugs, over-the-counter medicine, and herbal products
8. Environmental exposures
9. Psychosocial history including a history of physical, emotional, and/or sexual abuse
10. Family history including racial/ethnic background, medical problems, obstetric history, and substance abuse
11. Father of the baby: ethnic background and family's medical and obstetric history

LABORATORY TESTS TO CONSIDER:

CBC, rubella titer, varicella titer, Pap smear, TSH, HIV, syphilis, hemoglobin electrophoresis, hepatitis B, PPD for tuberculosis, gonorrhea, chlamydia, type-specific HSV serologic testing

❋ Conclusion

Box 1-12 summarizes the information to be obtained at the preconception interview and tests that may be indicated. Appendix D contains sample genetic history questions should an extensive history appear appropriate.

Conclude the preconception visit with a summary of what has transpired. Include 1) the plans that have been made to obtain additional information, 2) activities that have been recommended, and 3) concerns that have been addressed. Simple, written explanations for the client to take home are often helpful whether they are previously prepared handouts or hand-written directions and suggestions.

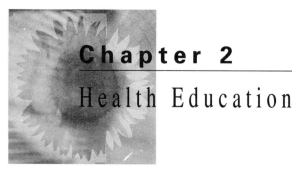

Chapter 2
Health Education

❋ Introduction

The preconception visit is an opportune time to discuss ways that the client and her family can promote a healthy pregnancy. Topics might include 1) the menstrual cycle and fertility, 2) the influence of contraceptive methods on conception, 3) important health practices while trying to conceive, and 4) general health recommendations. Midwives should take advantage of the visit to explore a couple's understanding of prenatal care and to initiate a discussion of options for the birth attendant and place of birth when appropriate.

❋ The Menstrual Cycle and Fertility

Women should know that their fertile period extends from about 5 days before ovulation through the day of ovulation. This constitutes the "fertile window." Recent data indicate that this window varies greatly among women, even those with regular cycles. Women with irregular cycles ovulate later and at more variable times than do women with regular cycles. The important lesson is that the fertile window can occur earlier or later than traditional guidelines indicate (Wilcox, Dunson, & Baird, 2000).

Keeping a menstrual history calendar can help to document cycle variations and identify the first day of the last normal menstrual period, facilitating the "dating" of pregnancy. Intermenstrual bleeding not related to a contraceptive method should be investigated.

❋ The Influence of Contraceptive Methods on Conception

Ovulation may be delayed after use of some contraceptives. Oral contraception seems to delay pregnancy longer than use of the intrauterine device (IUD). In one study, 90% of women whose IUDs had been removed were pregnant 14 months later, but it took 24 months for 90% of the pill users to conceive. Although a "significant delay" in conception was present for at least a year after oral contraceptives were discontinued, the mean length of time to conception for women using <50-µg estrogen pills was 4.01 cycles. The probability of conception increased with each cycle (Bracken, Hellenbrand, & Holford, 1990).

IUDs are not associated with temporary losses in fecundity. Depo-Provera users experience a delay to conception time of about 9 months after the last injection. By 18 months, 90% of users are pregnant. Ovulation returns promptly after Norplant removal (Speroff & Darney, 2001).

Women who stop taking the birth control pill to become pregnant should be advised to stop the pill at the end of a pill package and wait for one menstrual period before trying to conceive. This allows more accurate dating of the pregnancy, because some women do not menstruate immediately after discontinuing the pill. The approximate incidence of "postpill amenorrhea" is 0.7%–0.8%, which is equal to the incidence of spontaneous secondary amenorrhea, and there is no evidence to support the idea that oral contraception causes secondary amenorrhea (Speroff & Darney, 2001).

✳ Important Health Practices Before Conception

Prevention of Neural Tube Defects

Neural tube defects (NTDs) are defects of the spinal canal. They range in severity from anencephaly (when the cranial end of the neural tube fails to close) to spina bifida (when the distal end fails to close) to unnoticeable defects in the vertebrae. NTDs occur 3 to 4 weeks after conception when the neural tube fails to close. Epidemiologic studies have demonstrated that daily consumption of 400 µg of folic acid (folate), a B vitamin, periconceptionally, decreases by 50% to 70% the number of pregnancies in which the fetus has a NTD. Folic acid does not prevent these defects when taken later (Power, Holzman, & Schulkin, 2000). The recommendation for 400 µg was based not on randomized clinical trials, but on observational studies. "It is by no means certain that 400 micrograms is the critical level" (Mills, 2000, p. 1442).

Fortification of enriched grain products with folic acid—flours, breads, rolls, buns, corn grits, corn meal, farina, rice, macaroni, and noodles—began in the United States in January 1998, to supplement naturally occurring folate found in fruits, vegetables, and legumes. Folate levels in food are low and not as bioavailable as supplemental folic acid (Oregon Health Division, 2000a). The intent is to raise the folic acid intake of the average childbearing woman to 100 µg per day without exposing other individuals to levels that would mask vitamin B_{12} deficiency and pernicious anemia.

No controlled studies on the effect of the fortification program have been conducted. Additionally, analysis of the total folate content of enriched grain products has shown that "the actual folate levels were found to be significantly higher than either the amount required by federal regulations or the amount listed in the declaration of folate content on the label. Some products were found to contain 200% or more of the listed value. Thus, the U.S. population may be exposed to considerably more folic acid than the FDA planned or the Institute of Medicine considers safe" (Mills, 2000, p. 1443). Nevertheless, in 1998 the National Academy of Sciences revised its recommendation for folic acid intake for pregnant women from 400 μg per day to 600 μg per day. The safety of this recommendation has not been established. "Given the fact that folic acid fortification is exposing 274 million people to folic acid to prevent 2000 neural-tube defects per year, it is surprising that public health officials have not demanded a higher standard of proof that the current level of fortification is safe and effective" (Mills, 2000, p. 1444).

Most practitioners recommend that all women contemplating pregnancy take a prenatal vitamin, a multivitamin containing 400 μg (0.4 mg) of folic acid or, preferably, just 400 μg of folic acid from 4 weeks before conception through the first 7 weeks of pregnancy. Folic acid tablets are less expensive than prenatal vitamins, even the generic brands.

Women who have had a previous baby with an NTD or a family history of an NTD should take 4 *mg* daily. Also at increased risk for NTDs are women with diabetes and women with a history of seizures. They should also take 4 *mg* per day to bring their risk down to that of the general population. Women advised to take 4 *mg* daily, should not take four multivitamins each day, because dangerous levels of vitamins A and D can increase the risk of other birth defects. Instead, they should take four tablets containing 1 mg of folic acid or three tablets containing 1 mg of folic acid plus 1 prenatal multivitamin containing 1 mg of folic acid.

Consultation With a Specialist: DES Daughters and Women With Chronic Disease

In certain instances, consultation with a perinatologist and/or other medical specialist should be obtained before conception is attempted. Women in this category include daughters of women who took the drug diethylstilbestrol (DES) while pregnant, women with organic disease, and women with a history of repeated pregnancy loss.

Exposure to X-rays

Remind women that adequate shielding of pelvic structures should occur if an x-ray film is necessary. Diagnostic radiation techniques used in the United States today do not jeopardize fetal development or well-being as doses used are well below 5 rads. Current evidence suggests that below this dose, the risk of abortion, malformation, and growth restriction is not increased (Brent, 1999).

Cigarettes, Alcohol, and Drugs

Emphasize the importance of quitting smoking before pregnancy. This includes marijuana. Take advantage of opportunities to speak with cigarette-smoking partners about quitting as well. Certainly, the pregnant woman has prime responsibility for the health of her unborn child, but partners must also assume responsibility for supporting a woman trying to quit. This is best accomplished if the partner also quits. Children should be raised in a smoke-free home.

Women who consume alcoholic beverages should know the importance of drinking in moderation—no more than two drinks at a time and no more than seven drinks per week. This includes beer, wine, wine coolers, hard liquor, and cough and cold medicines that contain alcohol. Better yet, any woman contemplating pregnancy should avoid alcoholic beverages altogether as most women are initially unaware of a pregnancy. If alcohol abuse is suspected, serious discussions to determine whether additional information supports the suspicion should occur. Discourage pregnancy for a woman who drinks too much as well as for a woman whose partner drinks too much.

All illicit and recreational drugs, including marijuana, should be avoided by any woman contemplating pregnancy and by her partner as well.

Medicines and Dietary Supplements

To decrease any possibility of consuming a teratogenic agent, women wishing to become pregnant should avoid over-the-counter, prescription, and herbal or homeopathic medicines unless their use has been discussed with the health care provider. Recommend acetaminophen for pain relief and fever reduction rather than aspirin or a nonsteroidal anti-inflammatory agent (NSAID) such as ibuprofen (Advil). When supplementary vitamins are consumed, the vitamin A intake should remain below 5000 IU daily to avoid the possibility of a teratogenic effect from a high vitamin A intake (American College of Obstetricians and Gynecologists Committee on Obstetric Practice,1998d).

"Aspirin inhibits the platelet release reaction by acetylating platelet cyclooxygenase; this effect persists in the platelet for the duration of its life span and results in prolongation of the bleeding time and deficient platelet aggregation in the presence of collagen. Patients taking aspirin may note increased bruisability and minor bleeding problems, manifestations that persist for several days following a single dose. Ordinarily, these symptoms are inconsequential; during pregnancy and especially at term, however, hemorrhagic complications can be of more than trivial importance. Normal pregnant women given usual doses of aspirin within 10 days of delivery undergo increased intrapartum or postpartum blood loss, and their infants sustain a higher incidence of hemostatic abnormalities." (Kilpatrick & Laros, 1999, p. 955). NSAIDs also affect platelet function (by inhibiting prostaglandin synthesis), but they are "less powerful and shorter acting antagonists than aspirin." (Kilpatrick & Laros, 1999, p. 955).

Caffeine

Research conducted to determine the contribution of caffeine to poor reproductive outcome has produced conflicting results. While some studies have shown that "moderate" consumption doubles the risk of spontaneous abortion, other studies have found no risk even for women who consume "large" amounts of caffeine. In a study of 591 women who had spontaneous abortions, researchers compared them to 2558 women who carried their babies to at least 28 weeks' gestation. When serum paraxanthine concentrations (the primary metabolite of caffeine and a substance found to correlate with caffeine intake) were measured, only women with very high serum levels were found to be at increased risk for spontaneous abortion. The authors suggest that, using conservative guidelines, it would take five or more cups of coffee to put women at increased risk (Klebanoff, Levine, DerSimonian, Clemens, & Wilkins, 1999). While this study adds to the data addressing the association between caffeine intake and spontaneous abortion, definitive guidelines addressing daily caffeine intake have not been established.

Toxoplasmosis Infection

A primary infection with toxoplasmosis in pregnancy results in a one-third chance of fetal infection. The severity of fetal infection is greatest in the first trimester, but the rate of infection is higher in the third. Most infected infants escape the serious consequences of intracerebral calcifications, chorioretinitis, and hydrocephalus. Serious congenital infection is estimated to occur in 15% of cases (Gibbs & Sweet, 1999).

While the chances of toxoplasmosis infection in pregnancy are remote (as most of the population has already been exposed and are protected from further infection), women contemplating a pregnancy who have a cat as a pet should be advised to wash their hands after handling the cat, to have someone else change the litter box, and to keep the cat indoors to prevent it from eating an infected mouse. If it is not possible for a nonpregnant person to change the litter box daily, the client should wear protective gloves. A mask is probably not necessary because infection by inhalation is rare. Gardeners should wear gloves when gardening because cat feces may be in the soil.

Undercooked meat is a more common cause of toxoplasmosis than cats. To ensure that meat is done, observe the following temperatures:

- 145° for steaks and for beef, lamb, and veal roasts
- 160° for pork, ground meat, and wild game
- 180° (in the thigh) for poultry

Additionally, utensils used in food preparation as well as counters, cutting boards, and hands that have been in contact with raw meat, poultry, seafood, or unwashed fruits and vegetables should be washed with hot, soapy water.

Potentially Dangerous Pets

If there are pets in the home, such as ferrets and breeds of dog known to attack or bite babies or children, encourage women to find other homes for these animals. If sanitation is a problem because of many pets or animals in the house, encourage new homes for these animals as well. An alternative is close attention to appropriate hygienic procedures.

Exposure to Heat

High temperatures, particularly in early pregnancy, have been associated with congenital anomalies. Precise data on the timing and amount of heat exposure necessary to cause these problems are not available, yet sufficient concern exists to recommend avoiding hot tubs with a temperature above 100.4°F, particularly in the first trimester, and saunas throughout pregnancy.

Vaginal Douching

Vaginal douching for cleansing or to treat vaginal irritations or malodors is a common practice for some women. Because it may increase the risk for ectopic pregnancy (Kendrick, Atrash, Strauss, Gargiullo, & Ahn, 1997), women should be encouraged to avoid vaginal douching.

❋ General Recommendations for Good Health

Nutrition

A diet assessment can provide the basis for specific food recommendations. When discussing foods to include in a good diet, a discussion of the Food Guide Pyramid (Appendix E) and food labels are good places to start. The Food Guide Pyramid illustrates a range of servings of five essential food groups. A discussion of serving sizes can put the guidelines into context for everyday life (Appendix F).

The first line on a food label gives the serving size, and the second line gives the number of servings per container, an important feature to note because very few products come in single-serving packages. If not read carefully, a person could think the nutritional information on the label refers to the entire container when, in fact, there is more than one serving in the container. A woman's hand can be a helpful guide to portions. The palm compares to the size of a 3-oz portion of meat, fish, or poultry; the closed fist to a cup; the thumb tip a teaspoon, and the distance from the thumb tip to the joint, a tablespoon.

While eating patterns are hard to change, women contemplating pregnancy may be motivated to alter traditional eating habits. Among the suggestions that can be made are eating appropriately sized portions of a well-balanced diet and paying attention to the fat content of foods. Opt for lower-fat versions of milk, salad dressing, and cheese. Eat slowly and only when you are hungry. Stop eating when you are full. Rediscover water. Try it with a twist of lime or lemon! And don't deprive yourself of the foods you love—just eat less of them!

 HELPFUL HINT

Collect food labels from various products and place them in plastic sleeves in a three-ring binder. Choose labels that illustrate important differences in similar products. Use these labels to illustrate points you want to make about the value of reading labels.

Nutrition guidelines for the professional or elite athlete should be individualized, as diets of these women may not be nutritionally sound. Common problems include insufficient calories or consumption of large quantities of vitamins, which could be teratogenic. Athletes in the professional or elite category should discuss their training and competition programs with a perinatologist.

 HELPFUL HINT

Health education material illustrating and recommending food choices (including the Food Guide Pyramid) is often difficult for people to understand. With a wide range of readability levels, more than half the patient education material used today is too difficult for the average American to comprehend. Choose material with short sentences, a conversational style, commonly used words, a friendly cover graphic, and simple line drawings (Doak, Doak, & Root, 1996).

Exercise

An exercise program is an important part of staying healthy. Women without a regular program should be encouraged to begin one. Avoid precise recommendations about the amount, kind, and frequency of exercise, as most of these are daunting to women not accustomed to physical exertion. New evidence suggests that it is simplistic to rely on a single formula to recommend maximum heart rates for those in a regular exercise program. Chapter 15 contains suggestions for helping women initiate exercise programs.

Environmental Toxins

The exact dangers of environmental toxins are unknown. However, common sense dictates minimizing exposure. Toxicants in the home environment include indoor air pollution (tobacco smoke, woodstoves, gas ranges, building materials such as formaldehyde and asbestos); household cleaners, glues, lead paint, and paint stripper; pesticides and lawn care products; a tainted water supply; contaminated soil; and organic solvents used in some types of employment. Appropriate protection and adequate ventilation systems should be in place.

Immunizations

Immunizations should be up-to-date. Booster doses of tetanus and diphtheria toxoid (Td) are recommended every 10 years except when there is an injury and a tetanus-prone wound. In these cases, a booster dose is given after 5 years. The vaccine is 99% effective (Centers for Disease Control and Prevention, 1993).

Varicella (chicken pox) infection during pregnancy is associated with significant problems for both mother and baby. Women who have not had chicken pox should get the vaccine or have a blood test to see if they are already protected. Women who do not know if they have had varicella should be encouraged to have a titer drawn and a vaccine administered before conception if protection is not demonstrated. Nonpregnant women who receive the varicella vaccine should avoid pregnancy for 1 month after each injection.

Before administering any vaccine, know which ones can be given to patients who are allergic to eggs. "Influenza and measles-mumps-rubella (MMR) vaccines can be given safely in egg-allergic patients; however, the safety of other vaccines has not been established" (Steinberg, 2000, 875).

Seat Belts

Advise women to wear seat belts with both shoulder and lap belts. The lower strap should be placed as snug as is comfortable below the abdomen. Position the shoulder belt above the uterus. Make sure the headrest is at a height to protect the head from whiplash (Schoenfeld, Ziv, Stein, Zaidel, & Ovadia, 1987).

❋ Options for Birth Attendant and Place of Birth

Women or couples planning a pregnancy may or may not know that there are major differences in philosophy among health care providers in regard to prenatal care and birth. Certified nurse-midwives; direct-entry, community, licensed, or lay midwives; family practice physicians; naturopaths; and obstetricians all provide prenatal care and assist at birth, but the manner in which each goes about doing this work is highly variable. Clients should be encouraged to learn about practitioners in the community as well as in-hospital and out-of-hospital birth centers, hospital birthing units and levels of hospitals, and home birth. Policies and costs should be known. Health care professionals can offer clients a list of questions that might be asked of potential providers so that an informed choice about both provider and place of birth can be made. Because health plans are usually individually designed for an employee group, participants should study the provisions of the plan prior to conception to see what costs are covered and what restrictions, if any, may affect choices about prenatal care and birth.

Occasionally, newspapers publish updates on birthing services in a community. When this happens, save the report to share with people looking for this information. Clients with computers can be encouraged to use web sites to gather information about pregnancy and birth. A site such as *midwife-info.com* not only provides information about midwifery, but also contains information for parents on topics such as breastfeeding, birth centers, doulas, childbirth education, water birth, episiotomy, and epidurals.

Many women and couples will appreciate a list of books to read before and during pregnancy. Visit your public library and local bookstores to see what is available. Prepare an annotated bibliography listing your favorite references. Stores such as Goodwill and Salvation Army often carry used books at affordable prices. Your clinic or office may be willing to purchase these to lend to clients.

❋ Conclusion

Although preconception counseling is not widely used in the United States, all clinicians who care for women in the childbearing years should be prepared to ask the questions and provide the advice required by this kind of meeting. The issues raised are different from those encountered during a prenatal visit, and clinicians must be aware of the special concerns that should be addressed. Consider reviewing the health education guidelines in this chapter with any women of childbearing age who come for an annual examination or a gyne-cologic problem, whether or not a pregnancy is contemplated.

PART 2 The Initial Prenatal Visit

Early and consistent prenatal care improves the outcome of pregnancy. Fortunately, only 1% of pregnant women in the United States receive no prenatal care (Centers for Disease Control and Prevention [CDC], 2000). Data about the number of women who drop out of care are difficult to find. Early care, that is, care initiated by the thirteenth week of gestation, for 90% of pregnant women was a goal set as a national health objective for the year 2000. It was not achieved by any state.

The initial prenatal visit should convince the expectant mother that the time she spends getting ready for the visit, traveling to the clinic or office, and waiting for and interacting with clinic personnel is time well spent. Perhaps in no other situation is the importance of a holistic approach to clients more compelling than when counseling girls or women who are pregnant. To focus on obstetric markers and ignore the opportunity to assess psychosociocultural life influences, issues that can have an even greater effect on pregnancy outcome and quality of life for both mother and baby, is to abdicate our responsibility to the expectant mother and her family. On the other hand, to focus exclusively on the emotional components of pregnancy and birth is to subject the mother and her baby to potential harm. The goals of the initial prenatal visit, then, should be:

- To gather a database that looks at the client holistically
- To assess risks for obstetric complications
- To identify systems of stress and of support
- To determine knowledge about pregnancy
- To identify desires in regard to the birth of the baby
- To encourage modification of harmful beliefs and behaviors
- To initiate referrals to community resources as needed.
- To establish a mutually satisfying relationship

The initial visit consists of a history (Chapter 3) and a physical examination (Chapter 4). Laboratory tests are usually ordered (Chapter 5), and advice about having a healthy pregnancy is given (Chapter 6). While the visit is usually lengthy, it gives the clinician an opportunity to set the tone for the relationship in the weeks and months to come. As such, the visit is important from both an emotional and an obstetrical viewpoint. A calm, respectful, personal approach that indicates a desire to understand the client and provide her with competent, thoughtful care can be the beginning of an exciting journey.

Chapter 3
The Initial Prenatal Visit History

A theme throughout this book is the importance of taking time to obtain a complete database and to interact compassionately with the client and her family. To some, the lengthy history described here will be viewed as impractical in busy health care settings where "productivity" is emphasized. In many settings only 20 or 30 minutes are allotted for an initial prenatal visit, time merely to focus on the obstetric and medical history and perform a brief physical examination. Information about the psychosociocultural aspects of a woman's life is not elicited. Regardless of the restrictions imposed by the job setting, our commitment to women and their families demands that we do all we can to view them in the context of their lives, not just in the context of their uterus.

 HELPFUL HINT

When possible, provide clients with a history form to be completed at home and brought to the initial visit. You can review this form in 2–3 minutes, circling or highlighting the information about which you have questions or comments. It is most helpful if the form is devised by you if you work alone or by the group of midwives with whom you work if you are in a group practice. Typical ready-made forms do not address psychosocial issues and health-related practices. Women with low literacy skills may be unable to read or understand preprinted forms, and women who do not speak English will not be able to respond to forms written in English. In these instances, limit the questions asked at the first visit, saving some for subsequent visits.

 HELPFUL HINT

If your practice does not ask clients to fill out a complete history form before being seen by a clinician, or if the history form used in your practice is not thorough, laminate the list of topics that should be addressed at the initial visit. Keep the laminated list in a lab coat pocket so that you can refer to it as needed throughout the visit.

Following the "four E's"—engage, empathize, educate, and enlist— may help you as you start (Bayer Institute for Health Care Communication, date unknown). The first "E," engage, refers to establishing rapport with the client. A minute or two of social chitchat often puts the new client at ease, unless, of course, it is apparent that she is in either physical or emotional distress. If she is alone when you meet her, you might ask if someone came with her and, if so, whether she would like that person to be with her during the interview and/or physical examination. Be sure to add, however, that some of the questions you will ask are of a personal nature. Assure her that you ask the same questions of each person because they help anticipate problems, identify special tests and procedures that should be ordered, and determine if referrals should be made.

The second "E," empathize, involves assuring the client that her story is being heard, her fears acknowledged, and her feelings respected. You might begin by asking, "Is this a good time to be having a baby?" You can rejoice with women who are delighted with their condition and empathize with women who are not. Empathy can be a powerful tool, and listening, by itself, can be therapeutic.

The third "E," educate, can occur throughout the visit. An assessment of the client's knowledge base is an ongoing process. Interject small amounts of information pertinent to the topic being discussed throughout the interview as appropriate. Hopefully, by demonstrating your interest in a warm and personal manner, you will have accomplished the fourth "E," enlisting the client as a partner, by the end of the visit.

In a prenatal clinic, the reason for the first visit is almost always the initiation of prenatal care, but it might also be to discuss the clinic's philosophy of care, to obtain a referral for genetic counseling, or to consider options in regard to continuing the pregnancy. Once the purpose of the visit is identified, ask the client if there is anything else she wants to find out or discuss. Once it appears that the client's questions have been answered, encourage additional questions by asking, "Anything else?" so that other questions can be freely asked.

As in the preconception visit, be sure to find some time to speak with the client alone. This is often best done right before the client leaves. When alone with the client, ask if there is anything else you should know about her to give her good care, anything confidential she wishes to tell you, or anything she has a question about but was hesitant to ask in front of someone else. This is the time to ask specifically about physical, emotional, and sexual abuse if these topics have not been addressed.

✳ Cultural Competence

Cultural competence is a concept that addresses the ability of individuals and systems to 1) recognize and examine personal cultural values; 2) value and respect differences in people; 3) interact respectfully with people of all cultures, socioeconomic classes, ages, abilities, religions, ethnic backgrounds, political beliefs, sexual orientation, levels of literacy, and life experience; 4) acknowledge the complex dimensions of cross-cultural interactions; and 5) adjust one's practice style to meet the needs of different groups. Practitioners are most effective when they know the possibilities for discordance between their own beliefs and those of women with different backgrounds.

When clinicians work with families from differing racial or ethnic backgrounds, it is important to remember that there is no generic Native American, African American, Asian, or Hispanic population, even though each may be grouped that way. Our most important task is to convey respect to the families who come to us for care. Certainly, it is important to gather cultural "facts" about the cultural groups in our practices. But facts need to be intertwined with an awareness of the complexities of cross-cultural encounters and an understanding of the contextual systems within which families operate. Box 3-1 lists information that may help clinicians respond sensitively to clients of different cultures. Midwives, who often enter the profession because of their desire to "empower" women, may find it difficult to accept the importance of family and community decision making in some cultures and the lack of autonomy woman have in others.

"Informed consent" is a particular concern for some midwives as they recognize the dissonance between the legal requirements of informed consent in this country and the harm that providing this information might cause women from other cultures. What individuals in the United States generally view as their right to information about benefits, risks, side effects, and complications may be seen differently by others. The mere mention of complications associated with a procedure may, in some cultures, increase the likelihood that they will happen because of the cultural belief that discussing a complication makes it likely to occur. Something that those in the dominant U.S. culture must know may be something that those in other cultures must not know. "The formal specifications of informed consent—e.g., fixed disclosure requirements, isolated individual decision making, and signed, written consent forms—may faithfully advance individual autonomy and human dignity for many patients in dominant Western cultures. But this same formalism may be alienating and dehumanizing to those who view caring and healing not as a

---

Box 3.1

Information That Can Help Clinicians Respond Sensitively to Clients of a Different Culture

1. What is the appropriate form of address? (First names may not be appropriate.)
2. What greetings are appropriate? Should the greeting be different according to status? Should the greeting be lengthy? Is social chitchat appropriate?
3. Are there any restrictions on the sex of the person providing care?
4. Are there any customs to be observed in regard to eye contact?
5. To what extent should the partner, extended family, or community be involved in decision making?
6. Are there any restrictions on who may touch whom, body parts that should not be touched, or body contact between the sexes?
7. Are pelvic examinations likely to cause particular embarrassment? What can be done to lessen this embarrassment?
8. Should any special practices be observed during pregnancy, labor, or birth? Any rituals to follow, special clothes or amulets to wear, foods to eat or not eat, or taboos to observe?
9. Should special medicines, herbs, teas, poultices, or treatments be used?
10. Are any other practitioners consulted during pregnancy or after delivery? Who are they? What do they do?
11. Does pregnancy change the usual sexual practices, hygiene practices, or patterns of work?
12. What persons or practices are considered dangerous to either the pregnant woman or her baby? What is done about them?
13. What special practices should be observed after delivery? Special food? Special place for the mother?

From Cunningham, F. G., Gant, N. F., Leveno, K. J., Gilstrap, L. C., III, Hauth, J. C., & Wenstrom, K. D. (2001). *Williams obstetrics* (21st ed.; pp. 225–226). New York: McGraw-Hill.

bilateral contractual relationship with a physician, but within a mutually supportive, loving environment in the family and community" (Gostin, 1995, p. 844).

❖ Interpreters

Because language barriers have a profound effect on care, federal law mandates that all public and private entities that receive funds from the U.S. Department of Health and Human Services must ensure that patients with limited English proficiency (LEP) are provided with language assistance that results in accurate and effective communication at no cost. Interpreters then become an essential part of the health team. In ideal situations, this person is bicultural as well as bilingual, is familiar with medical terminology, is from the same country as the patient, and has had special training in cross-cultural interpretation. "The interpreter should also be of similar educational and social class. If the client is from a lower class, he or she may be intimidated, and if the client is from a higher class, the client may doubt the abilities of the interpreter or may refrain from full disclosure of health care issues" (Poss & Rangel, 1995, p. 44). "All people who speak the same language do not necessarily communicate well. For example, Spanish speakers from different countries or of different educational backgrounds will not necessarily understand each other. An interpreter who speaks Spanish as it is spoken in Spain will not communicate well with a person from rural Mexico. There are countless stories about misunderstandings between Spanish speakers from different countries. For instance, *guagua* means `bus' in Puerto Rico, but it means 'baby' in Chile. Misunderstandings can occur with the word *biscocho*, which means 'cake' to someone from Puerto Rico but is slang for female genitals to a Mexican" (Poss & Rangel, 1995, p. 44).

Interpreters have to straddle two worlds, the world of the client and the world of the clinician. They are not only a conduit for conveying information, but they also clarify information for both sides and advocate for the client. For example, interpreters can explain terms for which there is no linguistic equivalent, such as "domestic violence." They can provide the cultural framework that allows both client and practitioner to understand how to approach the encounter. For example, in some cultures the client expects the practitioner to "divine" the cause of the problem. Asking many questions in this instance could cause the client to lose faith in the practitioner.

The discussion with the client may involve choices with which the interpreter cannot morally agree, the subject may be one that makes the interpreter uncomfortable, the interpreter may be personally known by the client, or the interpreter may be from a country at war with the client's country of origin. These situations pose unique and difficult problems. For example, a clinician wanted to ask a client if she would like to use a method of family planning. After the clinician posed the question, the interpreter responded, "No, she doesn't," without asking the client. The interpreter and the client belonged to the same church, and the religious tenets of their faith prohibited birth control. Another clinician, wanting to ask a woman if she was in an abusive situation, spoke enough Spanish to understand that when the interpreter asked the question, he said, "Your husband doesn't hit you, does he?"

The following guidelines can facilitate communication during the visit.

1. The interpreter and the clinician should meet ahead of time to discuss the purpose of the meeting and exchange information that might help the clinician and the client have a productive meeting.
2. The clinician should look at the client, not the interpreter.

3. Side conversations between the clinician and the interpreter and the interpreter and the client should be avoided.
4. The clinician should pay attention to the length of the client's response and the tone of her voice to be sure the interpreter has not deleted client information that he or she may have considered irrelevant (such as attributing the cause of the problem to a spiritual force).
5. At the end, the clinician should conclude the interview by asking the interpreter, "Is there something else I should ask or be thinking about?"

If circumstances require that a family member, friend, or clinic or office staff member serve as an interpreter, the provider must remember that these circumstances involve potentially embarrassing situations for both the person interpreting and the client, may involve breaches of confidentiality, and can result in superficial or inaccurate information. A family member may try to shield the client from painful information or may not know the medical terms to convey the explanations of the clinician. Appendix G summarizes guidelines for working with an interpreter.

✻ Maternal Age

Young age at conception has traditionally been associated with low birth weight, anemia, stillbirth, preeclampsia, and preterm birth. However, a recent report from the United Kingdom, based on data from births to 5246 women who were less than 18 years old, showed that, except for preterm birth, those under 18 were at relatively low risk for obstetric complications. No association was found between young maternal age and low birth weight, operative vaginal delivery, cesarean birth, preeclampsia, or stillbirth. Anemia was more common (Jolly, Sebire, Harris, Robinson, & Regan, 2000).

A discussion of chromosomal and genetic risks to older pregnant women can be found in Chapter 1. Genetic counseling should be offered to all pregnant women who will be 34 or 35 years of age (depending on institutional policy) when their babies are born to discuss the incidence of chromosomal abnormalities in their age group and understand the benefits and risks of diagnostic procedures. When a genetic problem is identified, counseling includes a discussion of the diagnosis, prognosis, risk of recurrence, course of the disease, treatment options, and medical and social support.

✻ Menstrual History

The menstrual history is the first tool used to establish the baby's "due date." Strange as it may seem, by convention the "due date" is established based on menstrual age rather than fetal age. The estimated date of birth (EDB) (called the estimated date of delivery [EDD] or estimated date of confinement [EDC] in some places) is determined by following an internationally recognized and accepted calculation, Naegele's rule. The rule adds 9 months and 7 days to the first day of the last normal menstrual period (LNMP) or subtracts 3 months and then adds 7 days and 1 year. For example, if the first day of the LNMP was January 10, adding 9 months and 7 days gives a due date of October 17. If the first day of the LNMP was November 18, it is easier to count backwards, so subtract 3 months and then add 7 days and 1 year, for an EDD of August 25. At times you need to move into a new month. Suppose the LNMP was September 26. Counting back 3 months, you get June 26. Now add 7 days and 1 year. You get July 3. (June has only 30 days.) At times the LNMP may be misleading because of oligomenorrhea, implantation bleeding, hormonal contraceptive use, and conception following a recent birth or during lactational amenorrhea.

HELPFUL HINT

Pharmaceutical companies often distribute gestation calculators ("wheels") to facilitate determination of the EDB and gestational age in weeks. Some wheels also note mean fetal weight and length for each gestational week. These calculators should not be used to determine the EDB because the calculator-determined EDB will vary as much as 4 days from the EDB determined by Nägele's rule. While this may seem trivial, extensive testing for fetal well-being often begins at 41 weeks' gestation, and the EDB identified by a gestation calculator is likely to be earlier than the date arrived at using Nägele's rule. This discrepancy can result in unnecessary expense and anxiety. Everyone should use the same approach for determining the EDB, and Nägele's rule is the accepted standard. Save the wheel for calculating weeks' gestation at prenatal visits, because precision in determining gestational age at an uncomplicated prenatal visit is not as important as precision in determining the due date.

Women who have a history of long or short menstrual cycles (longer than 35 days or less than 21 days) require an adjustment in the EDB. A woman with 35-day cycles should have 14 days rather than 7 days added, and a woman with 21-day cycles would have 7 days subtracted. A last menstrual period that was shorter or lighter than usual makes determination of the EDB difficult without the help of an ultrasound examination. To be truly accurate, three consecutive regular and normal periods are required. Unfortunately, women are not always able to remember previous periods with certainty.

❊ Contraceptive History

Hormonal contraception at or near the time of conception can affect the EDB. For example, when a woman finishes the hormone-containing pills in a package of oral contraceptives, the menstrual period she will subsequently have is termed a "withdrawal bleed." It occurs not because of the woman's natural hormonal influences but because hormonal support of the endometrium supplied by the oral contraceptive has been withdrawn. Spontaneous menstruation may or may not occur subsequently. Women who become pregnant without a spontaneous menstrual period after stopping "the pill" should have a sonogram to accurately determine the EDB. A sonogram for accurate dating is also indicated when pregnancy occurs before resumption of spontaneous menses in association with or after use of other hormonal contraceptive methods (e.g., Norplant, Depo-Provera, Lunelle, hormone-containing intrauterine devices [IUDs]).

On rare occasions pregnancy will occur with an IUD in place. When this occurs, remove the IUD if the pregnancy is in the first trimester and the strings are visible. Refer the client to a physician for this procedure after the 13th week. Leaving the IUD in place increases the chances for a midtrimester septic abortion.

❊ Obstetric History

In every specialty there is a language through which specialists communicate important information. The language used to describe pregnant women is summarized in Box 3-2. Women pregnant for the first time as well as women who have not carried a baby beyond 20 weeks' gestation are sometimes erroneously termed "primips." Note that primipara should be used only to describe a woman who has given birth to one baby who weighed 500 g or reached 20 weeks' gestation (Cunningham et al., 2001), not to a woman with a first pregnancy.

 HELPFUL HINT

Speaking of pregnancy in terms of weeks of gestation may be confusing to women who are pregnant for the first time. While it is usually not possible to give each expectant mother a gestation calculator, you can place the gestation calculator on a copy machine and make a copy of the wheel to give to the client. Use a large calculator or set the copy machine to enlarge the image, making it easy for the client to read. Arrange the calculator so that the 40-week mark coincides with the EDB.

Women who have access to a computer can be told about Internet sites that allow women to track gestational age.

Essential information about previous pregnancies includes the month and year that the pregnancy ended, the gestational age at the termination of the pregnancy, the type of delivery (spontaneous, forceps, vacuum extraction, or cesarean), the length of labor (preferably from the first contraction), analgesia or anesthesia used, episiotomy or lacerations, birth weight, sex of each child, place of birth, type of health care provider, complications, and the current health of each child. When describing pregnancies that ended before 20 weeks, differentiate between spontaneous, elective, and therapeutic abortions, as well as ectopic and molar pregnancies. Note each child's name. Ask the client about her feelings and perceptions of each pregnancy and birth, as well as about the loss of any child. Send for the medical records when a complication of a pregnancy occurred.

Clinicians summarize the duration and outcome of pregnancy with a series of numbers beginning with the number of times a woman has been pregnant. The current pregnancy is included. The word that stands for the number of pregnancies is *gravida*. Outcomes are summarized by a 4-digit designation following the word *para*. The first digit refers to the number of term pregnan-

---

Box 3.2

Terms Used to Describe a Woman in Relation to Pregnancy

Gravida: A woman who is or has been pregnant

Nulligravida: A woman who has never been and is not currently pregnant

Primigravida: A woman who is pregnant for the first time

Para: A number that by itself refers to the number of babies delivered that were of sufficient size (500 g) or gestational age (20 weeks) to be considered viable, or a series of numbers that summarize the outcomes of previous pregnancies

Nullipara: A woman in her first pregnancy, as well as a woman who has not carried a pregnancy beyond an elective or spontaneous abortion

Primipara: A woman who has had only one pregnancy in which the fetus reached the age of viability

Multipara: A woman who has carried two or more pregnancies (as opposed to fetuses) to viability

From Cunningham, F. G., Gant, N. F., Leveno, K. J., Gilstrap, L. C., III, Hauth, J. C., & Wenstrom, K. D. (2001). *Williams obstetrics* (21st ed.). New York: McGraw-Hill.

cies (carried to the end of the 36th week), the second to the number of preterm pregnancies (those between 20 and 36 weeks' gestation), the third to the number of abortions (spontaneous and elective or therapeutic as well as ectopic pregnancies) through the 19th week of gestation, and the fourth to the number of living children. Remembering the mnemonic Tennessee Power and Light may be helpful (T for term, P for preterm, A for abortion, and L for living children) or Florida Power and Light (F for full term, P for preterm, A for abortion, and L for living children).

The final description should read *gravida,* followed by the number of times the woman has been pregnant, and *para,* followed by four numbers describing a different gestational age when the pregnancy ended. For example, the status of a woman who is pregnant for the third time and has had one first-trimester spontaneous abortion and one full-term pregnancy resulting in a living child would be gravida 3, para 1011 (or G3, P1011).

Interpregnancy Interval

Record the month and year of the births to determine interpregnancy interval. While data are conflicting, there *may* be a risk for preterm birth when the interval between birth and the next pregnancy in certain populations is less than 1 year. Anemia is more frequent when the interbirth interval is less than 1 year.

Gestational Age

Early pregnancy loss, though common, is usually sporadic. Extensive investigation into the cause of spontaneous abortion is usually withheld until a woman has had three consecutive, spontaneous abortions (two in an older woman, considering early pregnancy loss increases with maternal age and conception occurs less frequently). Recurrent early loss may indicate a need for testing and evaluation to identify causes such as uterine abnormalities, genetic abnormalities, and metabolic or endocrine disorders. For example, uterine fibroids, a uterine septum, or a bicornuate uterus may not provide enough room for the growing embryo to implant or grow. Some structural abnormalities may be correctable by surgery. Abnormal cervical development or trauma to the cervix from gynecologic procedures may render the cervix incapable of supporting the increasing weight of the growing baby. As a result, the "incompetent" cervix dilates, painlessly, in the midtrimester of pregnancy, and the immature fetus is expelled. A procedure in which a suture is placed through the cervix early in pregnancy can sometimes prevent the otherwise inevitable loss of the baby.

A history of one preterm birth increases chances for a second preterm birth by as much as 30%. The risk increases as the number of preterm births increases, and the risk decreases with the number of term deliveries (American College of Obstetricians and Gynecologists [ACOG], 1995). The causes of preterm birth are unknown. Single variables such as genital infection, abnormal cervical function, physical exertion, sexual activity, uterine volume and contractility, and vaginal bleeding have been studied, and preterm labor prevention programs have been established. These have not, however, "resulted in a decline in preterm birth. The failure of multiple trials of single risk factors provides substantial evidence that no single factor is responsible for such features of spontaneous preterm birth as its tendency to recur in subsequent pregnancies" (Iams, 1998, p. 55).

The chance for survival of premature babies increases as technology advances. While specialized neonatal intensive care units may save 40% of extremely small infants (those weighing less than 800 g) and extremely immature babies (those born at 26 weeks or less), major disabilities still occur in this group of survivors.

Place of Birth

Identification of the place where previous babies were born—home, birth center, hospital—helps the clinician begin to establish a picture of the birthing philosophy of the woman and her family. It provides a lead into questions about the birth experience and preferences for the present birth. Sometimes a woman is in a midwifery practice because it is her only option rather than because it is her first choice. In these cases, it is helpful to determine her feelings about lack of choice. If she *is* unhappy, talk about what it would take to make the current situation acceptable.

Type of Delivery

Note whether previous births were vaginal, cesarean, or assisted with forceps or vacuum. A woman who has had a cesarean birth may be a candidate for a vaginal birth. The decision usually depends on the location of the incision that was made into the uterus, the ability of the hospital birthing unit to respond promptly should uterine rupture occur, and the desires of the expectant mother once the risk of uterine rupture during labor has been discussed. Risks of 1.6 per 1000 among women with a repeat cesarean birth without labor, 5.2 per 1000 among women with spontaneous onset of labor, 7.7 per 1000 among women whose labor is induced without prostaglandins, and 24.5 per 1000 women with prostaglandin-induced labor have been reported (Lydon-Rochelle, Holt, Easterling, & Martin, 2001). If the uterine incision was made low in the uterus and cut horizontally (low transverse cesarean section) rather than vertically (classic cesarean section), an attempt can usually be made to deliver the baby vaginally. The direction of the skin incision may or may not reflect the direction of the uterine incision.

When possible, obtain copies of the medical records of both the labor and the surgery to identify the reason for a cesarean birth and to document the placement of the uterine scar. While lack of progress is often cited as the reason for a cesarean, unnecessary cesareans are common. A study of the births of 733 women delivering infants by unplanned cesarean section between March, 1993, and February, 1994, from 30 hospitals in Los Angeles County and Iowa found that 16% of the women were still in the latent phase of labor (according to ACOG criteria), and 36% of the women did not have a prolonged second stage prior to cesarean section (Gifford, Morton, Fiske, Keesey, Keeler, & Kahn, 2000).

Records should also be obtained whenever a birth was assisted with forceps or vacuum. This facilitates understanding the reason for an instrumental delivery and may help the birth attendant avoid problems during labor and birth with the present pregnancy.

Length of Labor

Length of labor is important because a long labor may also reflect a problem that could recur. Fortunately, long first labors are seldom followed by other long labors. It is a good idea, however, to request a copy of the labor and birth record whenever a woman reports a labor longer than 24 hours. Short labors also should be noted, as these often repeat. When a previous labor was short (<3 hours total), clinicians often request that women notify the birth attendant as soon as labor begins. Occasionally, induction of labor is appropriate so that the birth can occur under controlled circumstances.

Length of labor is often difficult to determine because clinicians vary in the point they choose to indicate the start of labor. Some choose the very first contraction, some like to select the time at which the contractions became "regular," some select the point at which contractions became painful, and some prefer 4-cm dilation. When questioning women about the length of previous labors, select the time at which contractions began as the starting point because almost every woman can supply this information.

Use of Analgesia and Anesthesia

Discussion of medication used to diminish or control labor pain should lead to questions about whether the medicine was helpful and whether the client is happy to have received it. At times this is a good opportunity to talk about the client's thoughts about pain in regard to the upcoming labor.

Episiotomy and Lacerations

It is difficult to anticipate how a woman will feel about an episiotomy or laceration at the time of birth. Women who have previously had an episiotomy or lacerations may have a preference either for or against the same in the future. If the episiotomy was mediolateral, postpartum pain may have lasted a long time. These women are not likely to want another episiotomy even when it is midline rather than mediolateral. On the other hand, women who have had an extensive laceration with prolonged repair may request an episiotomy.

For women having a first baby, the connotation of the word "tear" may lead to a request for an episiotomy. Women who have experienced childhood sexual abuse can also fear tearing, but can also be afraid of an episiotomy. Exploration of these feelings can occur during the pregnancy.

Birth Weight

Birth weight information identifies low-birth-weight babies and babies who were small for gestational age (SGA) or large for gestational age (LGA). These conditions tend to recur and are associated with increased morbidity and mortality. Low birth weight is defined as weight less than 2500 g (5½ pounds) at birth. SGA/LGA determinations are made at birth and compare birth weight with gestational age.

Long thought to be explainable by racial differences, the contribution of social and genetic factors to birth weight has not been determined. In the United States, African American babies have lower mean birth weights than White babies, a phenomenon commonly ascribed to racial differences with a genetic cause. However, attributing a genetic cause to the difference should be considered speculative. "To look for a genetic cause of the difference in birth weight between the races is premature until the sociocultural questions have been answered" (Foster, 1997, p. 1232).

When a vaginal birth has occurred, birth weight demonstrates that a baby of a certain size successfully traversed the maternal pelvis and provides some reassurance to clinicians that a baby of similar weight can be born vaginally.

 HELPFUL HINT

Two weights may be helpful for you to fix in your mind. The first is that healthy babies at 28 weeks weigh about 1000 g (2 lb, 3 oz). The second is that healthy babies at 36 weeks weigh about 2500 g (5 lb, 8 oz). If a woman tells you that she gave birth at 36 weeks to a baby that weighed 4½ lb, you will know that her baby was SGA.

Gender

Discussing the sex of previous babies provides an opportunity for the clinician to ask the client to share her feelings about having daughters and sons and her and her partner's preferences in regard to the sex of the present baby. This knowledge can be useful when the sex of the baby is different from a strongly expressed preference.

Type of Provider

Ask about the person(s) who provided prenatal care and attended previous births of the client. Identify what the provider did that was perceived as helpful or not helpful.

Complications

Any complication associated with a pregnancy should be known so that those complications known to repeat can be anticipated. Ectopic pregnancy, for example, tends to recur. Spontaneous abortion caused by chromosomal and genetic abnormalities and second-trimester losses also often recur. Other conditions that may recur include congenital anomalies, severe preeclampsia, intrauterine growth restriction, shoulder dystocia, postpartum depression, and postpartum hemorrhage (caused by uterine atony). When these conditions are reported, copies of medical records should be obtained whenever possible.

Pay particular attention to a previous shoulder dystocia. While permanent brachial plexus injury is rare (and not always associated with a traumatic delivery), a study from the 1970s noted a 14% recurrence rate (Gordon, Rich, Deutschberger, & Green, 1973). To determine whether there may have been shoulder problems at previous births, ask women to tell you about the birth itself. Did there seem to be any problem with delivering the baby? Was additional help requested? Was she asked to bring her legs back onto her abdomen? Women who report circumstances that point to a delay in delivery of the shoulders may have been traumatized by the measures taken to free the shoulder or the sudden invasion of the place of birth by multiple professionals arriving to help.

Current Health and Location of Children

The current health status of the client's children should be noted. Illness, disability, emotional problems, and discipline issues can create great stress in families. A helpful question may be, "Would you say that child is easy or hard?" Referrals for counseling, parenting skills, or physical or psychological evaluations may be indicated. Also ask about the location of each child, because the birth mother is not always the custodial parent.

Perception of Previous Pregnancy and Birth Experiences

Ask the client about previous pregnancies and births. What went well? Was she happy or unhappy with the experience? What would she like to do differently this time? How does she feel about any analgesia or anesthesia that was or was not administered? Is there something that worries her? Note in the record what the client says. It may be useful later in her pregnancy when discussing feelings about the upcoming labor and birth. Women who have had a traumatic birth experience may benefit from referral to a birth counselor or to a therapist. When help from one of these professionals is not possible, the clinician may be able to arrange extra time to listen, support, and help women prepare for the coming birth.

Loss of a Child

A woman who has lost a child, whether by miscarriage, an elective abortion, a stillbirth, a neonatal death, relinquishment of a baby for adoption or removal to foster care, or death of an older child, should be asked how that experience has affected her. What was it like? Does she still think about that baby or child? Was the relationship with her partner strained as a result of the loss? How are things now? Is she still grieving?

Women whose children live with another person, whether because of child custody arrangements or loss of the children to a child protective agency, should be given an opportunity to talk about that experience. Women who have relinquished a baby can be asked if they often think about the child. Expect tears when you ask this question, as there is often unhealed grief. Don't be afraid to ask, however, as women are usually grateful that someone is willing to acknowledge their continuing pain. Not all women, of course, will feel this way. Some have put their experience in the past and rarely or never return to it.

Women who have relinquished a child can also be asked if they have thought of "searching" for the child. The search issue in adoption exists for both the person who relinquishes a child and for the person who was relinquished. Each woman—and many clinicians—differ in their feelings about this process. Often a referral to someone who can help the client think through her feelings and consider the pros and the cons of searching will be appropriate. The International Soundex Reunion Registry (ISRR) provides a system for matching persons who desire contact with their next of kin by birth. Any adoptee 18 or older as well as any birth parent or adoptive parent of an adoptee younger than 18 can register, noting their willingness to be contacted. ISSR does not perform a search or provide search advice. The matching service is free (phone: 775-882-7755).

Almost all women who have lost a child for whatever reason experience profound grief, which they may or may not have been able to discuss. Often the mere fact that the clinician asks about and is willing to allow grieving mothers a chance to talk about pain, anger, and disappointment can be therapeutic. A referral to a support group may be helpful.

❖ Medical History

The medical history addresses organic disease and other conditions that may or may not have received a medical diagnosis. Chapter 1 discusses some of these diseases. A thorough review of past diagnoses and symptoms is the only way the midwife will be able to prevent or appropriately treat problems that can affect the outcome of pregnancy. Box 3-3 lists medical and surgical conditions to address prenatally.

Organic Disease

Women with chronic or debilitating health histories—uncontrolled chronic hypertension, autoimmune disorders, insulin-dependent diabetes mellitus, cardiac and pulmonary disease, and certain anemias, among other diseases—should receive their maternity care from an obstetrician or a perinatologist when possible. Chapter 1 discusses the possible influences of these diseases on pregnancy.

Pregnant women with hypothyroidism may need to increase the amount of thyroid medication they are taking. Thyroid-stimulating hormone (TSH) levels should be checked each trimester to see if the medication dosage should be adjusted. All states have mandatory newborn testing for congenital hypothyroidism.

Mental Illness

Mental illness should be identified for three reasons: there may be a genetic component to psychiatric illness, pregnancy may exacerbate the illness, and psychotropic drugs may be indicated or contraindicated in pregnancy. Remember that eating disorders and depression may be present but undiagnosed.

Depression

Depression is a relatively common finding in women. Many suffer needlessly because they do not recognize their symptoms as depression, they feel they should be able to "get through it" by themselves, they do not realize that psychotropic medicine and therapy can help, or they have no money to spend on professional help.

Some women taking psychotropic medicine for depression when the baby is conceived will stop the medicine fearing that it will harm the baby. Studies of pregnant women who took a tricyclic antidepressant or a selective serotonin reuptake inhibitor (SSRI), primarily fluoxetine (Prozac), have shown no increase in major birth defects. The development of children whose mothers took a tricyclic or fluoxetine seems to be no different than children of mothers

Box 3.3

Data To Be Obtained for the Medical/Surgical History

1. Headaches
2. Seizures/epilepsy
3. Anemia
4. Asthma
5. Arthritis
6. Diabetes
7. Bronchitis/pneumonia
8. High blood pressure
9. Urinary tract infection
10. Thrombophlebitis
11. Varicose veins
12. Cancer
13. Stroke
14. Lupus
15. Hepatitis
16. Tuberculosis
17. Skin problems
18. Eye problems
19. Thyroid problems
20. Heart problems
21. Lung problems
22. Gallbladder problems
23. Kidney problems
24. Gastrointestinal problems
25. Blood or clotting problems
26. Liver problems
27. HIV disease
28. Organ transplant
29. Varicella
30. Chlamydia
31. Condyloma
32. Gonorrhea
33. Hepatitis B
34. Herpes
35. Syphilis
36. Pelvic inflammatory disease (PID)
37. Abnormal Pap smear
38. Vaginal infection (yeast, trichomoniasis, bacterial vaginosis [BV])
39. Abnormal vaginal bleeding
40. Pelvic pain
41. Urinary incontinence
42. Incontinence of feces or flatus
43. Infertility
44. Surgery (when, kind, reason, complications)
45. Accidents, injuries, trauma

(continued)

Box 3.3

Data To Be Obtained for the Medical/Surgical History *(Continued)*

46. Blood products received (when, kind, reason)
47. Hospitalizations (when/reason, including for a nervous or mental problem/complications)
48. Medicines taken in the past
49. Bad reactions to prescription medicine, over-the-counter drugs, a vaccination, an anesthetic, x-ray dye, rubber, a blood product, or food
50. Depression
51. Anxiety
52. Feelings of panic
53. Mood swings
54. Nervous breakdown
55. Suicidal thoughts
56. Counseling
57. Participation in a self-help group
58. Medication for nerves or a mental problem
59. An eating disorder or history of dieting
60. Problems having or enjoying sex, including pain, lack of desire, and lack of orgasm
61. History of sexual, physical, and emotional abuse
62. Use of vitamins, teas, tinctures, salves or ointments, acupuncture, biofeedback, chiropractic services, energy healing, folk remedies, spiritual or religious healing, herbal or plant medicine, homeopathy, hypnosis, guided imagery, massage, or relaxation techniques, all to treat or prevent illness

who did not ingest these medications. "Behavioral teratologic effects" (learning problems, abnormal activity levels, and impaired problem solving) have not been studied (Wisner, Gelenberg, Leonard, Zarin, & Frank, 1999). Clinicians must weigh the severity of the depression and its potential for morbidity, including suicide, when discussing benefits and risks with patients. Involvement of a therapist knowledgeable about psychotropic drugs as well as a perinatologist and a genetics counselor is often appropriate.

Clinicians serving migrant, immigrant, and refugee populations should be aware of the high incidence of depression in these groups of women. Many are separated from their extended families and villages. Many have witnessed or experienced violence/atrocities, spent years in refugee camps, and walked hundreds of miles with inadequate food and water to arrive in the United States. Culture shock may be profound. Appropriate mental health resources for refugees, migrants, and immigrants are likely lacking. The concern, interest, and kindness of the midwife may be the most positive thing in the lives of these women.

Eating Disorders

Eating disorders occur across the life cycle. Women who have a history of an eating disorder are at risk for miscarriage, hyperemesis gravidarum (particularly bulimic women), low-birth-weight babies, and postpartum depression (Franko & Spurrell, 2000). These women may fear gaining weight while they are pregnant. This applies whether they are or have been diagnosed with anorexia nervosa, bulimia nervosa, or binge eating disorder. (A binge is defined as eating an excessive amount of food within a 2-hour period and feeling unable to control what or how much is consumed twice a week [on average] for at least 3 months. Binging is not characterized by vomiting, fasting, use of laxatives, or excessive exercise as is common in anorexia.)

Full-blown anorexia puts a woman at high risk for suicide—6 times greater than the norm. It has the highest lethality rate of any psychiatric illness. The lethality of bulimia is unknown. It is highly comorbid for other psychiatric illnesses and substance abuse, especially alcohol and marijuana, and is often difficult to recognize. Clients are reluctant to disclose their illness because of shame and embarrassment. Bulimia, but not anorexia, is associated with sexual abuse (Zerba, 2000).

Girls or women with these disorders often think only about eating or not eating. One approach to inquiring about eating disorders is to ask, "Do you worry a lot about your weight?" A positive response might lead to questions about what the client does to control or restrict her weight and whether she ever eats in secret. Inquire also about the exact amount and type of exercise the client is engaging in, as excessive exercise may be used to keep down weight.

❊ Gynecologic History

Certain gynecologic conditions have the potential for affecting the outcome of pregnancy. For example, pelvic inflammatory disease (PID) increases the risk for ectopic pregnancy, and an initial outbreak of herpes simplex type 2 late in pregnancy can cause severe neurologic damage and even death of the baby. Information about these occurrences, as well as a history of infertility, gonorrhea, chlamydia, syphilis, abnormal vaginal bleeding, and an abnormal Pap smear (and the date of the most recent Pap smear), should be obtained. A history of human papilloma virus (HPV) and herpes commonly causes anxiety when a woman discovers she is pregnant.

Human Papilloma Virus

Human papilloma virus (HPV) is a highly contagious virus that often causes condyloma acuminata (venereal warts). The warts can be found on the cervix and the vaginal wall, in the urethra, and on the buttocks, anus, and external genitalia. HPV is the most common viral sexually transmitted disease. In rare instances, babies born to mothers with HPV infection will have respiratory problems because the warts can grow in the baby's respiratory tract and cause recurrent respiratory papillomatosis. Lesions on the vocal cords or in the upper airway can usually be controlled with laser surgery, but lesions in the lungs can be fatal. Women with HPV types 16, 18, 45, and 56 have a higher incidence of cervical cancer (Ferenczy, 1995). Unfortunately, typing of lesions is not yet generally available. Therefore, regular Pap smears are particularly important for women with HPV.

Venereal warts can occasionally grow so large that a cesarean birth is required. When they enlarge significantly during pregnancy, look carefully at their point of origin. Although some may appear to obstruct the vaginal opening, they may arise from a single stalk that can easily be pushed aside as the baby's head is born. During pregnancy, venereal warts may be treated with liquid nitrogen or with weekly local applications of trichloroacetic acid after protecting surrounding tissue. Podophyllin is contraindicated in pregnancy because it is embryotoxic and teratogenic. Laser therapy, used to treat venereal warts in nonpregnant women, can lead to severe bleeding in pregnant women.

Although warts are generally benign, they may cause problems within a relationship because they are sexually transmitted and unattractive. Clinicians should emphasize that months and even years can elapse from the time the infection was acquired to the time the warts appear. Condom studies show little evidence that male condoms offer women protection from HPV (CDC, 2000).

Herpes

Genital herpes is usually caused by herpes simplex virus-2 (HSV-2). While some women are acutely aware of the initial infection and may even require hospitalization because of pain and inability to void, most women with HSV-2 do not know that they have been infected. Both cervical and perineal lesions are likely to go undetected. A prospective study of 53 men and women who had HSV-2 antibodies but reported no history of genital herpes showed that 83% had genital shedding of the virus, indicating that asymptomatic infection is common (Wald et al., 2000).

Neonatal herpes infection occurs when the virus gains entrance to the uterine cavity subsequent to rupture of the membranes or at delivery as the fetus passes through an infected cervix or lower genital tract. The fetus may also become infected in utero when the first episode of genital herpes occurs during pregnancy. HSV-2 infection can cause severe neurologic damage to the baby and neonatal death. The risk of transmission from an infected mother to the baby is 30% to 50% if the initial infection is acquired near delivery. The risk of transmission is low among women with a recurrent lesion at term and 3% among women who acquire the initial infection in the first half of pregnancy (CDC, 1998).

Most HSV-2 is transmitted among asymptomatic individuals. Instead of developing lesions with the primary infection, they have mild symptoms that resemble the flu. Individuals with these "silent" herpes infections appear to have lesions that occur less frequently and last a shorter period of time than individuals with clinical symptoms.

A pregnant woman who reports a history of herpes or a history of a partner with herpes should be counseled about notifying the clinician as soon as she thinks she is in labor so that an appropriate decision about route of delivery can be made. The patient should be instructed to remind the clinician of the history of herpes. An examination of the perineum, cervix, and vagina should occur early in labor. If prodromal symptoms—often a feeling of numbness, itching, or tingling where the external body lesion will appear—or a lesion are present when labor occurs or the membranes rupture, delivery is usually by cesarean section because of a high viral load in these instances.

Viral cultures at term are no longer a basis for management of women with a history of herpes infection because they do not predict who will be shedding the virus at the time of delivery. Antiviral medications (acyclovir, valacyclovir, and famciclovir) for women with recurrent lesions are not recommended at this time by the CDC (CDC, 1998). However, ACOG recommendations, based on consensus and expert opinion, state, "For women at or beyond 36 weeks of gestation who are at risk for recurrent HSV, antiviral therapy also may be considered," although such therapy may not reduce the likelihood of cesarean delivery (ACOG, 1999d, p. 7). Table 3-1 contains guidelines for antiviral treatment of HSV in pregnant and nonpregnant women.

In some practices, herpes lesions noted around the anus or other areas somewhat removed from the vulva may be covered with a gauze square during labor and at the time of birth. Whether a cesarean birth is truly indicated at all in the presence of prodromal symptoms or herpes lesions is currently being studied.

❋ Surgery, Accidents, and Hospitalizations

A thorough history includes information about operations, trauma, emergency room visits, and hospital stays. While some of this data may not relate to pregnancy or birth, important information such as the use of blood products

TABLE 3.1 Antiviral Treatment for Herpes Simplex Virus*

Indication	Valacyclovir	Acyclovir	Famciclovir
First clinical episode	1000 mg twice a day for 7–14 days	200 mg five times a day or 400 mg three times a day for 7–14 days	250 mg three times a day for 7–14 days
Recurrent episodes	500 mg twice a day for 5 days	200 mg five times a day or 400 mg three times a day for 5 days	125 mg twice a day for 5 days
Daily suppressive therapy	500 mg once a day (≤9 recurrences per year) or 1,000 mg once a day or 250 mg twice a day (>9 recurrences per year)	400 mg twice a day	250 mg twice a day

From Baker, D. A. (1998). Antiviral therapy for genital herpes in nonpregnant and pregnant women. *Int J Fertil 1998, 43,* 243–248.
   Reprinted with permission.

between 1978 and 1985 (when AIDS testing was not conducted) or pelvic trauma may be elicited. A woman who tells of frequent emergency room visits for accidents such as walking into doors or falling down stairs may be experiencing domestic violence.

Breast Surgery

Breast Reduction

Women who have had breast reduction surgery can have problems with breastfeeding. Older surgical procedures for breast reduction involved reimplantation of the nipple with complete circumferential nipple excision to make the nipple look anatomically correct. Unfortunately, nerves to the areola and nipple were often cut, interfering with messages from the breast to the brain. Women who have had this kind of breast surgery make colostrum and breast milk, but the volume of milk produced is usually insufficient to sustain the baby because the milk volume plateaus. When it will occur is not predictable. The baby's weight gain must be monitored closely. It may be possible to combine breastfeeding with a supplemental feeding system. Newer surgical procedures leave breast tissue and structures underneath the areola and nipple intact. A copy of the operative report may be helpful.

Breast Augmentation

Breast augmentation procedures may or may not affect the supply of breast milk. The location of the surgical incision influences the ability to lactate. Peri-areolar incisions are of greatest concern because they disrupt the ducts and the neurologic supply to the nipple. Innervation must be intact because sensation facilitates milk ejection (Friedmann, 2000). Be sure to ask about the appearance of the breast before surgery, as the augmentation procedure may have been done for mammary agenesis (no breast tissue), in which case exclusive breastfeeding will not support the infant.

✳ Pharmacologic Treatment

Prescription Drugs

Fortunately, only a few drugs are known to cause birth defects. Still, it is important to ask the client about use of past and present prescription and over-the-counter (OTC) drugs. Chapter 1 includes a list of drugs known to have adverse effects on the growing fetus. Box 3-4 lists the FDA's categorization of drugs in pregnancy.

To avoid anaphylactic reactions, inquire about adverse reactions to any diagnostic or therapeutic agent, to rubber, and to food. Because patients may not think of OTC medications as drugs, ask, "Have you ever had an allergic reaction or a bad reaction to a prescription medicine (like penicillin), an OTC medicine (like aspirin), a vaccination, an anesthetic, an x-ray dye, rubber, a blood product, or food?" A mild, upset stomach from an antibiotic is normal and should not be considered an allergic reaction (Steinberg, 2000).

Certain drugs have a potential for cross-reaction. For example, although the risk is small, cephalosporins given to a person who is allergic to penicillin may cause an anaphylactic reaction (and vice versa). Likewise, nonsteroidal anti-inflammatory drugs (NSAIDs) can cause an adverse reaction in patients allergic to aspirin (and vice versa). Every clinic or office should have a protocol for alerting the health care provider about previous bad or allergic reactions. This information must be prominently displayed, and providers should routinely ask about allergies before prescribing drugs and before recommending OTC products.

Pregnant women with upper respiratory infections while pregnant often inquire about medicine that is safe and effective. Box 3-5 identifies the FDA pregnancy category for medicines commonly used for symptomatic relief.

Box 3.4

FDA Categories for Drugs in Pregnancy

Category A: No risk to fetus in first trimester demonstrated in controlled studies and no evidence of risk in other trimesters.

Category B: No fetal risk shown in animal studies, but no controlled studies in pregnant women are available, or animal studies showed an adverse effect not confirmed in controlled studies with pregnant women in the first trimester. The penicillins are in this category.

Category C: Adverse effects on fetus found in animal studies but no controlled studies in women, or studies in women and animals are available. Give drug only if the benefit justifies the possible risk to the fetus.

Category D: Positive evidence of fetal risk exists, but the benefits may be acceptable despite the risk, as in life-threatening situations or serious disease. Phenytoin is an example.

Category X: Fetal abnormalities have been demonstrated or evidence for fetal risk exists, and risks from the drug outweigh any benefits. Isotretinoin is an example.

Source: U.S. Food and Drug Administration

Complementary and Alternative Medicine

Many people look outside the traditional health care system for alleviation of distressing physical symptoms. Nontraditional therapies include chiropractic, homeopathy, acupuncture and acupressure, massage, exercise, hypnosis, vitamin therapy, relaxation techniques and biofeedback, spiritual healing and prayer, lifestyle diets such as macrobiotics or veganism, imagery, herbs, weight-loss programs, self-help groups, energy healing, and folk remedies. These are commonly referred to as complementary and alternative medicine (CAM). Data from a national survey conducted in 1997 revealed that 42.1% of the U.S. White, adult population used at least one nontraditional therapy. Yet fewer than 40% of the nontraditional therapies were reported to the physician (Eisenberg et al., 1998). The reported use of CAM would likely be much higher if the survey had included representative numbers of other racial groups. Use the World Wide Web to keep up-to-date on the research generated in the field of CAM. Try the Office of Dietary Supplements' web site: http://odp.od.nih.gov/ods. *Complementary and Alternative Medicine at the NIH* is a 16-page newsletter published four times a year by the National Center for Complementary and Alternative Medicine (NCCAM). It is available on NCCAM's web site (http://NCCAM.nih.gov) or can be ordered free by calling 1-888-644-6226. The International Bibliographic Information on Dietary Sup-

Box 3.5

FDA Categories of Drugs Commonly Used for Symptomatic Relief of Upper Respiratory Infections During Pregnancy

Antihistamines
  Pseudoephedrine   Category C
    Studies have failed to confirm an association between
    pseudoephedrine and neural tube defects and gastroschisis, but
    ". . . it would be prudent to recommend avoiding the use of
    preparations containing psuedoephedrine during the first
    trimester."
  Loratadine   Category B
Nasal decongestants
Cough suppressants*
  Dextromethorphan   Category C
  Hydrocodone preparations
Expectorant
  Guaifenesin   Category C
Analgesic-antipyretic
combinations
  Aspirin   Category C first and second
                                     trimester, Category D third trimester
  Acetaminophen   Category B
  Ibuprofen
Vitamin C   Category A at RDA dosage
                                     Category C in large doses
Penicillins, including those   Category B
with clavulanic acid added
(e.g., Augmentin, Timentin)
Erythromycin, Zithromax   Category B
Cephalosporins (e.g., Keflex)   Category B
Ciprofloxacin   Category C but contraindicated in
                                     pregnancy, especially in first
                                     trimester because of reports of birth
                                     defects
                                     While these have not been
                                     confirmed, avoid Ciprofloxacin in
                                     pregnancy as ". . . better drugs are
                                     available that have minimal risk."
Trimethoprim-sulfonamide   Okay in second and early third
(e.g., Bactrim)   trimesters. Avoid in the last 4 weeks
                                     because of reports of an association
                                     with hemolytic anemia and
                                     hyperbilirubinemia. Not all studies
                                     confirm this association.

*Note alcohol content of cough suppressants. The range is from 0 to 12.5%.
OTC preparations commonly contain 1–2% alcohol.

Source: Farmer, R. (1999). Pregnancy and cold remedies: Teratogen counseling in pregnant women with upper respiratory infections. *Genetics Northwest, 13*(1), 6–7.

plements (IBIDS) database includes published international, scientific literature on dietary supplements (including vitamins, minerals, and botanicals).

Be sure to ask patients about nutritional supplements, particularly vitamins that are being consumed in lieu of or in addition to prenatal vitamins. The potential for teratogenicity or for suppression of trace elements with high-dose vitamins should be considered. Ask clients using nonstandard prenatal vitamins to bring vitamin containers to the prenatal visit to document their content.

❊ Family History

Information about the client's family identifies women at risk for a genetic disease that could affect the outcome of pregnancy or for having a child with a genetic disease. The family medical history is discussed in Chapter 1. If either the personal medical history or family medical history reveals that the client was adopted, this may be a good time to ask how that experience has affected her. For some people, adoption has been wonderful. For others it has always been painful. Pregnancy is often the factor that motivates or remotivates a man or a woman to wonder about family background and to want to know about their biologic family. Just as it is appropriate to discuss "searching" with a woman who has relinquished a baby, it is appropriate to ask the woman who has been adopted (and, when possible, the baby's father, if the father has been adopted) if she has thought of "searching" for her birth parents. People who have tried to try to find their birth parents probably know that much joy and much pain can come from reuniting. Often, support from a counselor who has experience in the field of adoption can be helpful in making a decision about whether to "search."

The family history should include questions about drug and alcohol use by close family members. Sometimes asking, "Have alcohol or drugs affected your life in any way?" opens the door to a fruitful discussion of this topic. Additional questions can be found in Chapter 1. Abuse of either drugs or alcohol by a close family member almost always has had some negative effect on family members, and it can be helpful to discuss this with clients.

❊ The Baby's Father

As discussed in Chapter 1, information about the baby's father should include racial and ethnic background and a family medical history to identify potential genetic problems. At times it may be necessary to discuss the father's involvement with another partner in which repeated pregnancy loss occurred.

The father's use of drugs and alcohol should be noted. Heavy marijuana users who consider this drug harmless are not likely to admit to a problem. Box 3-6 contains questions that can help heavy users evaluate their use.

❈ Foreign Travel Or Residence

A travel and residential history may suggest the need for certain kinds of testing. For example, in some countries, parasites, malaria, hepatitis or tuberculosis are endemic. Women who have visited or lived in these areas may benefit from testing.

❈ Sexual History

Screening for sexual dysfunction and providing information about sexuality is well within the abilities of midwives. We have an opportunity to help clients understand and appreciate the sexual part of their lives. New research recognizes that, for women, a desire for physical intimacy rather than sexual release probably begins the sexual response cycle, and nonsexual, interpersonal factors are extremely important (Leiblum, 2000).

Box 3.6

Questions to Ask to Facilitate Identification of a Problem With Marijuana Use

1. Has smoking pot stopped being fun?
2. Do you ever get high alone?
3. Is it hard for you to imagine a life without marijuana?
4. Do you smoke marijuana to avoid dealing with your problems?
5. Do you smoke pot to cope with your feelings?
6. Does your marijuana use let you live in a privately defined world?
7. Have you ever failed to keep promises you made about cutting down or controlling your dope smoking?
8. Has your use of marijuana caused problems with memory, concentration, or motivation?
9. When your stash is nearly empty, do you feel anxious or worried about how to get more?
10. Do you plan your life around marijuana use?
11. Have friends or relatives ever complained that your pot smoking is damaging your relationship with them?

Source: Marijuana Anonymous. (No date).

A sexual history provides opportunities to 1) offer information that may relieve anxiety and dispel myths; 2) offer suggestions to improve sexual functioning; (3) identify a client with a history of sexual abuse; and (4) make referrals when sexual dysfunction or emotional problems are noted. (See Box 3-7 for questions that contribute to a sexual history.) Remember to view sexual problems within the context of a relationship. Remember also that the meaning ascribed to sexual activities has great variation. A woman who says her partner wants sex "all the time" may be in a relationship in which the partner wants sex once a month.

How to Ask Questions About Sex

While sexual problems are common among both men and women who seek medical care, clinicians can have a difficult time initiating a discussion about sexual matters. They may hesitate because they have not received adequate preparation for addressing sexual issues or because they have inadequate time to address issues that may be revealed.

Box 3.7

Questions to Ask About Sex

1. Are you currently sexually active? Do you have more than one partner?
2. Is your partner male, female, either?
3. Are you having any problems with how often you have sex? Or, if client is partnered, you might ask, "Do you and your partner agree on how often you have sex?"
4. Do you have problems with whether or not you have sex?
5. Is there any pain when you have sex—with insertion, penetration, or thrusting? Is there any pain after intercourse?
6. Are there any problems having an orgasm?
7. Does your partner have any sexual problems?
8. Would you say you are satisfied or dissatisfied with the sexual part of your life? (You might ask her to rate this part of her life on a scale of 1 to 10.)
9. How satisfied do you think your partner is?
10. Is there anything you would like to change?
11. Is there something you think your partner would like to change?
12. Has your partner said anything about having sex with you since you've become pregnant?
13. Is there anything you are wondering about in regard to sex?
14. When a problem is identified, ask the client:
    "When did this seem to be a problem?"
    "Was there anything else going on at that time?"
    "Do both you and your partner perceive this as a problem?"

Beginners should remember they need to practice, practice, practice asking appropriate questions. To initiate a discussion about sexual activity, concerns, or problems, try a variety of approaches until you find one that fits your style. An approach during pregnancy is to say, "Most pregnant women have questions about sex while they are pregnant. I wonder if there is anything you would like to ask me." To her question(s), you could reply, "Many people wonder about that," and proceed to provide her with information. Another approach is to begin by addressing concerns that arise frequently during pregnancy. You could say, "Many pregnant women notice a change in their desire for sex when they are pregnant. Has this happened to you?" Occasionally, it is the male partner with decreased libido. A pregnant woman might feel relieved to know that some men prefer not to have sexual intercourse after a certain point in pregnancy because they are afraid it will hurt the baby.

Common concerns include frequency of intercourse, lack of sexual desire, dyspareunia, preorgasmia, vaginismus, anxiety about sexual orientation, posttraumatic stress from sexual abuse, noncoital sexual pain, and sexual problems within a relationship. If a problem exists, determine whether it is a long-standing or a recent problem. How much of a problem is it? Does the client's partner recognize the problem? Does the client know the cause? What has she done about the problem? Sometimes a concern can be solved by providing information, assuring the client that her concern is a common one, telling her that activities she may feel anxious about are considered "normal," or referring her to reading materials. A nonjudgmental attitude and an approach that conveys not only a willingness to discuss aspects of sexuality and sexual behavior, but also a belief that this information is important will go a long way.

A discussion of sex in pregnancy needs to include information about the danger of allowing air to be blown into the vagina during sexual play. One way to provide this information is to say, "There is one thing I always like to tell pregnant women . . ." and advise the client against allowing air to be blown in her vagina as this practice can cause a fatal air embolus. Because this practice is uncommon, clinicians may feel uncomfortable or embarrassed talking about it, yet it is important information to provide.

History of Physical, Emotional, and Sexual Abuse

Millions of women in the United States have experienced abuse as children or adults. The abuse may be physical, emotional, or sexual and may have affected multiple aspects of their lives. Screening for abuse is intended to stop ongoing abuse; prevent abuse in the future; anticipate issues that may arise during pregnancy, birth, and/or the postpartum period; and provide information and linkages to community resources so that, over time, healing may occur.

✻ Screening For Abuse

Physical Abuse

Study after study identifies routine screening of pregnant women for abuse as both appropriate and important. "There is reason to believe that violence may be a more common problem for pregnant women than preeclampsia, gestational diabetes, and placenta previa, conditions for which pregnant women are routinely screened and evaluated" (Gazmararian et al., 1996, p. 1920). ACOG suggests that pregnant women be screened every trimester and postpartally, the latter period being potentially the most dangerous (ACOG, 1999b). Clients are overwhelmingly receptive to screening questions. It only takes hearing one woman say, "I've never told this to anyone before," to know that a willingness to confront this difficult topic can be a life-changing event for abused women. Without your willingness to take this initial step, your clients may never have another opportunity to have someone point out "how strong they must be to be coping with the things they're coping with, how resourceful they must be just to get through a single day, or a single hour of a single day, and how intelligent they must be to have figured out how to survive in that situation. Since I can't rescue patients, I realize all I need to do is be empathetic and supportive, and this simple intervention can really help empower someone" (Family Violence Prevention Fund, 1999, p. 3).

This is of particular importance for women "immersed in cultures that grant men the implicit right to control and censure their behavior" (Olavarietta & Sotelo, 1996, p. 1937).

Little research on intimate partner violence has been conducted with ethnically diverse populations. A study of Hispanic women in New Mexico found more physical abuse in intimate relationships and more violence during pregnancy when compared with non-Hispanic women. Hispanic women in the study rarely reported the violence to authorities and sought help less frequently (Krishnana, Hilbert, VanLeeuwen, & Kolia, 1997).

Understanding the phases women go through as they move toward freedom from the abuser can be helpful: beguilement, where charm is a dominating characteristic; bewilderment, where the abused woman is baffled with the partner's behavior and hopes the partner will change; control, where the woman may experience stalking, destruction of property, separation from family members and friends, beatings, and derision or humiliation; escape, where the woman finds the courage to leave; and reflection, where women examine their feelings of guilt over staying in the relationship, learn slowly to trust again, and emerge stronger (Stewart, 2000). Predictors of violence in men include depression, alcohol use, illicit substance abuse, a personal history of childhood victimization, and the presence of a nonbiologic child in the home (Oriel and Fleming, 1998).

A woman's readiness to discuss abuse involves dealing with feelings of shame and embarrassment as well as fears of the police, family separation, and the clinician's reaction. These powerful emotional barriers to leaving also prevent women from leaving abusive relationships. Additional barriers are lack of financial support; poor job skills; fear of losing custody of children, the court process, loneliness, inability to survive alone, and formidable life changes; a belief that children should be raised in a family with a father; ties to home and belongings; religious doctrine that speaks against separation or divorce; guilt; love for the offender; feeling that the abuse is deserved; and a belief or hope that the offender will change. Perhaps most powerful is the realistic fear of retaliation. Items that should be gathered as part of an action plan to leave the relationship can be found in Chapter 1.

When interviewing women who have been or who are in an intimate relationship that involves violent or controlling behavior, determine whether children in the family have observed the behavior. A child who observes a family member being abused is automatically said to have experienced emotional abuse. "The deleterious effects on children who witness physical violence between their parents or caregivers has been well documented. Therefore, if children are living with the client, it is important to ask if the children have seen or heard threats or assaults or have been threatened or assaulted themselves by the abuser" (Alpert, 1995, p. 779). Finally, clinicians must also consider the possibility that the client herself is an abuser. Midwives may be reluctant to accept or consider this possibility and, although probably rare, it does occur.

Sexual Abuse

Evolving data suggest that a history of sexual abuse may influence a woman's ability to deliver vaginally. Powerful emotional forces may make women able to "shut labor down" so that they do not have to deal with people looking at their genitalia or feel the baby emerge from a place that is associated with pain, embarrassment, guilt, and humiliation. "The fear of losing control makes some laboring women with a history of sexual abuse struggle against their contractions. Relaxation may be impossible and suggestions from well-meaning childbirth educators or staff to 'relax,' 'surrender,' 'yield,' or 'open up,' may remind the survivor of the times when she was made to do these things and was hurt. Other suggestions, meant to reassure, such as 'trust your body' and 'do what your body tells you to do,' are incomprehensible to the survivor whose body has been a source of anguish and betrayal. Her efforts to keep labor under her control may actually slow or stop progress" (Simkin, 1994).

Asking about sexual abuse can occur at any time during the interview when there appears to be an opening. Some midwives wait until they feel the client has had time to become comfortable, and they introduce the subject toward the end of the interview. Some wait for a moment when it seems logical to introduce the topic, such as during the sexual history or when asking about other forms of abuse. Some midwives prefer asking the question face-to-face, while others feel that addressing the question on a written form makes it easier for the client to disclose an abusive history. Some find it helpful to substitute the words "disrespected" or "maltreated" for abuse. "How old were you when you had your first sexual experience?" can be a useful question with which to start. Follow with, "Was this with or without your permission?" You might continue by asking the client if she has had sex subsequently without her consent. Has she been forced to participate in any sexual activity against her will? When sexual abuse is acknowledged, three follow-up questions contribute to an understanding of the context of the abuse: "Whom did you tell? How did he or she respond? How did you make it stop?"

Asking, "Is any of this unfinished for you?" can help you decide whether a referral for counseling should be suggested. In many instances, the amazing resilience of human beings has worked well for women. It is inappropriate to pathologize, revictimize, or retraumatize women who have moved on in their lives.

Asking women with a history of childhood sexual abuse if they have a preference for the sex of the baby may help uncover conflicted feelings. These women might also be asked about their reaction to the daughters and sons they already have. "Some women react negatively to having a girl because they feel that they cannot possibly protect their daughter from abuse. Others do not want a boy, for fear that he will remind them of their perpetrator" (Heritage, 1998, p. 675).

❊ Environmental Exposures

Exposure to environmental toxins is probably caused by a combination of proximity to farmland, use of pesticides (school, home, and garden), occupation, hobbies, buildings, and ingestion of food and water. Whether there is increased risk of developmental problems from intrauterine exposure or exposure as an infant or toddler is under investigation. Additional information about environmental exposure can be found in Chapter 1.

Exposure to Lead

Prior to 1978, lead was added to paint because of its durability and antimildew properties. As lead-based paint deteriorates and repainting is planned, sanding, scraping, and power washing are often used to prepare the surfaces for repainting. This causes lead dust to settle in homes. Friction caused by opening and closing doors and double-hung windows adds to lead levels, as does lead tracked into the home on shoes or by pets who have stepped on soil laden with lead from exterior lead paint, leaded gasoline, and air pollution. Recently, 71% of 127 Oregon homes built before 1930 were found to have lead levels exceeding federal standards (Oregon Health Division, 2000b).

Other sources of exposure to lead include industrial sites and smelters that use lead; contaminated soil from target shooting; lead materials used in hobbies or crafts, such as assembling stained glass and casting lead fishing weights or bullets; some imported earthenware used for cooking; and some inexpensive vinyl window blinds (Oregon Health Division, 2000b).

Volatile Organic Compounds

While lead poisoning and asthma from indoor toxins are relatively well known by the health professional community, the carcinogenic volatile organic compounds (VOCs) have been pretty much ignored. "The sources responsible for indoor toxic emissions include household deodorizers, dry-cleaned clothes, air fresheners and cleaners, most insect repellent products, treated wood (e.g., furniture, wood paneling), incomplete combustion from cooking or from heating systems, and the single greatest source: environmental tobacco smoke (ETS)" (Spaeth, 2000, p. 632). Clinicians should be aware of these potential dangers and watch for research in the future.

Pesticides

"Pesticide" is a broad term referring to insecticides, herbicides, rodenticides, and fungicides. The nature and extent of detrimental health effects from pesticides is unknown. Those living in close proximity to farmland, including owners, producers, and field workers, appear to be especially vulnerable. Residential pesticide contamination, as measured by analysis of selected chemicals in house dust, may be worse than ground contamination by chemicals used outdoors where biochemical and physical processes degrade the compounds used. Acceptable levels of exposure, both indoors and outdoors, have not been determined.

Migrant workers who live in crowded conditions with poor ventilation, inadequate laundry facilities, and few changes of clothing are probably the most susceptible to increased risk for environmental contaminants. The normal "body burden" of pesticides for both adults and for children is unknown.

X-rays During the Current Pregnancy

Any exposure to radiation may carry the risk of genetic effects and birth defects. However, exposures that involve less than 5 rads are not associated with congenital malformations. Most diagnostic studies involve a low radiation exposure. Computed tomography (CT) scans give the most radiation. (An abdominal CT series equals 2.6 rads, while a chest x-ray equals .008 rads). However, CT is sometimes necessary to evaluate a client for trauma subsequent to an injury.

Significant exposures to x-rays in utero may increase the risk for childhood cancer. Research suggests that "the most sensitive period of exposure for developing leukemia is about the 7th month of pregnancy. The most sensitive period of exposure for developing all cancers, except leukemia, is the first 6 months of pregnancy" (Hanford Health Information Network, 1994, p. 5).

❋ Habits Undermining Health

Smoking Cigarettes

The mechanism by which cigarette smoking affects birth weight is unclear. Possibilities include the powerful vasoconstricting effect of nicotine, cell damage caused by carbon monoxide, lower calorie consumption by smoking women, and the complex interplay of the more than 3,000 chemicals in cigarette smoke. In the United States, 25% of women are smokers at conception, and as many as 40% of women who smoke will deny that they do. Approximately 40% of women who smoke and become pregnant will quit on their own once they learn they are pregnant.

The good news is that "women who stop smoking, especially by the 20th week of pregnancy, have babies of approximately equal size and health as women who never smoked. Women who stop smoking by the 30th week of pregnancy still have significant increases in the birth weight of their babies, compared with women who do not stop at all" (Goldenberg & Dolan-Mullen, 2000, p. 39). Women who quit on their own are likely to be lighter smokers, to have smoked for a shorter period of time, to be having their first baby, to have had more education, and to be of higher socioeconomic class (Goldenberg & Dolan-Mullen, 2000).

Because many women are willing to make sacrifices for their children and many women would like to quit smoking, pregnancy is an excellent time to ask women to stop—even those who think their labor will be easier or shorter because of a smaller baby, like the idea of having a smaller baby, or like the way smoking helps them decrease anxiety, relieve tension, or keep down their weight. Advice from a health care provider combined with support and self-help materials can be a powerful motivator. The first step is to assess the smoking status of every client. Box 3-8 contains questions to ask a pregnant woman about smoking.

Once you know that a client smokes, ask her, "What do you know about the effects of smoking when you are pregnant?" Many women do not know

---

Box 3.8

Questions to Assess a Pregnant Woman's Smoking Status*

Which of the following statements best describes your cigarette smoking?
1. I smoke regularly now—about the same as before finding out I was pregnant.
2. I smoke regularly now, but I've cut down since I found out I was pregnant.
3. I smoke every once in awhile.
4. I have quit smoking since finding out I was pregnant.
5. I wasn't smoking around the time I found out I was pregnant, and I don't smoke cigarettes now.

---

*From U. S. Public Health Service. (2000). *Treating tobacco use and dependence.* Washington, DC: U.S. Department of Health and Human Services, p. 95.

exactly what effects smoking can have on the baby. Some can be swayed toward quitting by learning that smoking increases the risk of spontaneous abortion, ectopic pregnancy, intrauterine growth restriction, placenta previa and abruption, stillbirth, prematurity, low birth weight, and sudden infant death syndrome (SIDS), which in turn increase and contribute significantly to maternal and perinatal morbidity and mortality. New evidence links in utero exposure to maternal smoking with decreased lung function in children (Gilliland et al., 2000), and long-standing evidence that environmental tobacco smoke during childhood contributes substantially to childhood health problems should be emphasized. You might convey this information to the client by saying, "If you smoke, your baby's lungs can be weak."

Although five medications have been approved by the FDA to treat tobacco dependence—sustained-release bupropion (Zyban), nicotine gum, the nicotine inhaler, nicotine nasal spray, and the nicotine patch—their safety in pregnancy has not been determined. Effective counseling strategies to help people stop smoking depend in part on the persistence of the clinician and the consistency of assessment and teaching among practitioners. A prenatal smoking cessation protocol can be useful. Just 1 to 3 minutes at each prenatal visit spent assessing the client's smoking habit and, for those wishing to quit, evaluating progress toward that goal can make a difference. The intervention program recommended by the U.S. Public Health Service is based on the "5 A Program": ask, advise, assess, assist, and arrange (Box 3-9).

When a client has made the decision to stop smoking, a discussion of obstacles to quitting—previous failures, fear of weight gain, smoking by other family members, and unpleasant withdrawal symptoms—is helpful. Aids that

---

Box 3.9

The "5 A's" for Brief Intervention*

Ask about tobacco use.	Identify and document tobacco use status for every patient at every visit.
Advise to quit.	In a clear, strong, and personalized manner urge every tobacco user to quit.
Assess willingness to make a quit attempt.	Is the tobacco user willing to make a quit attempt at this time?
Assist in quit attempt.	For the patient willing to make a quit attempt, use counseling and pharmacotherapy to help him or her quit.
Arrange follow-up.	Schedule follow-up contact, preferably within the first week after the quit date.

*From U.S. Department of Health & Human Services. (2000). *Treating tobacco use and dependence.* Washington, D.C.: U.S. Department of Health and Human Services, p. 26.

---

have helped some women quit smoking include inserting a picture of one of their children or a picture of the fetus from an ultrasound inside the cellophane wrapper of a cigarette pack or focusing on the rewards (such as saving $800 to $2,000 per year).

Innovative programs to promote smoking cessation during pregnancy continue to develop. Researchers in Oregon offered 200 low-income women $50 vouchers at a department store for every month they did not smoke. At the end of the study, 68 women had quit smoking. Twenty-one percent of the women were not smoking 2 months after giving birth, an encouraging statistic as most smoking cessation programs rarely result in more than a 14% cessation rate.

With impressive evidence that cigarette smoking is a powerful determinant of birth weight, clinicians may have a difficult time understanding why any woman would smoke while pregnant. Smoking may provide a harried mother with a few minutes each day to herself and the ability to stay calm; it may be the only thing that she does for herself all day. Women who are substance abusers may even use smoking to help keep them from using other drugs. "Noncompliance with medical advice may reflect not so much a failing on the part of the mother as her superior knowledge of the constraints of everyday family life" (Graham, 1988). Clinicians, then, must be sympathetic to the difficulties facing pregnant smoking women. This does not mean avoiding consistent messages of the importance of quitting. Rather, it means acknowledging the pain and sacrifice the effort to quit will require. It also means careful selection of health education material. Brochures with covers that show babies smoking are not likely to be read by the target audience, although I once had a woman tell me to get "the ugliest brochure you can find."

Substance Abuse

Alcohol

One out of 29 pregnant women engages in "risk drinking," seven or more drinks per week or five or more drinks on one occasion (CDC, 1997). The significant problems posed by children with fetal alcohol syndrome and alcohol-related neurodevelopmental problems make it imperative that clinicians ask about alcohol intake and remind women of the potential lifelong effect alcohol may have on the unborn baby. (See Chapter 1 for suggested questions.) While specific teratogenic effects occur between the third and eighth weeks of gestation, brain-affected consequences occur throughout pregnancy. Identifying women at risk for a child with fetal alcohol syndrome allows for counseling and, possibly, prevention.

Many approaches to determining alcohol intake during pregnancy have been proffered. Because pregnant women, particularly those who drink heavily, often underreport alcohol intake, you might simply ask the client, "How much do you drink?" To any response other than "never," ask her, "How much do you drink in a week?" Suggest a few amounts and start high: "A case, a few six-packs?" If it is obvious that the client drinks on a daily basis, try this question: "How much do you drink in a day—two packs? One?"

Another approach is to ask the three quantity-and-frequency questions:

On average, how many days per week do you drink alcohol?
On a typical day when you drink, how many drinks do you have?
What is the greatest number of drinks you've had at any one time in the past month. (Carlat, 1998)

Clinicians can look for opportunities to interject questions about alcohol consumption at any time during the patient interview. For example, a patient under a great deal of stress might be asked, "Given the stress you are under, I wonder if you've been drinking more lately?" (Henderson-Martin, 2000). Considering that alcoholism often leads to problems in many areas of the alcoholic's life, try to determine whether effects have been noticed in physical health, emotional well-being, relationships, the legal arena, on the job, or at school. Additional information about the effect of in utero exposure to alcohol and approaches to eliciting information about alcohol use can be found in Chapter 1.

Illicit Drugs

Identifying drug use in pregnancy is important for at least three reasons: to get help for women who wish to stop using; to identify fetuses and babies at risk; and to identify women at risk for HIV infection. However, determining whether a client is using drugs and assessing the extent of use can be difficult. Some clinicians feel it is important to *assume* that a client is using them. These clinicians will ask, "What recreational drugs do you use? How much? How many times a day, a week, or a month do you use them?" "When was the last time you used drugs?" Other clinicians prefer to ask a general question, such as, "Can you tell me how drugs have affected your life?" or "Have you ever used recreational drugs—marijuana, cocaine, acid, speed, or something similar?" Chapter 1 contains addition suggestions for eliciting information about drug use. Whatever approach you use, be sure to specifically mention marijuana, because some people do not consider it an illicit or recreational drug.

Women who use drugs put a high priority on keeping their world safe. They keep secrets, minimize the extent of their drug use, and may take an aggressive stance, particularly when they view the health care provider as an obstacle. Clinicians should keep in mind that pregnant women significantly underreport current use of illicit substances. Findings from one study of 789 pregnant women found that those who reported past use of tobacco, marijuana, and cocaine but denied current use had 25.2%, 23.9%, and 22.7% positive results of urinary assays, respectively (Markovic, Ness, Cefilli, Grisso, Stahmer, & Shaw, 2000).

If a new mother continues using drugs after her baby is born, risk to the baby continues. Not only are the babies born biologically vulnerable, but they also are born to mothers who face health and emotional problems of their own. These women are compromised in their ability to establish relationships and may be unable to respond to the baby's needs, particularly if they receive an infant who is medically fragile after an extensive hospital stay. Following are summaries of commonly used illicit drugs.

Cannabis

Cannabis, commonly known as marijuana, is one of three drugs that come from the hemp plant, Cannabis sativa L. Growing wild through most of the temperate and tropic regions of the world, cannabis contains delta-9-tetrahydrocannabinol (THC), the chemical believed to be responsible for marijuana's psychoactive effects. Cannabis is usually smoked in the form of loosely rolled cigarettes, often adulterated with chemicals that change both the effect and toxicity. Marijuana users are subject to the same problems with bronchitis, emphysema, and asthma that tobacco smokers experience.

Marijuana is the most commonly used illicit drug in this country. Thirteen percent of teenage girls have tried marijuana by the age of 13, and 50% have tried it by age 18 (Kosterman, Hawkins, Guo, Catalano, & Abbott, 2000).

Recently identified as an addictive drug, marijuana used short-term also causes "problems with memory and learning, distorted perception, difficulty in thinking and problem-solving, loss of coordination, increased heart rate, anxiety, and panic attacks" (National Institute on Drug Abuse, 2000, p.1), as well as respiratory problems (probably due to the absorption of 3 to 5 times the amount of tar and carbon monoxide as tobacco smokers [National Institute on Drug Abuse, 2000]), and "emotional unavailability" (Gold, 1999). "Additional effects include dry mouth, red eyes, impaired motor skills, inability to concentrate, and hunger" (U.S. Department of Justice, 1997).

Withdrawal symptoms from marijuana do not appear to be as pronounced as those with other drugs, possibly because of the long half-life (about 30 hours in humans). The physical dependence effects occur slowly and may be so subtle that they may be blamed on something else (Boyles, 2000). The effect of marijuana on the fetus is unknown, but concern does exist not only about the effects of secondhand smoke, but also about the mother's ability to parent the child if she is a chronic user.

Cocaine

Cocaine is distributed as a white crystalline powder that is snorted or is diluted prior to being injected. It affects the part of the brain that regulates feelings of pleasure, blocking the reabsorption of dopamine and causing neural impulses to keep firing. Pulse and temperature increase, the desire for sex is heightened, and illusions of mental alertness are present. However, euphoria, energy, and the aphrodisiac effect turn into anxiety, exhaustion, and depression. Snorting cocaine results in an effect in 3 to 5 minutes, while intravenous injection results in a rush in 15 to 30 seconds. "Crack" cocaine is the chunk or "rock" form of cocaine and is smoked. Because smoking delivers large quantities to the lungs, the effect is like that of an intravenous injection with intense feelings occurring almost immediately but rapidly subsiding. Smoking cocaine is associated with cough, shortness of breath and chest pain. One maternal death from vaginal use of cocaine has been reported (Greenland, Delke, & Minkoff, 1989). A small number of people lack an enzyme that breaks down cocaine. For them, one dose of cocaine can be fatal.

Cocaine is particularly dangerous to the growing fetus. It is associated with spontaneous abortion, preterm delivery, intrauterine growth restriction, cerebral ischemia, intracranial hemorrhage, abruptio placentae, and disturbances in the baby's sleep-wake cycle (Blatt, Meguid, & Church, 2000). There is disagreement about the long-term effects of cocaine on the baby. The neurobehavioral abnormalities originally described have not been found with more recent studies (Andres, 1999). Data are difficult to interpret because of small sample sizes, inappropriate developmental testing, and inability to distinguish between cocaine effects and other factors associated with cocaine use that affect child development. These factors include late and inadequate prenatal care, prematurity, lead poisoning, iron deficiency anemia, and lack of nurturing at home. Fortunately, many neurobehavioral effects decrease or disappear by 4 months of age (Blatt, Meguid, & Church, 2000).

Despite this fact, the abuse and neglect associated with cocaine when children remain with a cocaine-using parent threatens the hearts, minds, and bodies of the children. Cocaine-exposed children living with biologic parents are 5 to 6 times more likely to suffer from abuse or neglect and 14 times more likely to be placed in foster care. Infants placed with relatives continue to be at risk. "Kinship care comes with minimal oversight from social services, and it is not uncommon for the drug-abusing mother, against court orders, to reestablish custody while the child is in the care of relatives" (Blatt, Meguid, & Church, 2000, p. 79).

Amphetamines

Amphetamines are synthetic stimulants that can be injected, snorted, swallowed, or smoked. Long used to prevent sleep, control weight, improve athletic performance, and treat mild depression, amphetamines are highly addictive, produce strong cravings, and result in severe withdrawal symptoms. During the high, which lasts 4 to 16 hours, the user can feel aggressively smarter than others, becoming argumentative and violent. Feelings of euphoria and invincibility are common, as are hallucinations and feelings of paranoia. Users may not sleep for days, and then a crash occurs. Deep sleep ensues, during which time it may not be possible to rouse the user.

"Ice," named because it looks like crushed ice, is smokable methamphetamine (like "crack" is smokable cocaine). Although similar to that of cocaine, the onset of effect from amphetamines is slower, and the effect lasts longer. Psychotic, erratic, and violent behavior results from chronic abuse. The effect of amphetamines on the fetus is not known, but concern for parenting abilities remains.

LSD

Lysergic acid diethylamide (LSD) is the most potent hallucinogen known. It is taken orally and is usually sold in the form of impregnated paper, tablets, or thin squares of gelatin. Dilated pupils, decreased body temperature, nausea, perspiration, fast heart rate, and increased blood sugar are common physical reactions. Visual and mood changes occur within an hour of ingestion. Hallucinations affect perceptions of depth and time as well as the size and shape of objects and the user's own body image. Anxiety and depression are common aftereffects (U. S. Department of Justice, 1997). The effect of LSD on the baby is not known.

Heroin

The narcotic heroin is a powder that varies in color from white to dark brown (depending on impurities left from manufacturing or the presence of additives). Purity varies from 1% to 98%. "Black tar" (from Mexico), as its name implies, has the color and consistency of black tar. Purity ranges from 20% to 80%. In the past, heroin was injected intravenously, intramuscularly, or subcutaneously (skin-popping), but increasingly pure heroin allows users to snort or smoke it. Narcotics reduce tension and anxiety and thereby create a sense of well-being. At the same time, heroin can cause drowsiness, poor concentration, apathy, nausea and vomiting, and significant respiratory depression.

Maternal heroin use is associated with prematurity, intrauterine growth restriction, and withdrawal symptoms in the baby. Heroin complications in mothers are increasingly related to adulterants and to the use of contaminated needles for injection. Heroin users need the drug to prevent the withdrawal syndrome and require increasingly larger doses to achieve an effect.

❊ Social History

Each clinician should develop a list of questions suitable for obtaining the information needed for the social history. Some questions are essential to ask. Others are not *essential* but help you identify risk factors and understand the factors that affect the client's life. For example, knowledge of the client's socioeconomic status can be helpful. "African-American women with the same socioeconomic status as white women have twice as high a risk of giving birth to an infant weighing less than 2500 g and 3 times as high a risk of delivering a very-low-birth-weight infant (one weighing less than 1500 g)" (Foster, 1997, p. 1232).

If the client is homeless or in a temporary residence, flagging the chart can help you remember to verify her address and contact number at every visit. Box 3-10 lists questions that can serve as a starting point for obtaining the social history. Adapt them to your personal style.

Family Constellation

Information about the client's family should include her family of origin, place of birth, people with whom she is living, people that she considers "family," and people that she can count on for support. You might ask, "Could you tell me a little bit about the important people in your life?" or "Whom do you include in your immediate family?" Then continue with, "Do you live with a partner?" or "Are you single, partnered, married, separated, divorced, or widowed?," indicating that you are aware that not all pregnant women are involved in a conventional marriage arrangement. Ask about the quality of relationships with the partner or with the father of the baby if the baby's father is not the client's partner. The 1-to-10 scale can be helpful for some women: "On a scale of 1 to 10, with 10 being a wonderful relationship and 1 being an

Box 3.10

Questions to Ask to Establish a Psychosocial Database

1. Can you tell me a little about your childhood? Would you say that it was easy or hard?
2. Would you tell me a little about your mother, your father, your stepparent, or grandparent, as appropriate?
3. Did you ever live with someone other than your mother or your father? If yes, what was that like?
4. Have you had any big losses in your life—a family member, a relationship, a job, or a home?
5. What are the stresses in your life now?
6. Whom can you count on for support?
7. How would you describe your living situation?
8. Tell me a little bit about your job, being a homemaker.
9. What is the highest grade you've completed?
10. Do you have any plans to return to school?
11. What are your interests or hobbies?
12. How important is religion in your life?

awful relationship, where would you put your relationship now?" Unless the answer is "10," follow with "What would it take to make it a 10?" Another helpful question to ask is, "Can you count on your partner to be there for you?" Inquire about relationships with parents, siblings, friends, and with the partner's family as well.

If a lesbian woman informs you about her sexual orientation, ask whether her sexual preference is known to family, friends, and coworkers and whether she wants information about her sexuality in her medical record. Lesbians vary greatly in where they are in the "coming out" process and in their need for confidentiality. Nonjudgmental, sensitive health care by providers who are knowledgeable about lesbians, aware of their anxiety and vulnerability in traditional heath care settings, and willing to discuss their needs in regard to secrecy, support, and referrals will be appreciated.

Living Situation

Obtain information about where the client lives, how often she has moved, the kind of dwelling she lives in, the number of people with whom she lives, the safety of the area, and when indicated, whether there is sufficient food in the house. Without the advantage of a system of home visiting in this country, it behooves us to be as knowledgeable as possible about the context of the lives of our clients.

Sources of Support

Inquire about the people the client can depend on for support. Pregnant women may live far from significant female family members. At times women will report that no one is available to them. More frequent and longer visits that focus on providing emotional support and establishing linkages with appropriate community resources should be scheduled when possible.

Sources of Stress

Common sources of stress for pregnant women include money, housing, job, a difficult child, and relationship problems with a partner or a family member. Asking "What are the major sources of stress right now?" helps the clinician understand some of the factors impinging on the client's life.

Occupation

Knowing the client's occupation is important in order to know the client in a holistic way as well as to assess the potential for preterm birth and for exposure to occupational hazards. A recent meta-analysis of working conditions and the outcome of pregnancy showed a significant positive association between 1) physically demanding work, shift work, prolonged standing (more than 3 hours per day or the "predominant occupational posture"), and a "high cumulative work fatigue score"* and preterm birth; 2) physically demanding work and SGA babies; 3) and physically demanding work and hypertension or preeclampsia. Working long hours was not associated with an adverse outcome (Mozurkewich, Luke, Avni, & Wolf, 2000). Job requirements may expose employees to metals, dust, fibers, fumes, chemicals, biologic hazards, noise, vibration, and radiation.

Occupation is also important because it provides some information about income level. (See Box 3-11 for the Federal Poverty Guidelines effective through April, 2001. The guidelines change yearly. In addition, see Box 3-12 for suggested questions about occupation.)

Responses to inquiries about occupation can help the provider be aware of services and benefits that might be available to the client and her family. The Women, Infants, and Children (WIC) program, for example, is a health and nutrition program for pregnant women, breastfeeding women, and young

---

*"Standing position for more than 3 hours per day; work on strenuous industrial machines or conveyer belt; important physical exertion or load carrying; routine work or not stimulating task; and one or more of the following factors: noise, cold temperature, wet atmosphere, or manipulation of chemical substances" (Mozurkevich, Luke, Avni, & Wolf, 2000, p. 294).

Box 3.11

2001 Federal Poverty Guidelines

2001 POVERTY GUIDELINES FOR THE 48 CONTIGUOUS STATES AND THE DISTRICT OF COLUMBIA

Size of family unit*	Poverty guideline
1	$ 8,590
2	11,610
3	14,630
4	17,650
5	20,670
6	23,690
7	26,710
8	29,730

2001 POVERTY GUIDELINES FOR ALASKA

Size of family unit†	Poverty guideline
1	$10,730
2	14,510
3	18,290
4	22,070
5	25,850
6	29,630
7	33,410
8	37,190

2001 POVERTY GUIDELINES FOR HAWAII

Size of family unit‡	Poverty guideline
1	$ 9,890
2	13,360
3	16,830
4	20,300
5	23,770
6	27,240
7	30,710
8	34,180

*For family units with more than eight members, add $3,020 for each additional member. (The same increment applies to smaller family sizes also, as can be seen in the figures above.)

†For family units with more than eight members, add $3,780 for each additional member. (The same increment applies to smaller family sizes also, as can be seen in the figures above.)

‡For family units with more than eight members, add $3,470 for each additional member. (The same increment applies to smaller family sizes also, as can be seen in the figures above.)

Box 3.12

Questions to Ask About Occupation

1. Are you employed? Tell me a little about the job—what you do, the hours you work, and how many days a week you work.
2. How much standing does your job involve?
3. Do you get breaks? Where do you go when you get a break?
4. Do you do any heavy lifting?
5. Have you ever worked with or around anything that might be a health hazard? Have you ever had a job where you wore protective clothing?
6. Is there anything about your job that you think might be dangerous to you or your baby?
7. How do you like your job? Could you rate it on a scale of 1 to 10, with 1 being awful and 10 being terrific?
8. Do you make more than _____ each month? (See Box 3-11 and insert the figure that defines 100% of poverty based on the size of this woman's family.)

---

children. The program provides health and nutrition information, supplemental food, and access to health care services for pregnant women, nursing mothers (for up to 12 months after delivery), and children from birth to age 5. Pregnant women receive milk, cheese, eggs, vitamin C-fortified fruit juices, iron-fortified cereal, and peanut butter, dried beans or peas, or lentils. Breastfeeding mothers also receive carrots, canned tuna, peanut butter and peas, beans, or lentils for themselves. Women who are not breastfeeding receive infant formula for the first 12 months of the baby's life. Eligibility is based on a household income that is 185% or less of the federal poverty level.

Education, Interests, Hobbies, and Goals

Ask about the highest grade that the client has completed, as well as her interests, hobbies, and long-term goals. Her highest completed grade can give an approximation of her reading level. (Subtract 3 years from the highest grade.) Occasionally, potential hazards from hobbies such as painting, sculpting, welding, woodworking, piloting, auto racing, firearms, stained glass, ceramics, and gardening will be identified. Materials used in arts and crafts can contain silicon, talc, solvents, and heavy metals, all of which are potentially dangerous. Gardeners should be advised to wear gloves while digging in the soil to decrease the risk of toxoplasmosis. In warm, moist soil the oocysts can remain infectious for about a year (CDC, 2000d).

Religious Preference

Inquire about religious preference and any practices related to religion that should be observed during the pregnancy or at birth. This information can lead to a discussion about the importance of religion in the client's life, religious traditions surrounding pregnancy and birth, feelings about male health care providers, and in some cases, the use of blood products.

❊ Pets

Congenital toxoplasmosis can occur when women acquire primary toxoplasmosis while pregnant. A wide range of findings are found in babies with this disease. Among the effects are hepatomegaly, splenomegaly, intracranial calcification, chorioretinitis, and hydrocephaly. Toxoplasmosis can also cause abortion, prematurity, and growth restriction. Many women, particularly those who have had or have a cat as a pet, have protective antibodies and are not at risk for the disease.

Women in the United States are not routinely screened for Toxoplasma infections. However, all pregnant women in France are screened, and women who are nonimmune are tested monthly for seroconversion. Recent analysis of data from 591 live-born children whose mothers seroconverted during pregnancy showed that 29% had congenital infection; the risk for transmission rose as pregnancy progressed (2% at 8 weeks, 6% at 13 weeks, 40% at 26 weeks, 72% at 36 weeks, and 81% shortly before giving birth); severity is highest when maternal infection occurs in the first trimester; a negative amniocentesis cannot completely rule out infection; and a positive amniocentesis "almost certainly" rules in infection (Dunn, Wallon, Peyron, Peterson, Peckham, & Gilbert, 1999).

At the initial prenatal visit, ask about the kind and number of pets in the home. In most instances, women who have cats for pets can be reassured that the likelihood of acquiring a primary toxoplasmosis infection in pregnancy is small, unless they have had direct contact with cat feces that are 4 days old. It takes this long for the oocysts in the feces to become infective. Infection from undercooked meat is a much more likely source than infection from contact with a cat. Consequently, pregnant women who eat meat should eat well-cooked meat and should not give undercooked meat to cats.

In addition to assessing for toxoplasmosis, inquiring about pets allows the clinician to determine if potentially dangerous pets, such as ferrets and some breeds of dogs, are in the home (Rottweiler, Doberman). Additionally, an occasional client will be living in a home with such a large numbers of pets that it is unlikely that sanitary conditions exist. In these instances, clients should be encouraged to find new homes for the animals.

✼ Weapons

Weapons of all kinds can be found in many homes and are increasingly carried by individuals. A 1990 study found that almost 20% of 9th- through 12th-grade students had carried a weapon at least once in the preceding 30 days. Approximately 1 out of 20 students carried a handgun (CDC, 1991). Inquiring about the presence and storage method of firearms in the home should be a routine part of a history. All firearms should be kept in a locked box away from the eyes of children. Anyone who is depressed or who uses or lives with people using illicit drugs should be advised to remove weapons for the protection of everyone. The medical record should be flagged.

✼ Good Health Habits

Inquire about behaviors and practices known to promote health, to reinforce efforts already underway, and to begin planning for health education discussions as prenatal care continues.

Breast and Skin Examinations

Breast self-examination is a practice that all women should be encouraged to perform monthly. Women between the ages of 35 and 40 should have a baseline mammogram, although this examination is not recommended during pregnancy unless a suspicious mass is noted, as the increased blood supply to the breasts during pregnancy makes mammograms difficult to interpret.

A skin check at the same time breast self-examination is performed is an important health activity. Because of the association between solar rays and skin cancer, clients should be asked if they take any protective measures when they are in the sun. Use of tanning booths, another source of skin cancer, should be discouraged.

Immunizations

Information about previous immunizations determines the need for initial vaccination or booster doses of certain vaccines. The decision to administer a vaccine during pregnancy should consider the risk of vaccinating against the benefits of protection.

Risk from vaccination during pregnancy is largely theoretical. The benefit of vaccination usually outweighs the potential risk when 1) the risk for disease exposure is high, 2) infection would pose a special risk to the mother or fetus, and 3) the vaccine is unlikely to cause harm. "Generally, live-virus vaccines are contraindicated for pregnant women because of the theoretical risk of transmission of the vaccine virus to the fetus. If a live-virus vaccine is inadvertently given to a pregnant woman, or if a woman becomes pregnant within 3 months after vaccination, she should be counseled about the potential effects on the fetus, but it is not ordinarily an indication to terminate the pregnancy" (CDC Advisory Committee on Immunization Practices, 1998, p. 1).

It is common in certain developing countries to administer tetanus-diphtheria toxoid (Td) in the last trimester of pregnancy to protect babies against neonatal tetanus, the cause of an estimated tens of thousands of neonatal deaths each year. While Td is considered safe in the second and third trimesters (Gall, 1995), it is not commonly offered to pregnant women in the United States because neonatal tetanus is practically nonexistent. Hepatitis B vaccine is also considered safe in pregnancy. However, because pregnancy is a hypoimmune state with potential for infection of the fetus, some clinicians in developed countries prefer to administer the vaccine after the baby is born.

Consideration should be given to offering influenza vaccine (an inactivated virus) to women who will be in the third trimester of pregnancy or the puerperium during flu season (November to March), as well as to pregnant women of any gestation who are at risk for influenza complications (CDC, 1995). A 25% reduction in upper respiratory infections (URIs), a 43% reduction in URI-related absenteeism from work, and a 44% reduction in office visits has been noted when nonpregnant, healthy adults were vaccinated against influenza (Nichol et al., 1995). There is no evidence of fetal risk at any gestational period with this vaccine. Protective titers are achieved about 2 weeks after vaccination and decline after 4 to 6 months. This vaccine should not be given to women who are allergic to eggs. Table 3-2 summarizes recommendations from the CDC Advisory Committee on Immunization Practices (ACIP).

Health care providers should document all immunizations that clients have received so that appropriate recommendations can be made postpartally. Certainly, health care providers should follow immunization recommendations for themselves as well as for their clients. While health care workers often think primarily of HIV infection when they observe universal precautions, hepatitis B infection is about 40 times more likely than HIV infection to occur after a needle stick (Zuckerman, 1995).

Nutrition

Nutritional assessment is an important component of prenatal care. Perhaps most important during pregnancy is identifying women who will not or cannot consume enough calories to support good fetal growth. Women who fall into this category include women with hyperemesis gravidarum, women who are too poor to be able to buy enough food, women with an eating disorder, and some women who have a problem with body image.

A discussion of nutrition can be initiated by asking, "Is eating going to be an issue for you while you are pregnant?" This approach helps the clinician address what might be a concern for any woman.

Exercise

Concerns about exercise during pregnancy involve both mother and baby. These concerns include the potential for injury to mother and fetus should a fall occur. During pregnancy the influence of estrogen, progesterone, and elastin results in connective tissue laxity and joint instability. Some separation of the pubic symphysis is common. Nerve compression syndrome, as is found in carpal tunnel syndrome, may occur. These effects increase the likelihood of falling with resulting maternal injury and the possibility of premature separation of the placenta and preterm labor if abdominal trauma occurs.

Concerns about fetal well-being relate to the theoretical potential for

- Fetal teratogenicity from fetal hyperthermia subsequent to an increase in maternal body temperature
- Hypoxia and intrauterine growth restriction from blood being shunted away from the maternal viscera to working muscles
- Hypoglycemia
- Increase in stress hormones
- Preterm delivery

Few studies have examined hyperthermia in pregnant women. Skin temperature does reach high levels with exercise. However, "There seems to be enhanced thermoregulation during pregnancy, as compared with the nonpregnant state, that protects against hyperthermia" (Ezmerli, 2000, p. 263).

In general, most clinicians feel that mild to moderate exercise during pregnancy is not harmful. Certain sports, however, seem to be inherently hazardous to pregnant women. A fall during waterskiing could result in trauma to the abdomen or water under high pressure being forced into the vagina. Any contact sport could involve a fall or a blow to the abdomen. Orthopedic injuries from reduced joint stability and changes in equilibrium could also occur. Horseback riding, windsurfing, roller blading, and diving also seem to pose undue risks because of their potential for trauma to the maternal abdomen. It seems prudent to advise women to avoid these activities. Women who run should avoid running when the temperature or humidity is unusually high.

No data are available for pregnant women who have exercised at altitudes over 8,000 feet. Data do show that women who live at altitudes above 10,000 feet have more complications during pregnancy and give birth to babies with lower birth weights simply by virtue of living at the higher altitude. Conse-

Text continues on page 99

TABLE 3.2 Recommendations from the CDC Advisory Committee on Immunization Practices

"Risk from vaccination during pregnancy is largely theoretical. The benefit of vaccination among pregnant women usually outweighs the potential risk when a) the risk for disease exposure is high, b) infection would pose a special risk to the mother or fetus, and c) the vaccine is unlikely to cause harm." ACIP *General Recommendations on Immunization.* p. 20

Generally, live-virus vaccines are contraindicated for pregnant women because of the theoretical risk of transmission of the vaccine virus to

Vaccine	Should be Considered if Otherwise Indicated	Contraindicated During Pregnancy
Routine		
Hepatitis A		
Hepatitis B	✓	
Influenza	✓	
Measles		✓
Mumps		✓
Pneumococcal		
Polio (OPV and IPV)		
Rubella		✓
Tetanus/Diphtheria		
Varicella		✓
Travel & Other		
BCG		✓
Cholera		
Japanese		
Meningococcal	✓	

the fetus. If a live-virus vaccine is inadvertently given to a pregnant woman, or if a woman becomes pregnant within 3 months after vaccination, she should be counseled about the potential effects on the fetus. But it is not ordinarily an indication to terminate the pregnancy.

Whether live or inactivated vaccines are used, vaccination of pregnant women should be considered on the basis of risk vs. benefits—i.e., the risk of the vaccination vs. the benefits of protection in a particular circumstance. This table may be used as a general guide.

Notes

Safety in pregnancy not determined; theoretical risk low; weigh vaccination risk against risk of hepatitis.

Safety during first trimester of pregnancy not yet evaluated.

Avoid vaccination during pregnancy. However, if a pregnant woman requires immediate protection against poliomyelitis, she may be administered OPV or IPV in accordance with the recommended schedules for adults.

"No specific information exists on the safety of cholera vaccine during pregnancy. Its use should be individualized to reflect actual need."

"No specific information is available on the safety Encephalitis (JE) of JE vaccine in pregnancy. Vaccination poses an unknown but theoretical risk to the developing fetus, and **the vaccine should not be routinely administered during pregnancy**." "Pregnant women who must travel to an area where risk of JE is high should be vaccinated when the theoretical risks of immunization are outweighed by the risk of infection to the mother and developing fetus."

(continued)

TABLE 3.2 Recommendations from the CDC Advisory Committee on Immunization Practices *(Continued)*

Vaccine	Should be Considered if Otherwise Indicated	Contraindicated During Pregnancy
Plague		
Rabies	✓	
Typhoid (Parenteral and Ty21)		
Vaccinia		✓
Yellow Fever		

Author: Please provide source citation for table

Box 3.13

Topics for the Initial Prenatal Visit History

1. Maternal age
2. Menstrual history
3. Contraceptive history
4. Obstetric history
5. Medical/surgical history
6. Medicines: CAM, OTC, prescription
7. Family medical history
8. Pertinent information about the baby's father
9. Foreign travel
10. History of abuse
11. Environmental exposures
12. Use of cigarettes
13. Substance abuse
14. Psychosocial history
15. Pets
16. Weapons
17. Health habits including breast self-examinations, immunizations, nutrition, and exercise

Notes

"The effects of plague vaccine on the developing fetus ... are unknown. Pregnant women who cannot avoid high-risk situations should be advised of risk-reduction practices and **should be vaccinated only if the potential benefits of vaccination outweigh potential risks to the fetus.**" (15)

"No data have been reported on the use of any of the three typhoid vaccines among pregnant women."

"Although specific information is not available concerning adverse effects of yellow fever vaccine on the developing fetus, **pregnant women theoretically should not be vaccinated,** and travel to areas where yellow fever is present should be postponed until after delivery." "**Pregnant women who must travel to areas where the risk of yellow fever is high should be vaccinated**. Under these circumstances, for both mother and fetus, the small theoretical risk from vaccination is far outweighed by the risk of yellow fever infection."

quently, caution women about "skiing, biking, or hiking vacations at altitudes above 8,000 feet and certainly at or above 10,000 feet" (Clapp, 2001, p. 38).

❊ Conclusion

What a long time a thorough initial visit history takes! Box 3-13 lists the topics that should be covered. Some practices find that it is best to schedule the physical examination for a separate day. However, a written history form that the client completes before the visit usually makes efficient use of time and allows for the history to be obtained and the physical examination to be performed at the same visit.

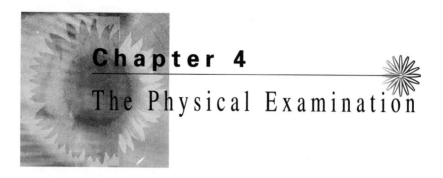

Chapter 4
The Physical Examination

✳ Introduction

The physical examination at the initial prenatal visit is intended to identify abnormalities or deviations from normal that could contribute to morbidity and mortality for either mother or baby. The examination can also identify bodily features that suggest a genetic disorder, and it contributes information that helps establish an accurate due date. Minimally, the examination should include determination of height and weight; measurement of blood pressure (BP) and pulse; an examination of the skin, thyroid gland, heart, lungs, breasts, extremities, and abdomen; and a pelvic examination.

The physical examination involves looking at and touching body parts considered intimate and private. Exposing these areas of the body to strangers can involve fear, embarrassment, dread, and occasionally, physical and emotional pain. The examination, then, requires both skill and sensitivity. A chaperone should be present whenever possible to protect the interests of both client and provider. The chaperone's presence protects the client from inappropriate sexual advances and protects the clinician from false charges of sexual impropriety. While most sexual impropriety occurs between male providers and female clients, same-sex boundary violations do occur.

✳ Height

Height should be obtained because it is necessary for the determination of body mass index (BMI). It also identifies women of short stature for their ethnic group (sometimes an indicator of a genetic disorder) and provides a baseline for subsequent height determinations as women age. Be sure to actually measure height; a client is often wrong when asked what her height is. When the client is shorter than expected for her family or when her height is more than two standard deviations below the mean, genetic counseling is appropriate. The role that height may play in pelvic size is unclear. Loss of height can be a sign of osteoporosis. Bone densitometry studies may be appropriate.

❊ Weight

Weight is obtained at the initial visit to determine BMI, recommend weight gain for the pregnancy, track weight gain or loss, and increase vigilance for women who fall into certain weight categories. The Institute of Medicine recommends the use of BMI to determine weight gain recommendations. The BMI is obtained by relating the client's height to her prepregnancy weight (Appendix H). Box 4-1 contains the Institute of Medicine guidelines for weight gain in pregnancy. Note that the weight gain goal is a range of pounds and uses the client's prepregnancy weight as the basis for measuring gain, even though the weight reported by the client may not be accurate.

Maternal obesity before pregnancy increases macrosomia and perinatal mortality. It also protects against preterm birth (half the rate of women with normal BMIs), and raises the incidence of post-term delivery. Researchers from Sweden examined birth certificates of 167,750 women and found that higher prepregnancy weight increases the risk of late fetal death independent of hypertension and diabetes (Cnattingius, Bergstrom, Lipworth, & Kramer, 1998). Maternal obesity is the most important determinant of birth weight in this group of women. Women with BMIs above 31 have a higher incidence of babies with spina bifida, great-vessel heart defects, abdominal wall defects, and intestinal defects. Women with low prepregnancy weight have a higher incidence of small for gestational age babies (Wolfe, 1998). In this group of women, weight gain during pregnancy is the major determinant of birth weight.

HELPFUL HINT

It can be fun for some women to weigh themselves and record the weight on a graph at each visit. Be careful, however, with some groups of women. Women with low literacy skills may find this activity difficult, and women who are obese or who have body-image problems may prefer not to participate.

❊ Blood Pressure

In normal pregnancy, BP declines slightly as early as the eighth week. It stays down through the second trimester and then moves back toward prepregnancy levels. Measurement in pregnant women should follow standard techniques. Use an appropriately sized cuff, a properly calibrated manometer, an intact inflating system, and a stethoscope with tubing of an appropriate length. Remember that hearing acuity, visual acuity, concentration, the angle at which

| Box 4.1 |

Institute of Medicine Guidelines for Weight Gain in Pregnancy

1. BMI less than 19.8 (underweight): 28 to 40 lb
2. BMI 19.8 to 26 (normal prepregnancy weight): 25 to 35 lb
3. BMI 26.1 to 29 (overweight): 15 to 25 lb
4. BMI greater than 29: at least 15 lb

From the National Academy of Sciences, Institute of Medicine. (1992). Nutrition during pregnancy and lactation: An implementation guide. Washington DC: National Academy Press.

the meniscus of the mercury column is observed, the rate of inflation and deflation of the cuff, digit preference, and placement of the manometer will influence the accuracy of the reading.

A large measuring cuff usually should be used whenever the client's upper arm measures more than 35 cm around. If no large cuff is available, a regular cuff can be placed on the forearm. In this case, the stethoscope should be placed over the radial artery. A small cuff used to determine BP on a woman with a large arm is likely to give an erroneously high reading. All BPs in pregnant women should be obtained with the woman in a sitting position. The same arm should be used each time, preferably the right arm for consistency. It is no longer accepted practice to have a woman with an elevated BP rest on her left side before or during the measurement. BPs obtained this way give a low reading that can lead to false reassurance that the BP is within normal limits. Women with an elevated or slightly elevated BP in the first half of pregnancy may have chronic hypertension or, if nulliparous with a systolic reading of 120 mm Hg or greater, may be at risk for preeclampsia (Sibai, 1996).

In many prenatal settings, BP is obtained by someone other than the clinician. Because BP is such an important parameter in pregnancy, personally measure all pregnancy BPs.

❖ The Skin

Common skin changes in pregnancy include hyperpigmentation of the face (chloasma), areola and nipples; striae gravidarum; spider nevi; and the linea nigra. Pathology may be noted as the skin is examined for color, rashes, growths, lesions, moles, scars, signs of physical abuse, or evidence of intravenous drug use. A rash on the palms of the hands or soles of the feet might be a sign of syphilis. Scars may be indicative of a surgical procedure or, in rare instances, of sexual practices associated with sadomasochistic rituals. When tattoos or piercings are present, ask about the needles used in the procedure. Shared needles can be a source of HIV infection. Six or more café au lait spots equal to or greater than 15 mm in diameter may indicate neurofibromatosis. Pay attention to possible manifestations of physical abuse: bruises, especially on the neck from choking; on the face; on the breasts; on the abdomen; or on the upper arm from grabbing. Injuries in various stages of healing, such as cigarette burns, should increase suspicion.

❋ The Thyroid Gland

The thyroid gland is slightly enlarged during pregnancy because of glandular hyperplasia and increased vascularity. These anatomic changes, however, do not produce significant thyromegaly, and any significant enlargement requires investigation. Hypothyroidism can be hard to detect in pregnant women because many of the symptoms of hypothyroidism—fatigue, weight gain, and constipation—mimic pregnancy. Hyperthyroidism is not common when tachycardia is absent.

❋ The Lungs

The lung examination should include observation for shortness of breath, shallow breathing, rapid breathing, irregular respirations, guarded respirations, wheezing, coughing, and dyspnea. Healthy women rarely have lung problems. Examination of the lungs is usually most helpful to aid in a diagnosis of bronchitis or pneumonia. Listen for crackles, wheezes, and decreased breath sounds.

❋ The Heart

Systolic heart murmurs are common in pregnant women. They are usually benign, as they result from the marked increase in blood volume that occurs in pregnancy—as much as 45% above a woman's nonpregnant level at the end of pregnancy (Pritchard, 1965). This increase nourishes the enlarged uterus and protects the mother when blood is lost at birth. However, murmurs may also be caused by abnormal cardiac structures as in aortic stenosis, ventricular or atrial septal defect, mitral regurgitation, mitral valve prolapse, pulmonary stenosis, and tricuspid regurgitation (Etchells, 2000). Systolic murmurs are categorized by their intensity (Table 4-1).

In an asymptomatic pregnant woman, a grade 1/6 or a grade 2/6 murmur is usually considered benign. When the systolic murmur is greater than 2/6, or

TABLE 4.1 Heart Murmurs Categorized by Intensity

Grade	Description
0	No murmur detected even after focusing on systolic interval
1	Murmur is not heard initially but is detected after focusing on systolic interval
2	Murmur detected immediately upon auscultation
3	Loud murmur detected immediately upon auscultation
4	Murmur associated with a thrill

Reprinted with permission from Etchells, E. (2000). The significance of systolic murmurs. *The Clinical Advisor, 3*(7/8), p. 44.

if any other murmur is heard, a cardiac workup may be indicated. Request both an electrocardiogram and an echocardiogram if resources are available. If the results are normal, a physician referral is not indicated.

The maternal pulse increases slightly during pregnancy, but it is rarely more than 100 beats per minute (bpm). Think of hyperthyroidism when it is more than 110 bpm, and order a thyroid-stimulating hormone (TSH) stimulation test. See Chapter 5 for information on thyroid testing.

❊ The Breasts

As many as 2% of breast cancers are diagnosed in pregnant women. Careful, thorough examination of the breasts is, therefore, a critical part of the physical examination during pregnancy. In addition to examining the breasts, inquire about breast pain, skin or nipple changes, and client detection of a breast mass or axillary lymph nodes. A breast that is warm or inflamed requires prompt referral to a surgeon to rule out inflammatory breast cancer. The approximate size, location, and consistency of any mass should be recorded. Location should also be diagrammed. Note any dimpling, retraction, erythema, or nipple scaling.

A clinically suspicious mass is one that is discrete, firm, unilateral, and typically nontender. While classical cancer tumors feel hard, fixed, and irregular, many cancer tumors mimic those usually found to be benign (cystic, mobile, regular). They may be mobile or fixed to adjacent tissue. Occasionally a cancer will present as an area of thickening, asymmetry, or focal persistent pain. Because breast cancer may present in such a variable manner, there are no physical exam features that reliably distinguish benign from malignant masses. All palpable masses require further investigation (Oregon Health Division, Oregon Breast and Cervical Cancer Program, 1999). During pregnancy, breast masses are usually evaluated by ultrasound and fine-needle biopsy because mammography is not generally helpful.

At the present time, there is no standardized technique for performing the clinical breast examination. In fact, there is no agreement on the extent to which the clinical breast examination (CBE) contributes to the detection of breast cancer. Only indirect evidence points to its effectiveness.

Begin the examination with an examination of the lymph node drainage of the breast. Seventy-five percent of lymphatic drainage from the breast is into the axillary nodes, and most of the rest of the drainage is into the infraclavicular nodes.

With the client seated and her shoulders lifted, use light pressure and small circular movements to palpate the supraclavicular lymph nodes from the sternoclavicular joints to the end of the clavicles. With the client's shoulders relaxed, palpate the infraclavicular lymph nodes along the underside of the clavicle in the opposite direction.

For examination of the axillary lymph nodes, face the patient while standing slightly to her side. Support the client's arm at the elbow while she rests her forearm on yours. With your examining hand reaching high into the axilla, palpate with the pads of your three middle fingers. "Proceeding down the midaxillary chest wall, lift the tissue with your examining hand and gently role [sic] it downward using circular finger movements, following along the pectoral node chain. Return to the axilla and check the subscapular and lateral nodes in the same way. When palpating the lateral nodes, hand position requires that the palm face the humerus" (California Department of Health Services, date unknown, p. 2). Repeat on the other side.

Lymph nodes in this region should not be palpable. If palpable, note their consistency, whether they are single or multiple, movable or fixed.

Common approaches to the examination of the breast itself have used the concentric-circles technique or the hands-of-the-clock/radial-spoke technique. Figure 4-1A illustrates the vertical-strip technique ("lawn-mower technique") recently advocated. With the client lying down, place the ipsilateral hand of the client (the hand on the same side as the breast to be examined) on her forehead or above her head. If the client's breasts are large, ask her to roll onto the opposite hip and rotate her shoulders back to a supine position. The boundaries of the breast to be examined are the clavicle (superiorly), midsternum (medially), midaxillary line (laterally), and bra line (inferiorly). Begin in the axilla and continue down the midaxillary line to the bra line, moving toward the center of the body once that line is completed. Overlap rows. Use the pads (Figure 4-1B) of the three middle fingers, using three different pressures: light, medium, and deep. Confine the area being examined to a dime-size spot. Do not neglect the area of the nipple. Palpation of the supraclavicular and axillary

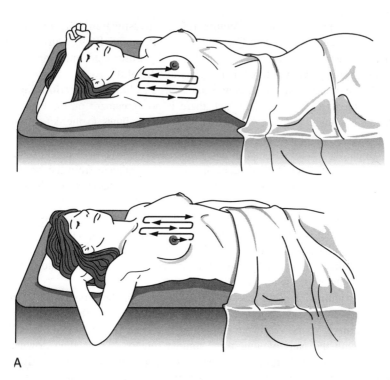

A

FIGURE 4.1 (A) "Lawn-mower" technique for breast examination. **(B)** Palpation technique for the clinical breast examination. Adapted from Barton, M.B., Harris, R., & Fletcher, S.W. (1999). Does this patient have breast cancer? The screening clinical breast examination: How should it be done? *JAMA, 282*(13), p. 1276.

regions can occur either before or after examination of the breast itself (Barton, Harris, & Fletcher, 1999).

Sensitivity of this technique correlates with the amount of time spent examining each breast. Careful examination of an average-size breast has been shown to require at least 3 minutes per breast. The current norm in practice is about 100 seconds and often includes instruction in breast self-examination as well (Barton, Harris, & Fletcher, 1999). Squeezing the nipple to see if fluid can be expressed is not a useful prognostic sign in women without spontaneous discharge. And data are lacking that support the value of inspection of the breasts with the woman's body or arms in a variety of positions. "In asymptomatic women clinicians should concentrate on careful breast palpation, all the while, of course, using their eyes. If the patient is symptomatic, or if an abnormality is discovered during palpation of an asymptomatic patient, careful inspection should be added" (Barton, Harris, & Fletcher, 1999, p. 1278).

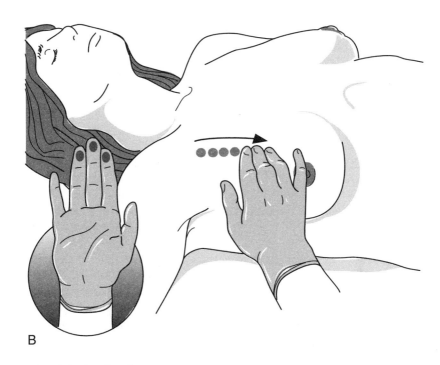

B

FIGURE 4.1 *(continued)*

Women who have had sexual abuse involving their breasts may become anxious when their breasts are examined. Asking permission to conduct this part of the examination is often appreciated. The lengthy breast examination advocated here could be disconcerting to women used to a more cursory examination (Barton, Harris, & Fletcher, 1999). Preface the exam with a statement about the time required with the new approach and a description of the technique that will be used.

If the clinician knows that the mother intends to breastfeed, it is appropriate to help her begin to think about her breasts as producers of milk.

Mammary Agenesis

Exclusively breastfeeding a baby is precluded when a mother has mammary agenesis, the absence or marked reduction of breast tissue. In this condition, the breasts have a conical appearance rather than a rounded one. On initial examination, a woman with mammary agenesis may be thought to be merely "flat-chested." However, close inspection and palpation will establish a diagnosis. Women with mammary agenesis will produce colostrum and, perhaps, a small amount of breast milk, but the amount will not be sufficient to nourish the baby. Women wishing to breastfeed can use a supplemental nutrition system, which allows formula to be delivered to the baby via a small plastic tube that is placed alongside the mother's breast and nipple.

The Nipples

In pregnant women, examination of the nipples is done primarily to assess protrusion should breastfeeding be desired. Size of the nipple is also important, as large nipples can be a problem when the infant's mouth is small. During the examination, ask the client if she has experienced any nipple discharge prior to becoming pregnant. A suspicious nipple discharge is one that is copious and spontaneous and comes from a single duct. Neither the client nor the practitioner needs to express the discharge manually for it to appear. Particularly worrisome is a clear or bloody spontaneous discharge. Referral to a surgeon is indicated (Oregon Health Division, Oregon Breast and Cervical Cancer Program, 1999). If the client reports spontaneous galactorrhea (persistent, milky discharge) prior to pregnancy, a medical workup that includes assessment of a prolactin level is needed. Common causes of nipple discharge include ductal ectasia, manual manipulation, an intraductal mass, pituitary adenoma, and of course, pregnancy and suckling.

Perform a "protractility" test for women who wish to breastfeed. With your thumb and forefinger, compress the breast tissue 1 to 1.5 inches behind the areola. If the nipple projects forward, the baby will probably have no difficulty latching on to the breast.

Inverted Flat Nipples

Breastfeeding is difficult with inverted or flat nipples. Inverted nipples can be "stretched" with the use of "breast shells." Use should start in the last trimester and may begin at the 28th week. If the client has symptoms of preterm labor (PTL) or has previously given birth to a preterm baby, delay breast shell use until 36 weeks' gestation because breast stimulation may provoke uterine contractions.

Large Nipples

Women with large nipples, sometimes defined as 2.5 cm or larger in width (about the size of a quarter), may or may not have problems breastfeeding. Babies with a small mouth may not be able to get behind the nipple to squeeze out milk. Manually expressing milk before putting the baby to breast may soften the nipple, making it easier to grasp, and using an electric breast pump before the baby nurses may help by "drawing the nipple into a teat" (Lawrence & Lawrence, 1999, p. 262).

❊ The Abdomen

Examination of the abdomen in the first half of pregnancy should be as thorough as the enlarged uterus permits. Eventually, the pregnancy progresses to a point where it becomes increasingly difficult to feel anything other than the uterus. In early pregnancy, evaluate for tenderness, masses, hernias, and enlargement of the liver, spleen, and lymph nodes. The presence or absence of fetal heart tones (FHTs) and determination of uterine size after the first trimester are important components of this examination.

Fetal Heart Tones

Most clinics or offices today use Doppler-type instruments for both early identification of FHTs and routine listening to FHTs at subsequent visits. Occasionally FHTs can be heard with these instruments as early as 8 weeks' gestation, but they are commonly heard initially at 10 to 12 weeks. To hear the baby's heartbeat at this time, exert a little pressure as you place the instrument immediately above the pubic symphysis. Slowly rotate it 360° until the beat is heard. If you hear nothing, move the instrument 1 cm at a time up toward the umbilicus until you are halfway between the symphysis and the umbilicus. If you have not yet heard the heartbeat, move 1 cm to either side of midline and proceed back down toward the symphysis (Figure 4-2). If FHTs are still not heard, follow the same procedure on the opposite side. Be sure to rotate the instrument at each new position, as the sound waves must be directed at the baby's heart valves. If no FHTs are heard with this instrument by 13 weeks, request a sonogram, as the "dates" may be wrong or the baby may be nonviable.

FHTs identified by fetoscope can first be heard by most people between 17 (more commonly 18) and 20 weeks' gestation. They are heard best when the tubing on the fetoscope is no longer than 10 inches and the metal headpiece is placed against the examiner's forehead. (Metal against bone helps conduct sound.) Some practitioners use the fetoscope without placing the headpiece against their foreheads. This practice may work late in pregnancy when the uterus is thin, but it is not helpful in the midtrimester of pregnancy.

Many practitioners today never listen to FHTs with a fetoscope. However, it is a useful skill to have in the first half of pregnancy when the "due date" is in question, and especially when ultrasound is not available. Be sure that the room is particularly quiet during your first attempts to use a fetoscope. You may need to turn off air conditioners, and it may help to have the client empty her bladder.

❊ HELPFUL HINT

If you cannot hear FHTs with a fetoscope at 18 to 20 weeks' gestation, find the FHTs with a Doppler instrument and then listen with the fetoscope.

Chart that you did or did not hear with a fetoscope when listening for early fetoscope FHTs (+FS [fetoscope] or −FS). Guidelines for listening to FHTs in the second half of pregnancy can be found in Chapter 7.

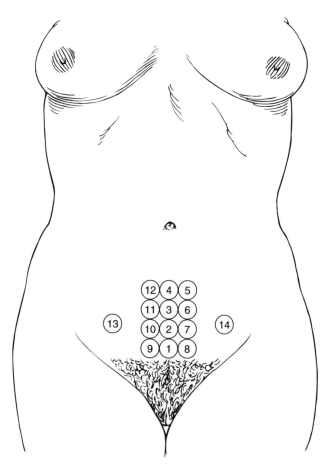

FIGURE 4.2 Technique for listening to early fetal heart tones.

Fundal Height

During the second trimester, uterine growth is often related to the location of the uterine fundus in relation to the umbilicus. Second-trimester guidelines to document uterine growth can be found in Box 4-2. Some practitioners start measuring fundal height with a centimeter tape between 16 and 20 weeks. At this time the centimeter measurement is less important than growth from one prenatal visit to the next, because it is common at this time for the centimeter measurement to be considerably greater than the gestational age.

In the third trimester, fundal height is measured in centimeters from the symphysis pubis. An approximate correlation between fundal height in centimeters and weeks of gestation is used for gestational ages of 26 to 36 weeks. Clinicians should keep in mind that multiple studies involving measurement of fundal height in both the second and third trimesters in varying populations have yielded conflicting results. Nevertheless, the cited guidelines are useful. Measurement of fundal height in the third trimester is discussed in Chapter 7.

❋ The Extremities

Examination of the extremities should include an assessment of deep tendon reflexes, examination of the legs for edema and varicose veins, and examination of the hands and feet for size, shape, and placement of the fingers and toes. Abnormalities may suggest a genetic disorder.

Hyperreflexia is a common finding, and it should be noted on the medical record so that the clinician will know what is normal for the client. Clinicians may think of hyperreflexia as a sign of preeclampsia. However, "Changes, or lack of changes, in deep tendon reflexes are not part of the diagnosis of preeclampsia" (Roberts, 1999, p. 838). The belief that increased deep tendon reflexes are associated with preeclampsia may come from the days when mag-

---

Box 4.2

The Relationship Between Fundal Height and the Umbilicus in the Second Trimester

16 weeks: 3 to 4 fingerbreadths (FB) below the umbilicus
18 weeks: 1 to 2 FB below the umbilicus
20 weeks: at the umbilicus
22 weeks: 1 to 2 FB above the umbilicus
24 weeks: 3 to 4 FB above the umbilicus

nesium sulfate was given intramuscularly to laboring women, and toxicity was evaluated by checking for the absence of reflexes.

❖ The Pelvic Examination

The final part of the physical examination is the pelvic examination. Although most practitioners have strong feelings about how to perform this examination, there is no "right" way (Brown, Wheeler, & Malby, 1999). While one practitioner may feel it essential to warn the client that the examination is about to begin by touching the back of the client's thigh, another equally sensitive practitioner may begin by merely informing the client that her genital area will be examined. The best approach seems to be one that works well for both client and provider.

HELPFUL HINT

Some clinicians begin by asking the client about her preferences in regard to the examination. You might ask, "Is there anything you would like me to know? Is there anything in particular that you want to have checked out?" and "Would you like me to do this examination slowly, explaining to you what I am doing, or would you like me to do it as quickly as possible so that it will be over?" Ask the woman who wants the examination over as quickly as possible whether it would help to know what you are doing as it is done.

HELPFUL HINT

Some women appreciate something to hold onto during the pelvic examination. A stuffed animal serves this purpose well. Keep one in the examining room and offer it as you feel it is appropriate.

You might begin by explaining that the examination has three parts: inspection of the genital area, insertion of the speculum, and examination of the uterus and ovaries with two of the examiner's fingers in the vagina and the other hand on the client's abdomen. Tell the client approximately how long the procedure will take. Offer to let her see and feel the speculum and the spatula, brush, or swab used to obtain the Pap smear and genital cultures. Tell her that you will stop at any time she wishes you to do so.

Occasionally, it will be appropriate to defer the pelvic examination because of the client's fear or anxiety. Although important information about gestational age (if the client is in her first trimester), cervical length and dilatation, and early identification of an abnormal Pap smear or sexually transmitted infection is gained from an early pelvic examination, deferring the examination may be in the best interest of the client and the client-provider relationship. If the provider feels that this may be the only opportunity to accurately determine gestational age or if a risk factor for preterm labor is present, an ultrasound examination can be requested to identify weeks of gestation and cervical length.

The "Educational" Pelvic

An "educational" pelvic is one in which the client has an opportunity to use a mirror to view her external genitalia and cervix. Some women appreciate this opportunity to become more familiar with their bodies. Figure 4-3 shows how

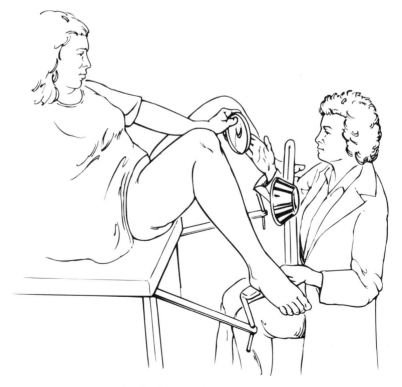

FIGURE 4.3 The educational pelvic examination.

to position the client so that she can see her external genitalia when she places a hand mirror between her legs.

Point out the labia majora, the labia minora, the hymen, vaginal opening, urethra, clitoris, and the perineum. Use both the anatomic name and a name that may be more familiar. For example, you might say, "These are the labia majora, the outer lips, and these are the labia minora, the inner lips." Avoid the use of the words "large" and "small" when you point out the labia because of the connotation these words may have and because, in some women, the labia majora, the big lips, are smaller than the labia minora, the small lips. Women who are learning about their own anatomy can be reassured that any asymmetry in the labia minora is normal and found in most women, similar to one breast being larger than another.

The External Genitalia

Examine the external genitalia by looking for lesions, growths, erythema, discoloration, swelling, excoriation, and bruises. Note any discharge and odor. A thorough examination usually requires separation of the labia minora from the labia majora and gentle retraction of the hood of the clitoris, looking carefully for lesions that might be syphilis or herpes. Be sure that all the movements of your fingers are purposeful. Avoid "fingering" the tissue as this could be interpreted as "sexual."

It is easy to confuse micropapillomatosis with venereal warts. "Smaller (micropapillary) condylomata should not be confused with the so-called micropapillomatosis labialis located on the epithelium of both labia minora. Unlike condylomata, in which multiple papillas converge toward a single base, each fingerlike papillomatous projection in micropapillomatosis labialis has its own base. Most clients with micropapillomatosis labialis have no symptoms and have sustained recurrent candidiasis, trichomonas, and chlamydia infections" (Ferenczy, 1995, p. 1334).

The first manifestation of syphilis is a small macule that becomes an ulcer. "The typical ulcer is usually solitary and painless and has a well-defined margin and an indurated base. Atypical chancres are common, however, and can be clinically indistinguishable from lesions with causes other than *Treponema pallidum*." "In women, the ulcer may be found on the vulva, vaginal walls, or cervix. Extragenital sites such as the anus or rectum are common. The ulcer is usually associated with enlarged inguinal lymph nodes, which tend to be bilateral, discrete, and nontender. If left untreated, the ulcer resolves spontaneously in 3 to 6 weeks, usually without leaving a scar" (Hoffman & Schmitz, 1995, p. 73).

Enlarged and raised flat lesions (condylomata lata) are manifestations of secondary syphilis. They are often found in the perianal region.

At some time you may examine a woman who has undergone female circumcision, "a cultural rite that serves to emphasize a people's identity and their belief system regarding sexuality, chastity, and the role of women in various matters including marriage and reproduction" (Meniru, Hecht, & Hopkins, 2000, p. 234). Worldwide, an estimated 130 million women and girls are affected, with more than 168,000 circumcised girls and women estimated to be living in the United States (Toubia, 1999). In one type of circumcision, the prepuce with all or part of the clitoris is excised (Type I). In these situations intercourse and labor occur without obstruction. Type II procedures excise the prepuce and clitoris with all or part of the labia minora. Types I and II constitute 80% of the procedures performed. The most extensive form of female circumcision (Type III), also known as infibulation or pharaonic circumcision, involves removal of part or all of the external genitalia and stitching of the vaginal opening. The incision of the labia majora creates raw surfaces that are either stitched or approximated with thorns so that the urethra and the vagina are covered. A small opening is left so that urine and menstrual blood can pass through it.

The type of procedure performed may not be apparent upon inspection of the genitalia, as the amount of cutting varies from one operator to another and complications can influence the appearance of the scar. When the most extreme type of circumcision has been performed, it may be impossible to insert even your little finger into the vaginal opening.

Obstructed labor and perineal tearing can be prevented with a reinfibulation procedure, optimally performed during the second trimester under local or regional anesthesia. If infibulated women do not agree to this procedure, an anterior episiotomy to cut the scar tissue may be necessary at the time a circumcised woman gives birth. Appendix I lists countries where female circumcision is practiced, prevalence rates and types of procedure by country, immediate and long-term complications, and a description of the Type IV procedure (unclassified).

Some women will ask to be reinfibulated (closing the vulva with a Type III procedure) immediately after giving birth. Health care providers in this country are likely to view this request with repugnance. But women who request reinfibulation may require it for their emotional and social health. A federal law passed in 1996 made performing any medically unnecessary surgery on the genitals of a girl younger than 18 years of age a federal crime. Cultural beliefs and practices do not justify exemptions. Reinfibulation is not included as a federal crime and can be performed with absorbable sutures in a running fashion (Nour, 2000). "Experience shows that informative and respectful counseling against reinfibulation removes the conflict between the woman's cultural orientation towards reinfibulation and the physician or nurses' orientation against the procedure. Most women agree not to reinfibulate once the potential health risks are explained to them. Clearly, avoiding legal measures and judicial intervention is always desirable. If the woman insists on reinfibulation despite adequate counseling, it is then left to the physician to consider whether to follow her request or abstain from performing the procedure on the basis of professional and ethical consciousness" (Toubia, 1999, pp. 69–70).

Practitioners usually have strong, personal feelings about female circumcision, also called "genital mutilation." Women in the United States are inclined to view ritual circumcision of women only as torture. It is difficult for most to understand that mothers of young girls in communities where ritual circumcision is practiced act out of love for their daughters. "In these societies, being a wife and a mother is a woman's livelihood; thus not circumcising one's daughter is equivalent to condemning her to a life of isolation. Infibulation safeguards her virginity, preserves her chastity, and ensures her eligibility for marriage, thus protecting her future" (Nour, 2000, p. 51).

A study of the birth experiences of 432 Somali women in Canada showed a cesarean rate of more than 50% (Chalmers & Hashi, 2000). Referral to or consultation with a nurse-midwife or physician who has experience assisting at the births of circumcised women can be helpful to anticipate possible problems.

The Vagina and Cervix

After the external genitalia have been examined, insert the speculum. It should be free of lubricant other than water. A dry speculum can often be inserted with ease when a woman is pregnant because the amount of vaginal discharge allows for easy entry. If using water for lubrication, use it sparingly to avoid cellular lysis and disruption.

Students are often taught the "oblique angle" approach to speculum insertion. In reality, no single technique works all the time. Just be sure that your fingers are placed in such a way that they open the vagina wide enough to accept the speculum. Once the speculum is in place, bring the cervix into view. Remove excess cervical mucus. If the pregnancy is advanced and the baby's weight has caused the body of the uterus to fall forward, the cervix may be posterior and the os difficult to visualize. It may also be difficult to obtain specimens for the Pap smear and cervical cultures. Elevating the client's hips by placing a towel under them can make visualization of the cervical os easier.

Look for vaginal discharge, venereal warts, mucopurulent cervicitis (a puslike discharge from the cervix that may be a sign of a sexually transmitted infection), and lesions that may be herpes or syphilis. Look also for evidence of exposure to diethylstilbestrol: cervical and vaginal ridging, hooding of the cervix, narrowing of the upper vagina, the cervix location flush with the vagina, and a wide transformation zone (Tedeschi, 1999).

If the client wishes to see her cervix, use an exaggerated semi-Fowler's position or ask the client to lean on one elbow. For the client to see her cervix clearly, the light must be properly placed between the client and the mirror. It may be helpful to have the client or the chaperone shine a flashlight into the mirror.

Obtaining Specimens

The Pap Smear

Opinions vary about the appropriate technique to use for obtaining Pap smear specimens. Opinions also vary about whether to obtain the Pap smear specimen first or the specimen(s) for gonorrhea and chlamydia testing first. Bleeding is common when obtaining a Pap smear from a pregnant woman and can occur whether a spatula, cotton swab, or brush is used. Sometimes the amount of bright red blood is frightening. Pressure against the cervix with a large swab for 60 seconds usually controls the flow of blood. When bleeding occurs, be sure to alert the client to expect additional spotting or bleeding over the next 24 hours. Reassure her that the bleeding is not harmful to the baby. An optimum specimen for Pap smear interpretation involves the absence of intercourse and douching for 24 hours prior to the test. Clients should be advised of this when they schedule their initial appointment.

A variety of new Pap tests are available. Aimed at increasing both sensitivity and specificity, these tests are still relatively expensive. Traditional Pap smear evaluation has a sensitivity of 50% and a specificity of 90% to 99% (U.S. Public Health Service, 1998).

The Specimen for Chlamydia

The specimen that will be tested for chlamydia should be obtained from the endocervix. If the laboratory procedure involves a DNA probe, a special, Dacron-tipped applicator should be used to obtain the specimen.

The Specimen for Gonorrhea

The specimen for gonorrhea should be obtained in the same manner that the specimen for chlamydia is obtained. The CDC recommends that the applicator used to obtain the specimen remain in the cervix for 10 seconds.

The Specimen for a Wet Smear

It is always a good idea to perform a wet smear on vaginal discharge at an initial prenatal visit. The three common causes of vaginitis are trichomonal infections, bacterial vaginosis, and candidiasis. Treatment of these infections is discussed in Chapter 5.

Bimanual Examination of the Uterus

Once the cervix and vaginal walls are inspected and laboratory specimens obtained, perform a bimanual examination to estimate uterine size, evaluate the adnexa if uterine size permits, and estimate the length and identify dilatation of the cervix, the latter to identify risk for PTL.

Determinations of uterine size by both internal and external clinical examination are imprecise. In the absence of other data, however, uterine findings may be of some use. First-trimester guidelines use bimanual examination of the uterus to relate its size to a tennis ball (8 weeks), an orange (10 weeks), or a grapefruit (12 weeks). These sizes are summarized in Box 4-3. Figure 4-4 illustrates the technique for evaluating uterine size in the first trimester of pregnancy.

Cervical length can be measured by placing the first phalanx of the index finger on the outside of the cervix (Figure 4-5). This measurement is usually about 3-cm long. If the cervix is 1 cm or less in length, the client should be referred for an ultrasound examination to determine cervical length. (See Chapter 5 for more information about ultrasound examinations for cervical length.) The client is also at increased risk for PTL if the internal cervical os is dilated before the 28th week or if it is dilated more than 2 cm between 28 and 34 weeks. Cervical length does not differ with parity.

Although adnexal evaluations for pelvic masses have been considered an integral part of any bimanual examination, significant limitations for both the detection of masses and accurate estimation of their size must be acknowledged. "No study has shown that routine pelvic examination increases detection of adnexal disease, whether benign or malignant" (Padilla, Radosevich, & Milad, 2000, p. 595).

❖ Clinical Pelvimetry

Evaluation of the bony pelvis to determine adequacy for a vaginal birth has been part of a routine initial pelvic examination for decades. Unfortunately, the subjective evaluation of pelvic bone structure rarely allows the clinician to predict with certainty which women will give birth vaginally and which will

Box 4.3		
Guidelines for Uterine Size in the First Trimester		
8 weeks: tennis ball	10 weeks: orange	12 weeks: grapefruit

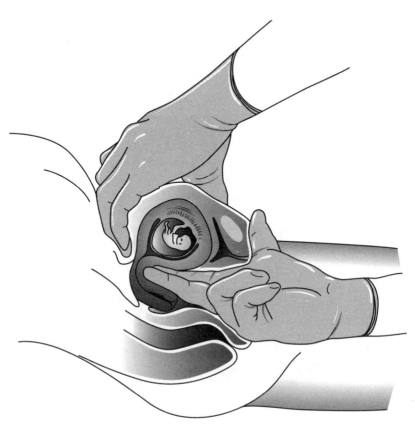

FIGURE 4.4 Technique to determine uterine size in the first trimester of pregnancy.

require surgery. Pelvic classification—gynecoid, android, anthropoid, or platypelloid—is based on the measurement of the pelvic inlet, yet "many pelves are mixed in that the various planes do not conform to a single parent type" (Oxorn, 1986, p. 34). In developed countries where nutrition is good and diseases are not likely to have affected the pelvis, true pelvic contracture or abnormality is rare. So many factors are out of the control of both mother and clinician during labor that it is appropriate to remain optimistic regardless of most clinical findings.

Some midwives feel it is important to encourage women by saying something such as, "I think your pelvis is just right for this baby." Other midwives feel that women who have been reassured about their pelvic adequacy and subsequently have a cesarean birth because labor did not progress have difficulty reconciling the prenatal information with the intrapartum surgery. These midwives prefer to make no comments about pelvic adequacy.

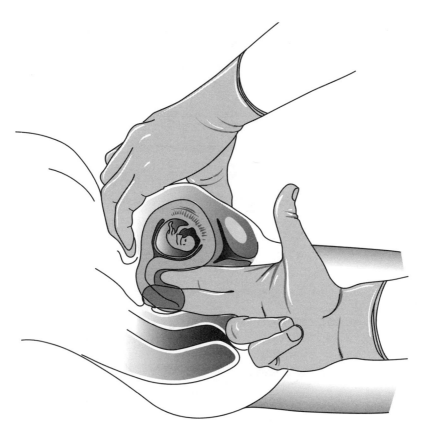

FIGURE 4.5 Measuring cervical length.

Box 4-4 lists accepted measurements for evaluating the maternal pelvis. If the pelvis feels small or "borderline" for accommodating the baby's birth, reevaluate the size at term. Measurements at this time may be within normal limits because of relaxation of the pelvic joints. A "trial of labor" is almost always indicated regardless of pelvic measurements, unless obvious deformities are present or pelvic fracture or surgery has occurred.

 HELPFUL HINT

Give the woman a soft or bony model of a pelvis to hold while you evaluate it. As you make your evaluation, show the client what you are examining.

Box 4.4

Norms for Clinical Pelvimetry

- Subpubic arch: round, 90°
- Sacrum: deep, hollow
- Diagonal conjugate: >11.5 cm (Cunningham et al., 2001), 12.5 (Oxorn, 1986)
- Ischial spines: blunt
- Sacrosciatic notch: about 2 fingerbreadths
- Sidewalls: parallel
- Biischial (bituberous) diameter: 8 cm

❈ Dating the Pregnancy

Estimating an accurate birth date is one of the most important clinician responsibilities. This date provides the expecting family with a framework for preparing for the baby's arrival and provides clinicians with landmarks for scheduling procedures (chorionic villus sampling, amniocentesis, tests of fetal well-being), performing laboratory tests (multiple serum marker), anticipating labor, evaluating fetal growth, and identifying problems such as PTL and postdate pregnancies.

Pregnancy dating begins with the menstrual history, but all parameters that support dating should be considered. In the past, much attention was paid to the presumptive, probable, and positive signs of pregnancy. The signs of Chadwick, Hegar, and Goodell as well as uterine ballottement were helpful for diagnosing pregnancy before the days of serum and urine pregnancy tests and ultrasound. Today they are primarily of historic interest.

The results of pregnancy testing and clinical landmarks (first-trimester bimanual examination of the uterus, initial hearing of the fetal heartbeat, the uterus at the umbilicus, and fundal height measurements) can strengthen or call into question information obtained from the menstrual history. Using such data, practitioners can determine whether an ultrasound examination is necessary for dating purposes. Information about the menstrual cycle and contraception at conception as well as the date of quickening can also be helpful. Box 4-5 summarizes findings that contribute to accurate pregnancy dating.

❈ Conclusion

Such important information can be derived from the prenatal physical examination that it deserves to be done in a thorough and skillful manner. At its con-

---

Box 4.5

Information That Contributes to the Accuracy of Pregnancy Dating

- Dates of last normal menstrual period, particularly if written down
- Menstrual cycle history
- Recent use of hormonal contraception
- Date of positive pregnancy test
- First-trimester bimanual examination
- Fetal heart tones at 10 to 12 weeks with a Doppler-type instrument
- Quickening at 16 to 18 weeks in a multipara or 18 to 20 weeks in a nullipara
- Fetal heart tones between 17 and 20 weeks with a fetoscope
- Uterus at the umbilicus at 20 weeks
- Ultrasound before 20 weeks' gestation

---

clusion, you are ready to evaluate your findings and either establish the estimated date of birth, schedule other visits to continue collecting information, or request an ultrasound examination to aid in your deliberations. You should also be ready to either reassure the client that the findings are within normal limits or recommend additional testing and/or referral to other health care professionals.

Chapter 5
Laboratory Tests and Diagnostic Procedures

✳ Introduction

Initial laboratory studies for low-risk pregnant women usually include urine and blood tests, cultures of cervical secretions, and a Pap smear. Urine tests typically include reagent strip testing and a urine culture. Table 5-1 summarizes time frames for performing selected tests during pregnancy and identifies normal findings.

Tracking results of laboratory testing is an essential component of clinical care. To avoid the adverse consequences resulting from failure to track, document, and report laboratory test results, a four-step method has been effective: 1) track all ordered tests by two people, 2) sign and date the laboratory sheet containing the test results, 3) copy the sheet and mail it to the client with a generic laboratory test explanation sheet, and 4) place the original laboratory test result sheet in the client's record (Mold & Dalbir, 2000).

✳ Routine Laboratory Tests in Pregnancy

Urine Testing With Reagent Strips

Reagent strips are used routinely to test a random sample of urine for protein and glucose at each prenatal visit to screen for preeclampsia, urinary tract infections (UTIs), and diabetes.

Proteinuria

Color changes in reagent strips distinguish between varying amounts of protein (1+ = 30 mg, 2+ = 100 mg, 3+ = 300 mg, and 4+ = >2000 mg). Unfortunately, both false-positive and false-negative results are common with reagent strip testing for protein. In a retrospective chart review of pregnant women hospitalized for high blood pressure (BP), 25% of the women who excreted 5

TABLE 5.1 Summary of Tests Commonly Used at Selected Gestational Ages During Pregnancy

Initial visit	15 to 20 weeks	26 to 28 weeks
1. Blood type and Rh 2. CBC (hematocrit, indices, platelets) 3. Antibody screen 4. Rubella titer 5. Syphilis 6. Hepatitis B 7. Chlamydia 8. Gonorrhea 9. Pap smear 10. Wet smear		1-h, 50-g glucose screen
Offer: HIV		
Consider: 1. Sickle cell screen 2. Hemoglobin electrophoresis 3. 1-h glucose screen 4. Urine culture 5. Urine drug screen 6. Thyroid screen 7. PPD 8. Varicella titer 9. CVS/amniocentesis 10. Ultrasound 11. HSV type-specific serologic testing	**Offer:** "Triple screen" Ultrasound (US) (18–20 weeks)	**Consider:** Hematocrit

g or more of protein in a 24-hour urine specimen had reagent strip values of 1+ or 2+, and only 36% of clients with reagent strips of 3+, excreted 5 grams of protein or more in a 24-hour urine specimen. Hour-to-hour variation in the amount of protein excreted in the urine, plus differences among observers interpreting reagent strip results, led the researchers to conclude that reagent strip testing for proteinuria "is an inaccurate test and should not be used as a substitute for 24-hour collections" (Meyer, Mercer, Friedman, & Sibai, 1994, p. 140). Any finding of 1+ or greater in a random sample of urine requires subsequent testing with a clean-catch specimen. A finding of 1+ or greater in the clean-catch specimen requires a 24-hour urine specimen to test for proteinuria,

35 to 37 weeks	Consider at various times
	Urine culture Herpes culture
	Urine drug screen

	Preeclampsia labs
	  Blood tests:
	    Hematocrit
	    Platelets
	    Creatinine
	    Uric acid
	    AST
	  Urine:
	    24-h for protein

Consider:

1. Group B beta-hemolytic streptococci
2. Hematocrit
3. Gonorrhea
4. Chlamydia
5. RPR
6. US if unable to assess fetal size
7. HIV

3-hour glucose screen
Repeat platelets

unless a UTI is suspected, as evidenced by a positive reagent strip test for leukocyte esterase and/or nitrites.

Glucosuria

Glucose in the urine of pregnant women can be caused by a lower renal threshold for glucose; it is also a symptom of diabetes. Unfortunately, it is impossible to know with certainty the origin of the glucose, even if the client recently consumed a food high in sugar content. If glucosuria is found before a 1-hour glucose screen is performed, the 1-hour screen should be performed regardless of the gestational age. If a 1-hour glucose has been performed between 26 and 28 weeks gestation and findings were in the range of normal, additional testing for diabetes is not necessary. Be sure to repeat the 1-hour screen in the third trimester when an early screen has been performed even if the results were within normal limits.

Asymptomatic Bacteriuria

Asymptomatic bacteriuria (ABU or ASB) is a common but nonpathologic condition in *non*pregnant women. In pregnant women, however, it can lead to pyelonephritis with its associated maternal morbidity. Pyelonephritis has also been associated with preterm labor (PTL). Treatment of ABU in pregnant women significantly decreases the incidence of acute UTIs.

Unfortunately, the best way to identify and treat pregnant women with ABU has not been determined. In many practices, a urine culture is performed routinely at the initial prenatal visit. However, the cost of a urine culture is relatively high and, as a result, reagent strip testing of antenatal urine specimens may be used instead. Despite problems with both the sensitivity and specificity of reagent strips, the leukocyte esterase/nitrite dipstick test has been found to be a useful substitute for the urine culture in populations without a high incidence of ABU (Rouse, Andrews, Goldenburg, & Owen, 1995). A urine culture may be advantageous prior to prescribing a medicine if a particular community demonstrates resistance. A culture will allow the clinician to determine sensitivity to the drug (Carson, Boggess, Colgan, Hooton, & Kerr, 2000).

The nitrite test may be falsely negative if bacteria in the bladder have not had time to produce a detectable level of nitrite. It may be negative despite the presence of *Staphylococcus saprophyticus* and *Enterococcus* (Carson et al., 2000). Whether to rely on the nitrite test or the leukocyte esterase test is unclear (Etherington & James, 1993; Carson et al., 2000). Women with a positive leukocyte esterase/nitrite reagent strip test can be treated for a UTI, and their urine can be tested again with a reagent strip after completion of therapy. In this approach, the urine is cultured only if the leukocyte esterase/nitrite test is positive after treatment.

Most (84%) pyelonephritis is cause by *Escherichia coli* (Millar et al., 1995). Traditionally, more than 100,000 colony-forming units/mL of a single pathogenic organism from a clean-catch, midstream urine specimen were considered necessary for treatment to be required. However, the American College of Obstetricians and Gynecologists (ACOG) suggests treatment when the colony count is between 25,000 and 100,000 units/mL (ACOG, 1998a). Some physicians feel that women with urine cultures that grow *Klebsiella* and *Proteus* should be treated when these organisms are found in any amount because they are not usually found in a sample of urine from a pregnant woman. Con-

---

Box 5.1A

Common Urinary Pathogens*

Gram-negative organisms
Escherichia coli
Proteus mirabilis
Klebsiella species
Enterobacter species
Gram-positive organisms
Enterococcus faecalis
Group B streptococcus

---

*A urine culture that reports a number of "mixed Gram-positive" colonies indicates that the specimen was contaminated with vaginal secretions.

---

sequently, their presence in any amount is considered significant. (See Box 5-1A for common urinary pathogens and Box 5-1B for common contaminants in a urine specimen.)

Urinalysis has not been found to be helpful in detecting UTIs (Bachman, Heise, Naessens, & Timmerman, 1993). Still, some clinicians feel that every pregnant woman should have a microscopic urinalysis performed to identify women with red blood cells (RBCs) in their urine. Red blood cells may indicate urinary tract cancer. However, almost all cases of red blood cells in the urine of pregnant women are attributable to a benign, familial condition that requires no therapy unless the hematocrit is dropping. Clinicians may, therefore, feel that a urinalysis is not cost-effective and refrain from requesting it.

Blood Tests

Blood tests include Rhesus (Rh) factor, antibody screen, complete blood count (CBC) or hemoglobin/hematocrit, rapid plasma reagin (RPR) or other test for syphilis, rubella titer, hepatitis B surface antigen (HB_sAg), and HIV. Routine

---

Box 5.1B

Common Contaminants in a Urine Specimen During Pregnancy*

Diphtheroids
Lactobacilli
Alpha-hemolytic streptococci

---

*No treatment should be instituted.

screening for toxoplasmosis and cytomegalovirus is not recommended (ACOG, 2000). As pregnancy advances, additional tests, such as the maternal serum triple screen and a 1-hour, 50-g glucose tolerance test are appropriate. Individual circumstances may require additional testing.

Rh Factor

The Rh factor is an antigen on the surface of an erythrocyte. While there are several Rh factors, the one most commonly identified is the antigen denoted "D." It is on the RBCs of about 85% of the White population and 93% of the African American population. Women who carry the Rh D antigen are said to be Rh-positive. Those without it are said to be Rh-negative. The Rh D antigen has been found on fetal cells as early as 6 weeks after conception. The Rh factor of the pregnant woman is determined to identify babies who could be sick or die from Rh disease (hemolytic disease of the newborn) and women who should receive anti-D immunoglobulin (Ig) to prevent this disease.

At the time of abortion and at the time of delivery, fetal blood, if Rh-positive, may enter the maternal circulation, causing Rh-negative maternal blood to become "sensitized." In this situation, the Rh-negative mother's immune system may produce antibodies against the Rh antigen that can pass from mother to fetus. In rare instances, sensitization will occur before delivery without any external evidence of bleeding.

Rh-affected babies may be mildly, moderately, or severely ill. Newborns in the mild group will have either mild or no anemia. Newborns with moderate disease will have hepatosplenomegaly and moderate anemia with jaundice after birth. Kernicterus may occur and cause mental retardation and even death. Severely affected infants will develop hydrops, often before 30 weeks' gestation. Death can occur in utero. Babies in this group usually require an intrauterine transfusion, as hemoglobin levels are commonly between 4 and 6 g/dL.

The first Rh-positive pregnancy is at low risk for sensitization. The risk of Rh sensitization in an Rh-negative woman who has ABO-compatible blood is 8% after the first pregnancy and 16% after the second pregnancy when anti-D Ig is not administered (Bowman, 1978). The percentages will be lower if the mother and baby have an ABO incompatibility because an ABO incompatibility appears to give some protection to the baby against the effects of an Rh incompatibility.

Anti-D Ig is used to counter the Rh D antigen. It contains antibodies to the Rh factor. The antibodies destroy any Rh-positive fetal cells in the mother's blood and prevent the development of the mother's own antibodies by her immune system. Rh Ig that has been administered within 72 hours of birth has almost eradicated Rh disease in developed countries, preventing the development of antibodies in 98% of the women who would have developed them.

Prenatal administration of anti-D Ig to unsensitized Rh-negative women at 28 weeks' gestation is aimed at the 2.0% of Rh-negative women who become sensitized in the last trimester of pregnancy (ACOG, 1999e).

Anti-D Ig is also administered to Rh-negative women after any prenatal bleeding episode, spontaneous or elective abortion, abdominal trauma, and certain obstetric procedures, such as a version late in pregnancy to turn a baby from a breech or transverse to a vertex presentation. Anti-D Ig comes in two dosages: 50 μg and 300 μg. The 50-μg dose will neutralize 2.5 mL of fetal red cells (ACOG, 1999e) and is given to Rh-negative women with an ectopic pregnancy, women having a first-trimester abortion (spontaneous, elective, or therapeutic), and women undergoing chorionic villus sampling (CVS). Whether to give anti-D Ig to women with threatened abortion and a live embryo/fetus up to 12 weeks' gestation is controversial, as data are limited and threatened abortion as a cause of alloimmunization is rare (ACOG, 1999e).

The 300-μg dose is used with Rh-negative women at 28 weeks' gestation (or later), after an amniocentesis, with an abortion beyond 12 weeks' gestation, and with suspected abruption. The American College of Obstetricians and Gynecologists notes that some authorities recommend a second dose of anti-D Ig when 12 or more weeks elapse after administration of the anti-D Ig and the baby has not been delivered, but ACOG refrains from recommending an additional dose because of limited data. ACOG also notes that the effect of the 300-μg dose is the same whether given at 28 weeks or 34 weeks (ACOG, 1999e). There appears to be no harm to either the mother or baby from the administration of anti-D Ig. Although it is a blood product, the donated blood is screened and treated for bacteria and HIV. No infectious diseases, including hepatitis and AIDS, have been associated with anti-D Ig. Because anti-D Ig is a blood product, members of certain religious groups may refuse it.

Protection from anti-D Ig lasts approximately 12 weeks. Considering most women give birth after their estimate date of birth (EDB), it seems sensible to give this product at 29 or 30 weeks' gestation, rather than at 28 weeks. However, the study demonstrating the effectiveness of prenatal Ig administered it at 28 weeks; therefore, 28 weeks is the standard of care.

Rh-negative women who plan a sterilization procedure need to consider whether they wish to receive postpartum anti-D Ig for protection should the sterilization procedure fail or a tubal reversal be performed at a later time. The American College of Obstetricians and Gynecologists states that use of anti-D Ig "should be guided by the patient's desire for protection against any chance of alloimmunization." ACOG further states, "Proponents of its use maintain that anti-D immune globulin administration will preserve the future option of transfusing Rh D-positive blood in times of emergency. Opponents of this view cite the low probability of sensitization with the previous pregnancy and the improbability of receiving Rh D-incompatible blood" (ACOG, 1999e, p.4).

Antibody Screen

The antibody screen identifies women with antibodies that can cause hemolytic disease of the newborn. While Rh disease is primarily responsible for this disease, approximately 2% of cases result from rare blood groups. Table 5-2 identifies some of these rare RBC antigens and the extent to which each may be a problem for the fetus or newborn. Note that many do not produce hemolytic disease. Women with a diagnosis of isoimmunization involving an antigen in a clinically significant group should be referred for physician follow-up (ACOG, 1996b).

Repeat antibody screening may be recommended prior to the administration of anti-D Ig to Rh D-negative women at 28 weeks' gestation to identify women who have become alloimmune since the initial antibody screen. However, the incidence of Rh D alloimmunization occurring prior to 28 weeks of gestation is reported to be as low as 0.18%, and the cost-effectiveness of routinely repeating the antibody test has not been studied. The consequences of antenatal Rh D alloimmunization can be severe, but the decision to obtain a repeat antibody screen should be dictated by individual circumstances (ACOG, 1999e, p. 4).

Complete Blood Count

In pregnancy, the CBC is used to identify two important conditions in pregnant women: anemia and thrombocytopenia (low platelet count). A CBC includes a numeric count of the RBCs, white blood cells (WBCs), and platelets; determination of the hemoglobin and hematocrit; and measurement of the RBC indices.

Anemia

In nonpregnant women, anemia is diagnosed when the hemoglobin falls below 12 g/dL or the hematocrit falls below 36%. During pregnancy, the cutoff values for nonsmokers depend on gestational age. Tables 5-3A, 5-3B, and 5-3C illustrate these values, along with adjustments that need to be made for women who smoke more than 10 cigarettes per day and women who live at altitudes above 3,000 feet.

Low hemoglobin or hematocrit levels should be evaluated in relation to the RBC indices: mean corpuscular volume (MCV), mean corpuscular hemoglobin (MCH), and mean corpuscular hemoglobin concentration (MCHC). Box 5-2 identifies normal values for RBC indices. MCV is a measurement of the size of the RBCs. Small RBCs (MCV less than 80 fL) define microcytic anemia. The most common causes of microcytic anemia are iron deficiency anemia, anemia of chronic disease, and some thalassemias.

Hemoglobinopathies are common when the MCV is in the 60s. Large RBCs (MCV greater than 100 fL) define macrocytic anemia. The most com-

TABLE 5.2 Antibodies Causing Hemolytic Disease*

Blood group system	Antigens related to hemolytic disease	Severity of hemolytic disease
CDE	D	Mild to severe
	C	Mild to moderate
	c	Mild to severe
	E	Mild to severe
	e	Mild to moderate
Lewis		Not a proved cause of hemolytic disease of the newborn
I		Not a proved cause of hemolytic disease of the newborn
Kell	K	Mild to severe with hydrops fetalis
	k	Mild to severe
Duffy	Fy^a	Mild to severe with hydrops fetalis
	Fy^b	Not a cause of hemolytic disease of the newborn
Kidd	Jk^a	Mild to severe
	Jk^b	Mild to severe
MNSs	M	Mild to severe
	N	Mild
	S	Mild to severe
	s	Mild to severe
Lutheran	Lu^a	Mild
	Lu^b	Mild
Diego	Di^a	Mild to severe
	Di^b	Mild to severe
Xg	Xg^a	Mild
P	$PP_1P^k(Tj^a)$	Mild to severe
Public	Yt^a	Moderate to severe
	Yt^b	Mild
	Lan	Mild
	En^a	Moderate
	Ge	Mild

table continues on page 132

TABLE 5.2 Antibodies Causing Hemolytic Disease* continued

Blood group system	Antigens related to hemolytic disease	Severity of hemolytic disease
	Jr^a	Mild
	Co^a	Severe
	Co^{a-b-}	Mild
Private antigens	Batty	Mild
	Becker	Mild
	Berrens	Mild
	Evans	Mild
	Gonzales	Mild
	Good	Severe
	Heibel	Moderate
	Hunt	Mild
	Jobbins	Mild
	Radin	Moderate
	Rm	Mild
	Ven	Mild
	$Wright^a$	Severe
	$Wright^b$	Mild
	Zd	Moderate

*Note that conditions listed as being "mild" only can be treated like ABO incompatibility. Patients with all other conditions should be monitored as if they were sensitized to D. Reprinted with permission from American College of Obstetricians and Gynecologists: Management of isoimmunization in pregnancy. Technical Bulletin No. 148. Washington, DC, ACOG, ©1990.

mon causes of macrocytic anemia are folate deficiency and vitamin B_{12} deficiency. Other causes are vitamin C deficiency, copper deficiency, certain drugs, renal disease, liver disease (as in alcoholism), hypothyroidism, and excessive red cell destruction. When normal size RBCs (MCV 80 to 100 fL) are present in conjunction with a low hemoglobin or hematocrit, the anemia is defined as normocytic. Causes of normocytic anemia include aplastic anemia, hypoplastic anemia, and myelodysplasia (defective formation of the spinal cord). These causes of anemia are summarized in Box 5-3.

TABLE 5.3A Cutoff Values for Anemia for Women

Pregnancy status	Hemoglobin (g/dL)	Hematocrit (%)
Nonpregnant	12.0	36
Pregnant		
Trimester 1	11.0	33
Trimester 2	10.5	32
Trimester 3	11.0	33

TABLE 5.3B Cutoff Values for Anemia for Women Who Smoke Cigarettes*

Cigarettes per day	10–20		21–40	
Pregnancy status	Hb (g/dL)	Hct (%)	Hb (g/dL)	Hct (%)
Nonpregnant	12.3	37	12.5	37.5
Pregnant				
Trimester 1	11.3	34	11.5	34.5
Trimester 2	10.8	33	11.0	33.5
Trimester 3	11.3	34	11.5	34.5

*No adjustment is necessary for women who smoke less than 10 cigarettes daily.

TABLE 5.3C Adjustments for Altitudes*

Altitude (feet)	Adjustment value	
	Hemoglobin (g/dL)	Hematocrit (%)
3,000–3,999	+0.2	+0.5
4,000–4,999	+0.3	+1.0
5,000–5,999	+0.5	+1.5
6,000–6,999	+0.7	+2.0

*To avoid underdiagnosis of anemia at high altitude, add the appropriate value from this table to the cutoff value given in Table 5-3A or 5-3B.

From CDC. 1989. CDC criteria for anemia in children and childbearing-aged women. MMWR 38:400–404

Box 5.2

Normal Values for Red Blood Cell Indices*

Mean Corpuscular Volume (MCV), a measurement of the average size of the RBC: 80 to 100 fL
Mean Corpuscular Hemoglobin (MCH), a reflection of the amount of hemoglobin per cell: 26 to 34 pg
Mean Corpuscular Hemoglobin Concentration (MCHC), a measurement of the mean total content of total hemoglobin: 31 to 36 g/dL

*Values vary according to laboratory.

During pregnancy, increases in plasma volume and RBC mass increase maternal blood volume about 45% over nonpregnant levels. However, the increase in red cell volume is less than the increase in plasma volume, and a "dilutional" or "physiologic" anemia occurs. Figure 5-1 illustrates the changes in blood volume during pregnancy. True anemia in pregnancy is usually caused by iron deficiency. The red cells become microcytic (low MCV) and hypochromic (low MCH). Mild iron deficiency anemia rarely poses a problem for either a pregnant woman or her baby. (Maternal hemoglobin levels are not related to fetal hemoglobin levels.)

Box 5.3

Common Causes of Anemia

Microcytic anemia (small RBCs, MCV less than 80 fL)
    Iron deficiency anemia
    Anemia of chronic disease
    Some thalassemias
    Hemoglobinopathies (common when the MCV is in the 60s)
Macrocytic anemia (large RBCs, MCV greater than 100 fL)
    Folate deficiency
    Vitamin B_{12} deficiency
    Vitamin C deficiency
    Copper deficiency
    Certain drugs
    Renal disease
    Liver disease (as in alcoholism)
    Hypothyroidism
    Excessive red cell destruction
Normocytic (normal size RBCs, MCV 80 to 100 fL)
    Aplastic anemia
    Hypoplastic anemia
    Myelodysplasia (defective formation of the spinal cord)

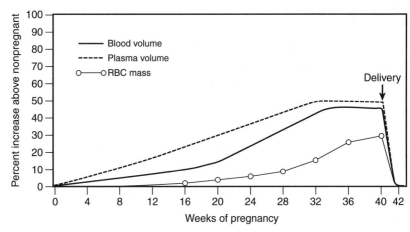

FIGURE 5.1 Blood volume changes in pregnancy. (From Scott, D.E. (1972). Anemia in pregnancy. Obstetric & Gynecology Annals, 1, p. 219.)

Thrombocytopenia

Platelets are required for blood clotting. In nonpregnant women, normal platelet counts range from 150,000 to 400,000/uL with severe thrombocytopenia identified as less than 50,000/μL. In pregnant women, the mean platelet count is lower. Also, in pregnant women, "The definition of thrombocytopenia is somewhat arbitrary and not necessarily clinically relevant. Clinically significant bleeding usually is limited to patients with platelet counts less than 10,000/μL" (ACOG, 1999f, p. 2). A recent study showed that platelets counts above 115,000/μL in healthy pregnant women should be considered normal (Boehlen, Hohlfeld, Extermann, Perneger, & de Moerloose, 2000).

In pregnancy, the most common cause of thrombocytopenia is gestational thrombocytopenia, also known as essential, incidental, or benign thrombocytopenia of pregnancy. It can occur in the first trimester but is more likely to be found later. In this condition, the platelet count is usually more than 70,000/μL, there is no history of bleeding, low platelet counts have not been found prior to pregnancy, and the low count returns to normal within 12 weeks of birth (ACOG, 1999g). If the platelet count is less than 70,000/μL, the diagnosis is likely to be immune thrombocytopenic purpura (ITP). Box 5-4 lists the differential diagnoses for thrombocytopenia in pregnancy.

Platelet counts are reassuring when they are more than 150,000/μL. When the count is less than 100,000/μL, the workup should include a peripheral smear to "rule out platelet clumping that may be associated with pseudothrombocytopenia" (ACOG, 1999f, p. 2). "In general, in a woman with no history of thrombocytopenia or the milder the thrombocytopenia, the more likely she is

Box 5.4

Differential Diagnoses for Thrombocytopenia in Pregnancy

Gestational thrombocytopenia
Idiopathic thrombocytopenic purpura
Preeclampsia
Thrombotic thrombocytopenic purpura
Hemolytic uremic syndrome
Acute fatty liver
Disseminated intravascular coagulation

Source: ACOG. (1999g). Thrombocytopenia in pregnancy (ACOG Practice Bulletin No. 6). Washington, DC: Author.

to have gestational thrombocytopenia. If the platelet count is less than 70,000/µL, ITP is more likely to be present, and if the platelet count is less than 50,000/µL, ITP is almost certainly present. During the third trimester or postpartum period, the sudden onset of significant maternal thrombocytopenia should lead to consideration of PIH [pregnancy-induced hypertension], thrombotic thrombocytopenic purpura, hemolytic uremic syndrome, acute fatty liver, or disseminated intravascular coagulation, although ITP can present this way as well" (ACOG, 1999f, p. 3).

Limited data are available to determine what platelet level indicates a danger of an epidural hematoma after epidural anesthesia.

Syphilis

Fetal infection with the spirochete, *Treponema pallidum*, can occur at any stage of pregnancy and during any stage of maternal disease. Infection is transmitted through sexual contact or in utero. Primary syphilis occurs when the organism enters the body via mucous membrane or compromised cutaneous surfaces, spreading to nearby lymph nodes. After 10 to 20 days, a chancre appears and lymph nodes enlarge. During this time the open lesion(s) is/are highly infectious. Without treatment, spirochetes disseminate through the blood system to many organs. Initial manifestations of this hematogenous spread are a rash and mucous membrane lesions (secondary syphilis). After 10 to 30 years, tertiary syphilis with a wide spectrum of clinical manifestations will develop in 10% to 20% of those infected.

There were 801 reported cases of congenital syphilis in the United States in 1998. These cases can be attributed to no prenatal care, testing performed too late in pregnancy, delayed treatment, or inadequate follow-up. Half of all reported cases of syphilis are in 28 counties, most of which are in the South and selected large, metropolitan areas. The 10 cities with the highest number of reported syphilis cases in 1998 were (in descending order by number of cases) Baltimore, Chicago, Memphis, Nashville, Phoenix, Detroit, Indianapolis, Atlanta, Dallas, and Los Angeles (Prevention Connection, 2000).

All women with syphilis should be offered HIV testing, and in areas with a high prevalence of HIV, patients who have primary syphilis should be retested for HIV after 3 months if the first test is negative (Centers for Disease Control and Prevention [CDC], 1998). A campaign to eliminate syphilis by 2005 and address the larger social issues that increase the risk for syphilis (e.g., racism, poverty, sexism, homophobia, illegal drug use, prostitution) by promoting community involvement and support activities was initiated in 1999 (CDC, 1999).

Untreated syphilis during pregnancy causes infant death in up to 40% of cases (Prevention Connection, 2000). "An untreated, infected mother can transmit syphilis to her fetus at delivery, but the majority of infants are infected in utero. The risk of transmission to the baby is extremely high during the first 2 years after the mother's initial infection and declines to low levels after 4 years" (CDC, 1999, p.759).

In areas where syphilis rates are high, the CDC recommends treating a pregnant woman with syphilis as a medical emergency. In these areas, immediate on-site testing of women with a positive pregnancy test should occur, and testing should be repeated in the last trimester (CDC, 1999). Because it may take weeks for antibody titers to become elevated, infection contracted late in pregnancy can be missed if the screening test is not repeated. Serologic titers may be performed monthly, as reinfection can occur between tests.

The tests commonly performed to screen for syphilis, the RPR and the Venereal Disease Research Laboratory (VDRL) test, are nontreponemal tests. This means that they are not specific for *T. pallidum,* and false-positive results from causes not related to syphilis (as chronic infection and autoimmune disease) may occur. Accordingly, a positive RPR or VDRL requires confirmation with a treponemal test, such as the fluorescent treponemal antibody-absorption (FTA-ABS) test, which is 90% to 95% sensitive, or the microhemagglutination assay for antibody to *T. pallidum* (MHA-TP), which is 80% to 85% sensitive. If the confirmatory test is negative, the treponemal test result was a false-positive. In this instance, a test for antinuclear and anticardiolipin antibodies should be ordered because the false-positive test could be caused by a connective tissue disorder such as systemic lupus erythematosus. Infectious mononucleosis can also give a false-positive result.

Nontreponemal test antibody titers are reported quantitatively, with a fourfold change in titer (e.g., from 1:16 to 1:64) indicating clinical significance. The same test should be used to determine the titers because RPR titers may be slightly higher than VDRL titers (CDC, 1998).

Treatment of syphilis during pregnancy depends on the stage of the disease. Box 5-5 outlines the current recommendations. Parenteral penicillin G is the only documented effective treatment for syphilis during pregnancy. Penicillin resistance has not occurred. Treatment may trigger a rare reaction (Jarisch-Herxheimer reaction) characterized by headache, muscle aching, rash, and hypotension that may precipitate PTL and fetal distress for women treated for syphilis in the second half of pregnancy. "A fourfold decrease in titers 6 months after treatment is reassuring. Unchanged titers 6 months after treatment signal individuals at risk for treatment failure. Individuals who continue to have symptoms or who have increasing titers should be considered to have treatment failure or reinfection" (Roe, 1999, p. 641).

Rubella

The devastating effects of congenital rubella—eye lesions, heart disease, deafness, central nervous system (CNS) defects, anemia, hepatitis, pneumonitis, bone defects, and chromosome abnormalities—were first described in the 1940s. These defects are most likely to occur when rubella infection is present

---

Box 5.5

Recommendations for the Treatment of Syphilis During Pregnancy

Syphilis stage	Therapy
Primary, secondary, or early latent	Benzathine penicillin G, 2.4 million units single dose IM (1.2 million units in each buttock). In patients with history of penicillin allergy, confirm allergy by skin testing; if confirmed, desensitize and treat with penicillin.
Late latent, cardiovascular or gummatous disease	Benzathine penicillin G, 2.4 million units IM weekly for 3 weeks
Neurosyphilis	Aqueous penicillin G, 2.4 million units per day IV for 10–14 days
	or
	Aqueous procaine penicillin G, 2.4 million units IM daily, plus probenecid, 500 mg orally 4 times per day, for 10–14 days

From Reyes, M.P., & Akhras, J. (1995). Dealing with maternal and congenital syphilis. *Contemporary OB/GYN, 40,* 52+

in the first trimester. Data from the late 1970s show that rubella is most teratogenic in the first half of pregnancy, affecting about 80% of fetuses at 12 weeks, 50% at 13 to 14 weeks, and 25% at the end of the second trimester (Miller, Craddock-Watson, & Pollock, 1982).

The rubella titer identifies women who have antibodies against rubella. Immunity exists when the titer is more than 1:10. Rubella immunization is contraindicated during pregnancy because an attenuated live virus is used, although follow-up of women who conceived within 3 months of receiving the vaccine has not demonstrated any congenital malformations.

Outbreaks of rubella in the United States still occur in both native-born and foreign-born individuals. Women from countries without national immunization programs for rubella or from countries where such programs are recent developments are particularly vulnerable (CDC, 2000). Women with nonimmune rubella titers (less than 1 in 10) should receive rubella vaccine soon after delivery to protect them should they become pregnant again.

Hepatitis B

The hepatitis B virus (HBV) affects the liver. It is found in blood, semen, and vaginal secretions and is 100 times more infectious than the virus that causes AIDS. Many people infected with the virus do not feel sick. Screening of all pregnant women for hepatitis B is recommended by both ACOG (1991) and CDC (1998).

The screening test commonly used is the hepatitis B surface antigen (Hb_sAg), which is contained in the outer capsule surrounding the virus' inner core. The Hb_sAg is the first hepatitis test to become abnormal and indicates either active infection or, if it persists, indicates that the patient is a chronic carrier. A positive test documents a need for additional testing (Figure 5-2) to identify:

• Women who have had hepatitis in the past but are not contagious now
• Women with active disease
• Women who are chronic carriers
• Babies at risk for perinatal transmission of hepatitis B who should receive hepatitis B Ig and hepatitis B vaccine
• Families that should be tested, receive immunoprophylaxis, and be instructed in hygienic measures that decrease transmission of the disease

While pregnancy rarely alters the course of hepatitis B infection, infants born to HB_sAg-positive women are at risk for developing chronic active hepatitis and have an increased chance of dying from liver cirrhosis, hepatoma, hepatocellular carcinoma, or fulminant liver failure (Holst & Ritter, 2001).

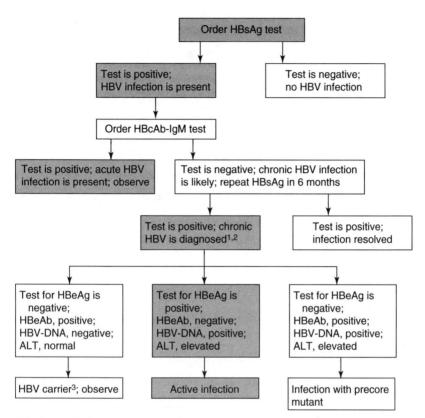

HBV, hepatitis B virus; HBsAg, hepatitis B surface antigen; HBcAb-IgM, hepatits B core antibody-IgM; HBeAg, hepatitis B e antigen; HBeAb, hepatitis B e antibody; ALT, alanine aminotransferase.

1. Chronic HBV infection may result in carrier status or active chronic disease, the latter associated with progressive liver disease.
2. All patients with chronic HBV infection should be evaluated for liver disease, hepatitis C virus, delta hepatitis virus, HIV, and hepatocellular carcinoma.
3. Evaluate carriers for viremia and elevation of liver enzymes every 6 months as the disease can reactivate at any time. Long-term carriers are at risk for hepatocellular carcinoma.

FIGURE 5.2 Diagnostic approach to the patient with suspected HBV infection. (Adapted from Smith, J.R., & Herrera, J.L. (2001). Chronic Hepatitis B: Diagnosis and current treatment options. *Consultant, 41*(5), 782–786.

"Fewer than 5% of acutely infected adults in the U.S. become chronic carriers, compared with some 25% . . . to 90% . . . of perinatally infected infants" (Oregon Health Division, 1994). "Approximately 10% to 20% of women who are seropositive for Hb$_s$Ag transmit the virus to their neonates in the absence of immunoprophylaxis. In women who are seropositive for both Hb$_s$Ag and

Hb_eAg, the frequency of vertical transmission increases to approximately 90%.

"In patients with acute hepatitis B, the frequency of vertical transmission also depends on the time during gestation that maternal infection occurs. When maternal infection occurs in the first trimester, up to 10% of neonates will be seropositive for Hb_sAg, In women acutely infected in the third trimester, 80% to 90% of offspring will be infected" (ACOG, 1998c, p. 2).

Infants born to HB_sAg-positive women should receive the first dose of HBV vaccine within 12 hours of birth, the second between 1 and 2 months of age, and the third at 6 months. They should also receive hepatitis B Ig within 24 hours of birth. Breastfeeding is not contraindicated in women with hepatitis B (Fagan, 1999).

When HB_sAg is positive, order the test for HB_eAg, as this test is the best marker of infectivity. Liver function studies, aspartate aminotransferase (AST) and alanine aminotransferase (ALT), should also be requested, although they are typically normal in chronic infection.

Human Immunodeficiency Virus

The Institute of Medicine, the American Academy of Pediatrics, and ACOG recommend screening all pregnant women for HIV. Early identification of HIV-positive status gives women the opportunity to take advantage of treatment, make informed decisions about their own high-risk behaviors, make timely decisions about continuation of the pregnancy, and when a decision is made to continue the pregnancy, initiate therapy to reduce the risk of perinatal transmission. Testing also identifies HIV-exposed infants. High-risk, HIV-negative women tested in early pregnancy who do not practice safe sex should be encouraged to be tested again in the third trimester.

Decisions about terminating or continuing a pregnancy in the face of HIV disease are complex. Information that can help a woman make a decision about continuing the pregnancy includes the nature of HIV disease in infants, adults, and children; the transmission rate; and support that is available now and likely to be available in the future.

Pregnant women who receive antiretroviral chemotherapy reduce the risk of giving birth to an HIV-infected baby from 25% to 5%–8%. When this therapy is combined with scheduled cesarean birth, the risk drops to 2%. The American College of Obstetricians and Gynecologists recommends that HIV-positive women be offered scheduled cesarean delivery at 38 completed weeks of gestation to reduce the chance of labor and/or spontaneous rupture of membranes and prevent vertical transmission of HIV to the baby. However, maternal morbidity with cesarean birth is increased. Discussion of the maternal risks and neonatal benefits should begin as early in pregnancy as possible (ACOG, 1999c).

Initial laboratory screening usually consists of an enzyme immunoassay (EIA) followed by a confirmatory test, either the Western blot analysis or immunofluorescence assay (IFA). The Western blot analysis is more commonly done. A false-positive result is extremely rare. More likely to occur is an EIA-positive, Western–blot-indeterminate result. The IFA test results are usually accurate. Liver function studies should be part of the initial laboratory evaluation of an HIV-infected woman.

Tests of Cervical and Vaginal Secretions

Chlamydia

Research studies have been inconclusive about complications for pregnant women from chlamydia. A recent study of 2929 symptom-free pregnant women found a twofold to threefold increased risk of preterm birth when chlamydia infection was present at 24 weeks' gestation (Andrews et al., 2000). Babies born to women with chlamydia infections are known to be at risk for chlamydial conjunctivitis and chlamydial pneumonia, the latter manifested up to 3 months after birth.

The drug of choice to treat chlamydia infections in pregnant women has been erythromycin, but amoxicillin (500 mg taken orally 3 times a day for 7 to 10 days) has been shown to be as effective and to have fewer gastrointestinal side effects (Turrentine & Newton, 1995). Because experience is limited with azithromycin, another drug of choice in nonpregnant women, it is not presently recommended by the CDC for use during pregnancy. It is, however, on the alternative regimen list (CDC, 1998). ACOG lists azithromycin along with erythromycin base/erythromycin ethylsuccinate and amoxicillin as appropriate medications for treatment, the advantage being that a single oral dose of 1 g is effective. Additionally, there are fewer gastrointestinal side effects with azithromycin. No adverse fetal effects have been attributed to the drug (ACOG, 1998). Box 5-6 contains recommendations for treating chlamydia in pregnancy.

Doxycycline, one of the drugs of choice for the treatment of chlamydia in *non*pregnant women, is a tetracycline. It generally is avoided in pregnant women because of reports of yellow-brown discoloration of the deciduous teeth and acute fatty liver changes in certain pregnant women with renal problems.

Routine test-of-cure for chlamydia during the immediate posttreatment period is not recommended by CDC when "highly active drugs" are used because there are no resistant strains of *Chlamydia trachomatis*. Azithromycin is considered a highly active drug, but erythromycin and amoxicillin are not. In these cases, CDC recommends repeat cultures 3 weeks after therapy is completed, as neither is highly effective and the side effects of erythromycin result in poor compliance (CDC, 1998). Even with "highly active drugs," an indi-

---

Box 5.6

Recommendations for the Treatment of Chlamydia During Pregnancy: Comparison of CDC* and ACOG** Guidelines

CDC-recommended regimens:
Erythromycin base (E-Mycin) 500 mg orally 4 times a day for 7 days
or
Amoxicillin 500 mg orally 3 times a day for 7 to 10 days
Alternative regimens:
Erythromycin base (E-Mycin) 250 mg orally 4 times a day for 14 days
or
Erythromycin ethylsuccinate (E.E.S.) 800 mg orally 4 times a day for 7 days
or
Erythromycin ethylsuccinate (E.E.S.) 400 mg orally 4 times a day for 14 days
or
Azithromycin 1 g orally in a single dose
Note: Because of the risk of drug-related hepatotoxicity, erythromycin estolate is contraindicated during pregnancy.

  ACOG-recommended regimens:
Erythromycin base 500 mg orally 4 times a day for 7 days
or
Erythromycin ethylsuccinate 800 mg orally 4 times a day for 7 days
or
Amoxicillin 500 mg orally 3 times a day for 7 to 10 days
or
Azithromycin 1 g orally in a single dose

*From CDC. (1998). 1998 Guidelines for treatment of sexually transmitted disease. *MMWR 1998, 47* (RR-1).

**From ACOG Educational Bulletin No. 245, *Antimicrobial Therapy for Obstetric Patients*, 1998, p. 6.

---

vidual woman's history may suggest the need for retesting. Women at risk for chlamydia should have a repeat test at 36 weeks.

Because current DNA detection tests for chlamydia detect both living and dead organisms, and dead organisms can persist for at least 1 month, testing done soon after completion of drug therapy may result in a false-positive test. CDC recommends waiting 3 weeks after completion of treatment before retesting (CDC, 1998).

Recent epidemiologic evidence suggests that *Chlamydia trachomatis* infections increase the risk for cervical squamous cell carcinoma (SCC). A study from Finland noted that serotype G is most strongly associated with SCC, and increasing numbers of exposures to varying serotypes increases risk as well (Anttila et al., 2001).

Gonorrhea

Gonorrhea infections during pregnancy are associated with septic, spontaneous abortion (Cunningham et al., 2001); premature rupture of the membranes; prematurity; intrauterine growth restriction (IUGR); chorioamnionitis; disseminated gonococcal infection; and postpartum endometritis. *Neisseria gonorrhoeae* also causes neonatal gonorrheal ophthalmia that, untreated, can lead to corneal ulceration, scarring, and blindness (Gibbs & Sweet, 1999). Women with gonorrhea symptoms usually develop them within 10 days of infection, but most gonorrhea infections are asymptomatic. A single sexual encounter with a man with gonorrhea carries an 80% to 90% risk of infection (Landers, 2000).

The incidence of gonorrhea declined significantly between 1974 and 1997. For this reason, some clinics or offices routinely screen for chlamydia but not gonorrhea infections. However, the number of gonorrhea cases in the United States increased by 9% from 1997 to 1998. While changes in the test used for diagnosis, screening criteria, and the number of persons tested account for some of the increase in cases, true increases in the incidence have occurred.

A single, oral dose of cefixime, 400 mg, is one of the recommended treatments for gonorrhea in pregnant women. Recommendations for follow-up after treatment are conflicting. Because drug resistance to cefixime has not been demonstrated, CDC does not recommend a test-of-cure unless reinfection is suspected (CDC, 1998). Gibbs and Sweet (1997) recommend culturing again in 2 to 3 months to identify reinfection. Landers (2000) recommends follow-up cultures 4 to 7 days after completion of therapy during pregnancy. Sexual contacts within the previous 120 days should be treated presumptively. Women at risk for gonorrhea should have a repeat test at 36 weeks. Box 5-7 contains recommendations for the treatment of gonorrhea during pregnancy.

A Wet Smear

Wet smear examinations can diagnose bacterial vaginosis and candida and trichomonal infections, providing useful information at the initial visit in addition to occasions when symptoms of vaginitis are present.

Trichomoniasis

Trichomonal infections are caused by *Trichomonas vaginalis*, a highly contagious protozoal flagellate that is sexually transmitted. Symptoms include pruritus, malodorous discharge, dyspareunia, and in some women, lower abdominal pain. A frothy gray or yellow-green discharge is frequent, although clinicians are notoriously unable to make a correct diagnosis based only on the appearance of the discharge. The strawberry-like cervix described in textbooks is seldom seen with the naked eye. More useful is microscopic examination of

Box 5.7

Recommendations for the Treatment of Uncomplicated Gonorrhea During Pregnancy

A single dose of ceftriaxone 125 mg IM or cefixime 400 mg orally
plus
Treatment for chlamydia if chlamydia testing was not done, because up to 40% of people with gonorrhea are also infected with chlamydia.

the vaginal discharge on a saline wet mount that reveals the motile, pear-shaped flagellates. The sensitivity of this test has been estimated to be 45% to 60% "by an average microscopist" (Wang, 2000, p. 150). The Pap smear is not acceptable for diagnosing trichomoniasis in asymptomatic women and ". . . should be presumed to be falsely positive until it is confirmed by a wet mount and/or culture" (Wang, 2000, p. 150).

Trichomonal infections are associated with premature onset of contractions, PTL, and premature rupture of membranes (CDC, 1998) as well as low birth weight and preterm delivery (Cotch et al., 1997). Treatment (Box 5-8) is recommended in women with symptoms and risk factors for preterm birth. Sexual partners should also be treated, although studies have not been conducted to determine if treatment reduces risk of adverse outcomes (Cotch et al., 1997). The most common side effects of metronidazole, the drug of choice for treating trichomoniasis, are minor nausea, epigastric distress, and anorexia. Clients should be advised not to drink alcohol while taking metronidazole because some people will experience abdominal cramps, nausea, vomiting, and flushing.

 HELPFUL HINT

Motile trichomonads noted on a wet smear indicate the diagnosis of a trichomonas infection. Having clients look at the moving organism under the microscope can be useful.

Bacterial Vaginosis

Bacterial vaginosis (BV) is the most common cause of vaginal odor. It becomes particularly noticeable after intercourse (due to the release of amines when alkaline semen is present). BV is probably caused by a disturbance in the vaginal ecosystem, with a reduction in lactobacilli and an overgrowth of

---

Box 5.8

Treatment of Trichomonal Infections in Pregnancy

OPTION 1*
Metronidazole 500 mg b.i.d. for 7 days

OPTION 2†
Metronidazole 2 grams orally in a single dose

OPTION 3*
Metronidazole 250 mg b.i.d. for 7 to 10 days

---

*From CDC. (1998). 1998 guidelines for treatment of sexually transmitted disease. *MMWR, 47*(RR-1).

†From Gibbs, R. S., & Sweet, R. L. (1999). Maternal and fetal infectious disorders. In R. K. Creasy & R. Resnik (Eds.), *Maternal-fetal medicine* (pp. 659–724). Philadelphia: W. B. Saunders.

anaerobic bacteria, probably *Mobiluncus* species, *Bacteroides* species, and *Mycoplasma hominis.*

Guidelines (Box 5-9) for treating BV with oral metronidazole were issued after studies noted preterm birth decreased when BV was treated during pregnancy (CDC, 1998). Recent data suggest that treatment does not decrease the preterm birth risk and may, in fact, be harmful (Carey et al., 2000). The CDC Division of STD Prevention "will consider removing this treatment option with its STD treatment guidelines" (STD Prevention Letter p.6).

BV is diagnosed when three out of four of the following are present: a nonirritating, thin, homogenous gray or white discharge; vaginal fluid pH at or greater than 4.5 (determined by touching a swab moistened with the discharge to a pH reagent strip); an amine, "fishy" odor when potassium hydroxide is added to the vaginal secretions (whiff test); and "clue cells" (epithelial cells with a stippled appearance) found when the discharge is examined microscopically. BV should not be diagnosed solely by the presence of clue cells during the wet smear examination or the finding of *Gardnerella vaginalis* on a Pap smear.

Candidiasis

Vaginal discharge may also be due to candidiasis. Most candida infections are caused by *Candida albicans,* although *C. tropicalis* and *C. glabrata* are also causative agents. Typical symptoms include pruritus, dyspareunia, and a thick, white discharge sometimes similar in appearance to cottage cheese. The cervix and walls of the vagina may be covered with the cheesy discharge. While diagnosis can often be made by noting hyphae or budding spores on a wet smear,

---

Box 5.9

Treatment of Bacterial Vaginosis in Pregnancy*,†

RECOMMENDED FOR HIGH-RISK, ASYMPTOMATIC WOMEN

Metronidazole 250 mg t.i.d. for 7 days
The alternatives:
  Metronidazole 2 grams orally in a single dose
  or
  Clindamycin 300 mg orally b.i.d. for 7 days

RECOMMENDED FOR LOW-RISK SYMPTOMATIC WOMEN

Metronidazole 250 mg t.i.d. for 7 days
The alternatives:
  Metronidazole 2 grams orally in a single dose
  or
  Clindamycin 300 mg orally b.i.d. for 7 days
  or
  Metronidazole gel 0.75%, one applicator intravaginally b.i.d. for
5 days‡

---

*CDC's Division of STD Prevention ". . . will consider removing this treatment option for pregnant women with its STD treatment guidelines" (STD Prevention Letter, 2000, p.6).

†Clinicians commonly use 500 mg of oral metronidazole for 7 days despite CDC recommendations.

‡Limited data in pregnant women

Source: Centers for Disease Control and Prevention. (1998). Guidelines for treatment of sexually transmitted diseases. *MMWR; 47*(No.RR-1): p.4.

---

absence of these findings does not mean that candida is absent from the vagina. Treatment on the basis of symptoms alone is ill-advised, because of data indicating that vaginal pruritus is often due to genital herpes. Candida infections have not been associated with PTL.

Azole vaginal creams, tablets, and suppositories are effective in the treatment of candidiasis. These include butoconazole (Femstat), clotrimazole (Mycelex), and miconazole (Monistat). No one brand is significantly more effective than another. During pregnancy, the 7-day regimen is usually recommended over the single-dose or 3-day regimens. Only nystatin vaginal tablets (Mycostatin), FDA pregnancy category A, are recommended for use in the first trimester. However, vaginal tablets appear to be less effective than cream preparations (Medical Letter, 2001) and should be used for 14 days (American Medical Association, 1994).

Oral medication for vaginal candidiasis is not recommended during pregnancy (Medical Letter, 2001). Some clinicians, however, do use oral, single-dose fluconazole (150 mg). It can cause nausea, vomiting, diarrhea, abdominal pain, and headaches (Medical Letter, 2001).

Serum Screening for Birth Defects

The "Triple Screen"

Since the early 1980s when pregnant women were first offered serum screening to detect risk for neural tube defects, additional tests have demonstrated the ability to identify women also at risk for delivering babies with Down syndrome and trisomy 18. The multiple marker screening test analyzes maternal serum for levels of alpha fetoprotein (AFP), human chorionic gonadotropin (hCG), and unconjugated estriol (uE3) to identify women at increased risk for having a baby with Down syndrome, trisomy 18, or a neural tube defect. Originally, only one analyte (AFP) was measured. Elevated levels were found to correlate with neural tube defects. Further research showed that measurement of two additional analytes, hCG and uE3, could demonstrate increased risk for Down syndrome and trisomy 18—hence the name "triple screen." The triple screen is sometimes erroneously referred to as the AFP test. The test is most sensitive when performed between 16 and 18 weeks' gestation, although most laboratories are able to test between the 15th and the 22nd week (Scioscia, 1999). Because the test is only a screening test, false-positive results will occur. These are estimated to occur 2% to 5% of the time.

Women who have not had an ultrasound before the test is performed should know that most of the positive tests are the result of inaccurate dating. Most women with positive results have normal, healthy babies. All women also need to know that the test does not detect all cases of anomalies.

When an abnormal test is reported, it is important to tell a woman more than the following: "The test is abnormal. You need to go for genetic counseling." Interpret the risks in a way that will be best understood by the client. A helpful approach may be to translate the numbers into a percentage that reflects the chances for a healthy baby. For example, if a woman's chances of having a baby with Down syndrome are 1 in 267, she has a 99.5% chance of having a normal baby. A 1-in-50 chance of having a baby with a chromosomal abnormality is still a 98% chance of having a healthy baby.

Serum Screening for Neural Tube Defects

The screening test for open neural tube defects uses only one analyte, AFP, a glycoprotein synthesized by the fetus and excreted by the fetal liver. When the neural tube fails to close, the nonintact fetal skin allows AFP to leak from the fetal capillaries into the amniotic fluid. From there it crosses fetal membranes and enters the maternal circulation. The incidence of neural tube defects is not related to maternal age. The etiology is multifactorial.

Reliable test results depend on an accurate assessment of gestational age and maternal weight, as maternal serum alpha fetoprotein (MSAFP) values normally increase as pregnancy progresses, and a dilutional effect resulting in an incorrectly low value could occur in heavy women. Abnormal values will be obtained if gestational age is inaccurate or if more than one fetus is present. Accordingly, before amniocentesis is performed, an abnormal multiple marker screen should be followed by an ultrasound examination for gestational age and structural abnormalities, if one has not been performed previously.

If an ultrasound examination has already determined gestational age and the number of fetuses, a second ultrasound examination to look for anatomic abnormalities should be requested, as a number of these are associated with elevated MSAFP levels. Clinicians should be aware that a variety of third-trimester complications could occur in association with unexplained MSAFP elevations. These include low birth weight, prematurity, IUGR, preeclampsia, and placental abruption (Scioscia, 1999). Screening for open neural tube defects uses only AFP. The level of AFP in maternal blood is expressed as "multiples of the median" (MOM). Levels of 2.5 MOM or greater indicate increased risk for open neural tube defects.

Serum Screening for Down Syndrome

The risk for Down syndrome (and other chromosome abnormalities) increases with maternal age, yet only 20% to 30% of babies with Down syndrome are born to mothers 35 years of age or older when their babies are born. Children with Down syndrome have characteristic features and mental retardation. Congenital heart abnormalities occur in about 40% of cases (Grant, 2000). While elevated AFP levels screen for neural tube defects, low levels can predict up to one fourth of Down syndrome cases in women under age 35 at the time of delivery. When unconjugated estriol (uE3) and human chorionic gonadotropin (hCG) are measured at the same time MSAFP levels are determined, sensitivity in identifying Down syndrome is increased to approximately 60% (Busch & Himes, 1995). The concentration of hCG, a placental hormone, is nearly twice as high when Down syndrome is present. Maternal serum concentration of uE3 is about 25% lower.

The screening for Down syndrome uses all three analytes: AFP, hCG, and uE3. Sixty percent to 70% of babies with Down syndrome in women under age 35 can be detected with multiple marker screening. Only 20% can be detected if only MSAFP is used. Women who will be 34 or 35 years of age (the cutoff age depends on institutional recommendations) at the time of the birth should be offered chorionic villus sampling (CVS) or amniocentesis to test for chromosome abnormalities. Those who refuse CVS or amniocentesis may wish multiple marker screening. Women with a positive MSAFP screen for Down syndrome should have an ultrasound examination for dating. If the gestational age determined by ultrasound varies from the gestational age determined by menstrual history, the risk should be recalculated.

Serum Screening for Trisomy 18

Trisomy 18 is a syndrome associated with a third number 18 chromosome. Some of the abnormalities are not compatible with more than a few months of life, and most infants die within the first year. Babies with trisomy 18 commonly have polyhydramnios, low birth weight, low-set and malformed ears, congenital heart disease, and hand abnormalities. The screening for trisomy 18 uses all three analytes. Estriol is the most sensitive. Positive test results cannot be explained by incorrect dating, and therefore, recalculation of risk is not indicated for trisomy 18.

The "Quadruple (Quad) Screen"

Maternal serum inhibin A concentration has been recently identified as another useful marker for Down syndrome. When combined with maternal age and the triple screen markers, the detection rate of Down syndrome may increase to 75%, with a false-positive rate of 5% (Haddow, Palomaki, Knight, Foster, & Neveux, 1998). With the addition of this fourth analyte, the triple screen becomes the "quad screen." It will probably be available nationally in the near future.

Screening for Gestational Diabetes Mellitus

Gestational diabetes mellitus (GDM) is a diagnosis made when any degree of glucose/carbohydrate intolerance begins or is first recognized during pregnancy. It can be caused by a number of factors unmasked by pregnancy: the anti-insulin effect of human placental lactogen secreted by the placenta; slower release of insulin from the pancreas (impaired beta-cell secretion) as pregnancy advances; and insulin resistance due to increasing levels of estrogen, progesterone, cortisol, and prolactin. GDM is associated with macrosomia, birth trauma, cesarean section, preeclampsia, and neonatal hypoglycemia. An association between GDM and perinatal mortality has not been demonstrated (Greene, 1997).

Conflicting recommendations pervade many areas of GDM diagnosis and management: whom to screen, the threshold for diagnosis, how to manage when a diagnosis is made, what test(s) to use during pregnancy to evaluate management, how often to perform the test(s), and how to follow up after pregnancy. Arguments against screening at all include lack of reproducibility on retesting (50% to 70% of the time), no clear reduction of perinatal morbidity or mortality with treatment, and the high-risk designation that diabetes confers, with attendant expenses and interventions (Enkin et al., 2000). However, some experts fear that high fasting blood sugars increase the incidence of stillbirths, and Coustan (2000, p. 100) counters the argument against screening with this statement: "It is true that benefit to the population from screening programs has not been unequivocally demonstrated, but it is not true that a lack of benefit has been proven." Fortunately, an international, randomized, controlled trial of the management of abnormal glucose tolerance test values is under way, and we can hope that the data will resolve differences in opinion.

Who to Screen

The American Diabetes Association Expert Committee on the Diagnosis and Classification of Diabetes Mellitus does not recommend universal screening of low-risk women for GDM.

"This low-risk group comprises women who are 25 years of age and of normal body weight, have no family history (i.e., first-degree relative) of diabetes and are not members of an ethnic/racial group with a high prevalence of diabetes (e.g., Hispanic, Native American, Asian, African-American). Pregnant women who fulfill all of these criteria need not be screened for GDM" (American Diabetes Association Expert Committee on the Diagnosis and Classification of Diabetes Mellitus, 1997, p. 1188). The American College of Obstetricians and Gynecologists recommends selective screening (Box 5-10) in some clinical situations and suggests that ". . . in certain Native American populations the prevalence of GDM is so high that pregnant women in these populations can be considered to have a positive screen. They may proceed directly to diagnostic testing" (ACOG, 1994, p. 363).

Some practitioners feel it is unnecessary to screen adolescents for GDM because the overall prevalence is low. A recent study of adolescents with GDM

Box 5.10

Historic and Clinical Risk Factors for Gestational Diabetes Mellitus

- 25 years of age or older
- High BMI (27 or greater)
- First-degree relative with diabetes
- Hispanic, Native American, Asian, or African American
- History of unexplained reproductive loss
- History of a macrosomic baby
- Previous GDM
- Previous congenital anomaly
- Chronic hypertension
- Polyhydramnios
- Glucosuria

reported that a body mass index (BMI) of 27 or more in an adolescent "... might be a useful criterion for identifying patients likely to benefit from diabetic screening" (Khine, Winklestein, & Copel, 1999, p. 742). Another study involving pregnant women under the age of 20 found that only 10% of the macrosomic infants were born to women with glucose intolerance and concluded, "Although macrosomia is an important consequence of gestational diabetes mellitus and glucose intolerance, there are probably other factors predisposing to macrosomia, such as maternal obesity and cumulative weight gain, that play a more important role in this population" (Lemen, Wigton, Miller-McCarthey, & Cruikshank, 1998, p. 1253).

When to Screen

Screening should ordinarily occur between 24 and 28 weeks' gestation to allow time for diet guidelines to keep blood levels within a normal range. Obese women and women with a previous history of GDM should be screened at the initial prenatal visit. A woman with glucosuria should also be screened before 24 to 28 weeks' gestation when glucosuria is found and a screening test has not previously been performed.

The Screening Test

The glucose screening test for pregnant women requires that the client drink a special liquid containing 50 g of glucose. Blood is drawn 1 hour later. Fasting before the 50-g screening test is not required. Thresholds commonly used to identify women requiring further testing vary by institution. They include glucose levels of 130 mg/dL, 135 mg/dL, and 140 mg/dL. Values above 190 mg/dL in Hispanic women and above 225 mg/dL in White women are considered diagnostic, and the 3-hour glucose tolerance test is contraindicated.

Alternatives to the 50-Gram Liquid

Some clients are averse to swallowing the glucose-intense liquid used in the screening test. While special foods thought to be the equivalent of the 50-g dose have been suggested, the only alternative actually studied and accepted as an alternate choice is eating 28 Brach's jelly beans within a 10-minute period. The blood glucose level is measured 1 hour after the Brach's jelly beans have been eaten. (A previous study concluding that 18 Brach's jelly beans could be substituted for the screening liquid was found to have mistakenly determined the amount of glucose in the 18 jelly beans.) Jelly beans cannot be used for the diagnostic test (Lamar, Kuehl, Cooney, Gayle, Holleman, & Allen, 1999). Side effects associated with the sweet 50-g liquid— nausea, vomiting, sweating, and headache—are fewer when jelly beans are used. Chapter 8 discusses the management of GDM once a diagnosis is made.

The Diagnostic Test

After fasting for 8 hours (except for water) and not smoking for 12, the client drinks a liquid containing 100 g of glucose. (European medical communities use 75 g.) No smoking, eating, or drinking should occur during the test. Norms commonly accepted for the 3-hour test are shown in Box 5-11. Gestational diabetes is diagnosed when two or more values are met or exceeded.

If a woman vomits after ingesting the glucose, do not ask her to repeat the test. Instead, follow her fasting glucose levels at each prenatal visit. Do not use random glucose testing to screen or diagnose GDM, as it provides no pertinent information.

Many labs recommend a high-carbohydrate diet (150 g) for 3 days prior to the test because the insulin of women on carbohydrate-restricted diets may be slower to respond to the glucose, and a false-positive result is more likely. However, a recent prospective pilot study involving 20 subjects given two glucose tolerance tests, one with no dietary restrictions and one after a 3-day diet containing 150 g of carbohydrates, showed no significant differences between the groups in test results. This finding led investigators to conclude that dietary preparation for a 3-hour test is unnecessary (Crowe, Mastrobattista, & Monga, 2000). Because of the very small number of subjects in this study, changes in practice should await additional investigation. An easy way for some women to eat sufficient carbohydrates is to consume four extra slices of bread for each of the 3 days prior to the test.

Box 5.11

Norms for the 3-Hour Glucose Tolerance Test for the Diagnosis of Gestational Diabetes*,†

Fasting	105 mg/dL
1 hour	190 mg/dL
2 hours	165 mg/dL
3 hours	145 mg/dL

*Two abnormal values are necessary for a diagnosis.

†Some practices will use other values, especially for the fasting level.

From American College of Obstetricians and Gynecologists. (1994). *Diabetes and pregnancy*, Washington, DC: Author, p. 1.

❊ Special Laboratory Tests

Sickle Cell Screening

Approximately 1 out of 12 adult African Americans in the United States is heterozygous for hemoglobin S and, consequently, has sickle cell trait (hemoglobin AS). A child born to two parents who are heterozygous for hemoglobin S has a 50% probability of inheriting the trait and a 25% probability of having sickle cell trait. All Black women should be screened for hemoglobin S at the first prenatal visit. Women with sickle cell trait are not at risk for poor perinatal outcome.

Hemoglobin Electrophoresis

Hemoglobin electrophoresis identifies abnormal forms of hemoglobin in the blood (the thalassemia syndromes and the structural hemoglobinopathies, including sickle cell anemia). Each major hemoglobin type (A, A_2, F, S, and C) is electrically charged, to varying degrees. "When the hemoglobin from lysed RBCs is placed on electrophoresis paper and placed in an electromagnetic field, the Hgb [hemoglobin] variants migrate at different rates and, therefore, spread apart from each other. The migrations of the various forms of Hgb make up a series of bands on the paper. Therefore, the bands correspond to the various forms of hemoglobin present. The pattern of bands is compared to normal and other well-known abnormal patterns. Further, each band can be quantitated as a percentage of the total Hgb, indicating the severity of any recognized abnormality" (Pagana & Pagana, 1999, p. 467). Table 5-4 identifies the hemoglobin contents of common hemoglobinopathies. Request hemoglobin electrophoresis when women at risk for thalassemia have a low MCV and when African American women have a positive sickle cell screen.

Varicella

Varicella during pregnancy can cause congenital varicella syndrome, characterized by various eye abnormalities (cataracts, chorioretinitis, microophthalmia), microcephaly, and limb hypoplasia in the first half of pregnancy and skin scarring in the second half.

A pregnant woman with varicella may deliver prematurely and/or develop varicella pneumonia, a serious and often life-threatening disease (Katz, Kuller, McMahon, Warren, & Wells, 1995). Even in the presence of full pulmonary support, if hemoptysis occurs, the maternal death rate can be as high as 50%.

If maternal infection occurs around the time of delivery, after the mother has become infected but before she has had time to mount an antibody response, the baby will receive a high viral load. The neonatal death rate is

TABLE 5.4 Hemoglobin Contents of Some Common Hemoglobinopathies*

	Percentage range					
	Hgb A1	Hgb A2	Hgb F	Hgb S	Hgb H	Hgb C
Sickle cell disease	0	2	2	80–100	0	0
Sickle cell trait	60–80	2–5	2	20–40	0	0
Hemoglobin C disease	0	2–5	2	0	0	90–100
Hemoglobin H disease	65–90	2–3	0	0	5–30	0
Thalassemia major	5–20	2–3	65–100	0	0	0
Thalassemia minor	50–85	4–6	1–3	0	0	0

*Reprinted with permission from Pagana, K. D., & Pagana, T. J. (1999). Hemoglobin electrophoresis. In *Mosby's diagnostic and laboratory test reference* (4th ed., p. 469). St. Louis: Mosby.

high when maternal disease develops ". . . from 5 days before delivery up to 48 hours postpartum as a result of the relative immaturity of the fetal immune system and the lack of protective maternal antibody" (ACOG, 2000c, p. 4). "If possible, delivery should be delayed until 5 to 7 days after the onset of maternal illness to allow passive transfer of protective antibodies. If delay is not possible, the neonate should receive varicella zoster immune globulin (VZIG)" (Chapman, 1998, p. 342).

A woman who knows she has had varicella in the past can be assumed to be immune. Household contacts who receive the vaccine do not endanger the expectant mother. While counseling is recommended if pregnancy occurs within 1 month of receiving the vaccine, ". . . in most circumstances, the decision to continue a pregnancy should not be based on exposure to the varicella vaccine" (Gibbs & Sweet, 1999, p. 686). Breastfeeding is not contraindicated ". . . as long as vesicular lesions are not present in the area where the infant suckles" (Chapman, 1998, p.342.)

Type-2 Herpes Simplex Virus

Type-2 herpes simplex virus (HSV-2) infection frequently is unrecognized. In the National Health and Nutrition Examination Survey (NHANES) only 9% of persons who were seropositive for HSV-2 stated that they had genital herpes (Fleming et al., 1997). And as many as 85% of persons with HSV-2 antibodies shed the virus when there are no symptoms of infection, meaning that most HSV-2 positive individuals can spread HSV to their uninfected sex partners, even when a couple has been in a long-standing monogamous relationship. This new information about HSV-2 combined with the development of diagnostic type-specific serologic tests may mean that identification of "HSV-discordant" couples will eventually become part of routine prenatal laboratory testing, allowing for counseling couples about the risks of genital and orogenital sexual practices (Corey & Handsfield, 2000).

Thyroid-Stimulating Hormone

Maternal thyroid requirements increase 25% to 50% in pregnancy (Murdock, 1999). Because signs and symptoms of thyroid disorders are nonspecific and can range from one to several (Box 5-12), thyroid dysfunction may be difficult to recognize. A thyroid-stimulating hormone (TSH) test is the most sensitive test for the initial assessment of both hypothyroidism and hyperthyroidism and is recommended by the American Association of Clinical Endocrinologists (AACE) as the primary test for diagnosis (AACE, 1996). Normal TSH levels range from 0.23 to 4.0 mU/L, with a borderline high ranging from 4.1 to 9.6 μIU/mL (Gardiner & Holahan, 1999). The TSH level is increased in

> **Box 5.12**
>
> ### Symptoms of Thyroid Disease
>
> | | |
> |---|---|
> | Hypothyroidism | Periorbital swelling |
> | Fatigue or lethargy | Hyperthyroidism |
> | Weight gain | Increased appetite |
> | Cold intolerance | Weight loss |
> | Hair loss or coarse hair | Insomnia |
> | Dry skin | Heat intolerance and increased |
> | Constipation | perspiration |
> | Joint stiffness, pain, myalgias | Palpitations |
> | Flat affect or depression | Frequent bowel movements |
> | Impaired memory | Tremors, nervousness, anxiety |

hypothyroidism and decreased in hyperthyroidism. If the TSH is either increased (>9.6 μIU/mL) or decreased (<0.23 μIU/mL), request a serum-free T_4 (FT_4) and refer the client to a physician for management. (Some clinicians request the TSH and FT_4 tests at the same time.) In addition to awareness of symptoms of thyroid dysfunction, clinicians should measure TSH levels each trimester when pregnant women have a personal or family history of thyroid disorders (Murdock, 1999).

Tuberculosis

Screening for tuberculosis (TB) is appropriate for any woman who is symptomatic, HIV-positive, a close contact of a person with pulmonary tuberculosis, an alcoholic or IV drug user, from a country with a high prevalence rate, a resident of a correctional institution or a long-term care facility, a health care worker, or poor and medically underserved. The purified protein derivative (PPD) test, 90% to 99% sensitive in detecting active TB in healthy individuals, is the standard method for TB screening (Vo, Stettler, & Crowley, 2000). An intradermal injection of 0.1 mL of 5 tuberculin unit strength is placed in the forearm, and the test is interpreted 48 to 72 hours after the injection.

A positive PPD indicates infection or disease. The distinction between infection and disease can be difficult to remember as most clinicians equate infection and disease. But infection in regard to TB is "a state in which the tubercle bacillus has become established but produces no symptoms, radiological abnormalities, or recoverable bacilli on culture or body fluids. Active TB is defined as a proliferation of the organisms, either from a recent exposure or a reactivation, causing signs and symptoms of active disease. The chance that a patient with a positive PPD will subsequently develop the disease is 5% to 10%, provided his or her immune system is intact" (Vo, Stettler, & Crowley, 2000, p. 246).

Prior vaccination with bacillus Calmette-Guérin (BCG) vaccine should not preclude a tuberculin skin test (PPD) for anyone who received this vaccine in infancy or childhood, because sensitivity decreases 10% per year without repeated doses. "In persons vaccinated with BCG, sensitivity to tuberculin is highly variable, depending on the strain of BCG used and the group vaccinated. There is no reliable method of distinguishing tuberculin reactions caused by BCG from those caused by natural infections" (CDC, 1994, p. 64).

To identify women with active disease, a positive PPD (Appendix J) requires follow-up with a chest x-ray, whether or not BCG vaccination has occurred. Women with a negative chest x-ray should receive isoniazid therapy postpartally, although neither the CDC nor ACOG state when therapy should be initiated. Although isoniazid is used during pregnancy to treat active TB, treatment delays for pregnant women with latent TB come from fear that pregnancy might increase the risk for isoniazid-induced hepatitis. "In a retrospective analysis of isoniazid use in women, a 2.5-fold increased risk of isoniazid hepatitis and fourfold increased risk of death was noted in pregnant Hispanic women compared with previously collected Public Health Service data on over 3900 pregnant women. Although this difference was not statistically significant, the authors urged caution and further study on the use of isoniazid during pregnancy" (Boggess, Myers, & Hamilton, 2000, P. 757).

Group B Streptococcus

Streptococcus agalactiae, Group B streptococcus (GBS), is a common cause of severe morbidity and mortality in newborns. The CDC, in collaboration with ACOG, the American Academy of Pediatrics, and other professional organizations, has published guidelines for the prevention of GBS in newborns. Clinicians are free to choose from two approaches: the screening-based approach and the risk-based approach.

The screening-based approach uses prenatal screening at 35 to 37 weeks' gestation to determine which women should receive intravenous antibiotic prophylaxis in labor. The risk-based approach involves administering intravenous antibiotics to laboring women who have a condition that increases their risk for GBS infection. The main disadvantage of the risk-based approach is that asymptomatic colonization is not recognized. Colonization rates for GBS vary across the United States, from 3% or 4% in some Latina populations to 40% in populations with high rates of sexually transmitted diseases (STDs). An estimated 30% to 50% of early-onset GBS in newborns occurs in women with no risk factors (Hager et al., 2000).

Figures 5-3A and 5-3B illustrate these two approaches. Unfortunately, neither strategy has been evaluated extensively in clinical practice or compared in randomized controlled trials (ACOG, 1996c).

The GBS specimen should be obtained from both the vaginal introitus and the rectum. This procedure increases the recovery rate by 25%. Insertion of a speculum is not necessary to obtain the vaginal specimen. Specimens obtained more than 5 weeks before delivery do not accurately predict colonization at delivery. Whether a second specimen should be obtained when birth has not occurred within 5 weeks of the first test is unknown. Administering oral antibiotics prenatally eradicates GBS, but only temporarily. There is a high spontaneous recolonization rate after antibiotics are discontinued.

Genetic Testing

When a pregnant woman is at increased risk for having a child with a birth defect, she should be offered a referral to a center for genetic counseling. (The risk of a birth defect in any pregnancy, regardless of maternal age, is 3% to 5%.) It may be difficult to talk with pregnant women about genetic counseling, as the clinician's own feelings about less-than-perfect babies and about abortion can affect a discussion as much as the client's own feelings about these issues. Some women feel certain that they will have an abortion if they find out they are carrying a baby with a specific genetic/chromosomal problem. Other women are just as certain they would never have an abortion under any circumstances. But time, experience, and information can change people's minds. Therefore, it is important to offer counseling to all women. Avoid assumptions about what any one woman will choose to do, and support women when their choice is made.

Prenatal diagnosis to identify chromosome abnormalities, gender, and single-gene conditions is hindered by timing problems. Amniocentesis is performed at 16 to 18 weeks' gestation, but 2 to 3 additional weeks are required before an analysis of the cells is available. By this time the pregnancy is likely to be apparent, and the mother has probably felt fetal movement. "Women often postpone the normal process of preparing to become parents until the testing has been completed and the results are known. The delay in testing is especially difficult for couples who are as a high risk for having a child with a severe genetic condition and who face a 25% chance of having an affected child" (Himes, 1999).

Chorionic Villus Sampling

Chorionic villus sampling (CVS) was developed as an early prenatal diagnostic tool. In this procedure chorionic villi are aspirated from the placental bed

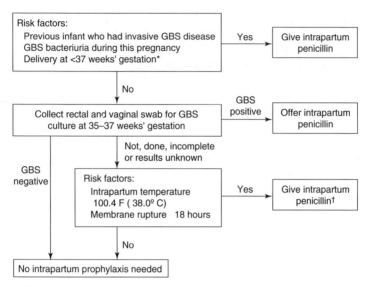

* If membranes ruptured at <37 weeks' gestation, and the mother has not begun labor, collect group B streptococcal culture and either a) administer antibiotics until cultures are completed and the results are negative or b) begin antibiotics only when positive cultures are available. No prophylaxis is needed if culture obtained at 35-37 weeks' gestation was negative.

† Broader spectrum antibiotics may be considered at the physician's descretion, based on clinical indications.

A

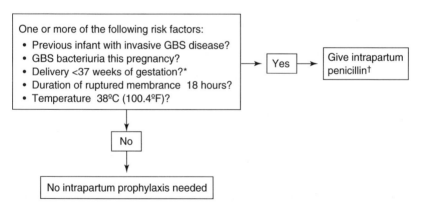

*For ruptured membranes without labor at <37 weeks, collect GBS culture and either:

a) give antibiotics until cultures are completed and negative, or

b) begin antibiotics once positive culture results are available

†Broad-spectrum antibiotics may be considered at the discretion of the physician based on clinical indicators.

B

through a soft catheter inserted into the cervix between 10 and 12 completed weeks' gestation. Then they are cultured to determine the fetal karyotype. The risks of the procedure are somewhat difficult to assess because the procedure is performed in the first trimester in older gravidas, both situations already associated with increased fetal loss. "There appears to be a 2% risk of spontaneous abortion after sonographically confirmed viability, and the loss seems to be slightly higher in older women" (Scioscia, 1999, p. 55).

A second complication is limb reduction defects such as absent fingers and toes or missing portions of fingers and toes. The association between these defects and the CVS procedure is disputed. Nevertheless, CVS should be avoided before 10 weeks' gestation, and clients should be counseled about the controversy and the possibility of limb deformities (ACOG, 1995a).

Amniocentesis

Amniocentesis is the most common prenatal diagnostic procedure performed in the second trimester. Fetal cells for karyotyping are obtained from the amniotic fluid via a spinal needle inserted through the maternal abdomen and uterus. Approximately 20 mL of amniotic fluid is removed. The procedure is performed between 16 and 18 weeks' gestation. It is preceded or performed concurrently with an ultrasound examination to identify fetal number, confirm or establish gestational age, localize the placenta, and estimate amniotic fluid volume. The risk for a complication (miscarriage, infection, bleeding, or, in rare cases, fetal damage) from the procedure is estimated to be 1 in 100 to 1 in 150 when performed after 15 weeks' gestation. When the mother is age 35, the risk of giving birth to a baby with Down syndrome is approximately 1 in 370, and the risk of giving birth to a live-born baby with any chromosome abnormality is approximately 1 in 200.

Early Amniocentesis

CVS problems led to early performance of an amniocentesis as a way to provide a safer alternative for early prenatal diagnosis. The definition of "early" amniocentesis varies, generally ranging between 9 and 15 weeks. Risks associated with the procedure have been difficult to establish with accuracy. Associations with pregnancy loss, postprocedure leakage of fluid, talipes equino-

◀ **FIGURE 5.3** Prevention strategy for group B streptococcal disease. (A) Using the screening-based approach. (B) Using the risk-factor approach. From Centers for Disease Control and Prevention. (1996). Prevention of perinatal group B streptococcal disease: A public health perspective. *Morbidity and Mortality Weekly Report, 45*(RR-7), 20.

varus (clubfeet), and increased respiratory problems in children have been noted (Himes, 1999).

Fetal Fibronectin

A recently developed test, the fetal fibronectin (fFN) assay, has the ability to significantly reduce hospital admissions and hospital stay for suspected PTL, as well as reduce the use of tocolytic agents. Fetal fibronectin is a substance thought to play an important role in binding fetal trophoblastic tissue to maternal decidual tissue. Significant concentrations are found in vaginal secretions until the chorion has fused with the decidua (22 weeks' gestation). Investigators hypothesize that elevated levels of fibronectin after this time (τ50ng/mL) signify disruption of the chorion-decidual interface with an accompanying increased risk for PTL (Joffe, Jacques, Bemis-Hates, Burton, Skram, & Shelburne, 1999). The test is appropriate to perform between 24 and 34 weeks' gestation (ACOG, 1997b).

The specimen for the fFN assay is obtained from the posterior vaginal fornix before a digital examination of the cervix is performed. Manipulation of the cervix may cause fFN to be released. If intercourse has occurred in the preceding 24 hours, defer obtaining a specimen because semen and/or sperm increase the likelihood of a false-positive test. In addition, amniotic membranes must be intact, and cervical dilatation must be less than 3 cm. A negative result indicates that the patient is unlikely to go into labor in the next 7 to 14 days. A positive result is difficult to evaluate and, therefore, is not helpful in making management decisions. Directions for obtaining the specimen for the fFN assay are summarized in Box 5-13.

❖ Ultrasound Examinations

Despite ACOG's conclusion that ultrasound examinations should be performed only for specific indications in low-risk pregnancies (ACOG, 1997), a routine examination at some point in pregnancy is common practice in the United States. Ultrasound can determine the EDB, confirm an EDB based on menstrual history, determine whether a multiple gestation is present, identify structural abnormalities in the baby, locate the placenta, measure amniotic fluid volume, assess fetal growth (see Chapter 8), measure the length of the cervix, reassure families about fetal well-being, and perhaps, facilitate bonding. Incidental findings may include identification of uterine leiomyomas (fibroids) and vasa previa. Box 5-14 lists the components of a basic ultrasound examination according to the trimester in which the examination is performed. Pretest counseling before any ultrasound examination is important, particu-

Box 5.13	

Directions for Obtaining the Specimen to Test for Fetal Fibronectin

Before obtaining the specimen, determine that
1. Gestational age is no less than 24 weeks, 0 days, and no greater then 34 weeks, 6 days.
2. Amniotic membranes are intact.
3. No intercourse has taken place in the last 24 hours.
4. Cervical dilatation is less than 3 cm.
5. No digital examination of the cervix has been performed recently.

To obtain the specimen
1. Perform a sterile speculum examination.
2. Lightly rotate the swab across the posterior vaginal fornix for 10 seconds.
3. Immerse the swab into the buffer solution provided.
4. Break the wooden shaft at the score.
5. Place the shaft of the swab in the hole of the cap and press down tightly.
6. Store the specimen in a refrigerator or on ice until testing.

Interpretation of results:
1. Negative: the patient is unlikely to go into labor in the next 7 to 14 days
2. Positive: difficult to evaluate

larly as the examination relates to structural anomalies (i.e., imperfect ability to identify all abnormalities).

Ultrasound Examination for Dating

The most common use of ultrasound in pregnancy is for "dating" purposes. Ultrasound examinations to date pregnancy infer age from fetal size. The optimum time to determine gestational age by ultrasound is from 7 to 9 menstrual weeks (Hadlock, 1994). The range of error at these times is plus or minus 8%, meaning that the variability in crown-rump length, the "measurement of choice" for determining menstrual age in the first trimester, would be only 0.64 weeks (Hadlock, 1994). Because of increasing biologic variability in fetal size as pregnancy progresses, third-trimester ultrasounds have severe accuracy problems. Due date variability ranges from 2½ to 4 weeks. Consequently, clinicians must avoid changing the due date when a later ultrasound suggests a different EDB from one obtained in the middle of the first trimester (Hadlock, 1994).

It seems logical that a first-trimester ultrasound should be obtained as soon as a problem with menstrual history dating is noted. However, some

---

Box 5.14

Components of a Basic Ultrasound Examination

FIRST TRIMESTER

- The location of the gestational sac
- Identification of an embryo and the crown-rump length
- Evaluation of uterus (and cervix) and adnexa
- The presence or absence of fetal life
- Number of fetuses

SECOND TRIMESTER

- Cardiac activity
- Number of fetuses
- Presentation
- The location of the placenta
- Estimate of the volume of amniotic fluid
- Gestational age and interval growth assessment if a previous ultrasound examination was performed
- Fetal presentation
- Anatomy survey
- Evaluation of uterus and adnexa

---

insurance plans pay for only a single ultrasound examination unless there is an obstetric indication for more. When insurance plans or health care systems pay for a single ultrasound during pregnancy, wait until 18 weeks when other important parameters can also be assessed (cervical length, placental location, some anomalies, amniotic fluid volume [Filly, 1994]) . Table 5-5 outlines the limits of variance for estimating the date of birth by ultrasound performed at varying gestational ages. (These guidelines for estimating due date and/or changing the due date based on ultrasound findings may vary from one institution to another.)

Anomalies

Ultrasound examinations are able to detect some structural abnormalities. Ideally, ultrasound department technicians know their detection rates (sensitivity). An expectant mother should understand that ultrasound is used for screening purposes, and as many as one third of structural anomalies are not detectable by the examination. Ultrasound ". . . may be helpful in ruling out anomalies, but it is not particularly reliable in detecting them" (ACOG, 1997d, p. 1051). Box 5-15 summarizes the information that should be provided to a pregnant woman before an ultrasound examination.

TABLE 5.5 Limits of Variance for Ultrasound Examinations in Pregnancy

Week of gestation	Due date variance
6–12 weeks	± 3 days
12–20 weeks	± 7 days
20–24 weeks	± 12 days
24–30 weeks	± 15 days
32+ weeks	± 2.5 weeks

Concern about risks of miscarriage and birth defects associated with CVS and early amniocentesis have encouraged researchers to look for alternative methods of assessing risk for a chromosome abnormality. At 11 to 13 completed weeks' gestational age the fetus has a small, fluid-filled space that separates the muscles at the back of the neck (nuchal translucency). Increased width of this region due to subcutaneous accumulation of fluid has been associated with three serious chromosomal defects—trisomies 13, 18, and 21 (Down syndrome)—and with defects so severe that the infants do not survive after birth. "By combining ultrasound measurement of the nuchal translucency with maternal age it is possible to identify pregnancies at increased risk for chromosome abnormalities and some congenital heart defects. These women can then be offered chorionic villus sampling or amniocentesis for definitive diagnosis of chromosome abnormalities. If the chromosome evaluation is nor-

Box 5.15

Information To Be Provided Before an Ultrasound Examination*

1. Ultrasound examinations are for screening rather than diagnostic purposes.
2. Major anomalies are likely to occur in 2% to 3% of pregnancies.
3. One third of major anomalies are undetectable by ultrasound.
4. A woman who has one negative ultrasound examination in the second trimester has at least a 1% to 2% risk of a major anomaly.
5. If the ultrasound examination suggests an anomaly, women are likely to experience anxiety that may or may not be relieved as the pregnancy progresses.

*From Dooley, S. L. (1999). Routine ultrasound in pregnancy. *Clinical Obstetrics and Gynecology, 42*(4), 737–748.

mal, another ultrasound is performed in the second trimester to examine the fetal heart and other organs. When combined with maternal age and appropriate maternal serum biochemistry, some have reported a sensitivity of almost 90% with a false positive rate of 5%. This form of screening requires skilled operators and is prone to operator variability" (Grant, 2000, p. 7). Ultrasound for nuchal translucency at 11 to 13 completed weeks of gestation cannot rule out Down syndrome and is not used interchangeably with the multiple marker screen or amniocentesis.

Cervical Length

A recent development in obstetric use of ultrasound is measurement of cervical length. Increasing evidence suggests that decreased cervical length as measured by transvaginal ultrasound helps predict preterm birth (Goldenberg et al., 1998). (The ultrasound measurement of cervical length is different from the measurement obtained by a clinician on pelvic examination, as clinicians can only feel that portion of the cervix that extends into the vagina. One half to two thirds of the cervix may not be palpable.) A prospective, observational study of 760 pregnant women who had cervical length measured at ultrasound examination between 16 and 22 weeks' gestation found that ". . . the risk of early delivery, before 35 weeks, was increased fivefold to 10-fold over women with normal cervical lengths, and the risk increased by 10.3% for every millimeter decrease in cervical length below the mean. Multiparas were at greatest risk" (Hibbard, Tart, & Moawad, 2000, p. 976).

Increasing use of this parameter is likely to be useful once more data are gathered on which guidelines can be based. Preliminary data suggest that a cervical length of 2.5–3.0 cm predisposes the client to PTL.

Vasa Previa

Additional information found at ultrasound may include the presence of vasa previa, a condition in which the umbilical cord inserts itself into the placental membranes that cover the cervical os. Vasa previa is one of the most lethal conditions in obstetrics. If the fetal blood vessels rupture, the baby usually rapidly bleeds to death. Perinatal death can also occur if the presenting part compresses the vessels and compromises fetal circulation.

A retrospective study of ultrasound examinations of the internal cervical os of more than 93,000 women over an 8-year period found 18 cases of vasa previa on initial examination. The earliest case identified was at 15.6 weeks' gestation. Risk factors for vasa previa included an edge of the placenta over the os, a multifetal gestation, velamentous insertion of the umbilical cord, biloba or succenturiate placenta, and suspicion of a blood vessel across the internal os. Antepartum bleeding at a mean gestational age of 31.3 weeks was found in one third of the women (Lee, Lee, Kirk, Sloan, Smith, & Comstock, 2000).

Uterine Leiomyomas

Fibroids may also be found on ultrasound examination. Another retrospective study found an association between uterine leiomyomas and complications of pregnancy, labor, and delivery. These uterine tumors were associated with breech presentation (a fourfold increase compared with a control group), abruptio placentae (a fourfold increase), premature rupture of the membranes, dysfunctional labor, cesarean birth (66%), low birth weight, and low Apgar scores (Coronado, Marshall, & Schwartz, 2000).

Ultrasound for Psychological Reasons

In some instances, midwives have been slow to see some of the psychological advantages of ultrasound examinations. While little scientific data are available, experience demonstrates that ultrasound examinations may facilitate maternal and/or paternal bonding with the baby, and as such, ultrasound should be viewed with its potential for contributing to psychological well-being.

With increasing frequency, parents want to know the sex of their baby in utero. While some parents may still be enthralled with the suspense of waiting to know if it is a girl or a boy, others may have compelling as well as seemingly noncompelling reasons to know sex prior to birth. In some instances, knowing the sex of the baby ahead of time gives family members who are disappointed with the sex time to adjust.

✽ Antepartal Fetal Surveillance

Antepartum assessment of the baby's condition is sometimes required. Antepartal testing usually consists of a nonstress test (NST) or a contraction stress test (CST), as well as an amniotic fluid index (AFI) or biophysical profile (BPP).

The Nonstress Test

The NST evaluates the fetal heart rate without "stressing" the baby with uterine contractions. (Contractions decrease perfusion of the placenta and may cause signs of distress in compromised babies.) While the pregnant woman reclines in a chair or in a semi-Fowler's position in bed, two straps attaching a pressure transducer and an ultrasound device to a fetal monitor are placed across her abdomen. Tracing paper documents the fetal heart rate and any contractions that are present. While contractions are not required for this test, their presence provides additional information about the baby's well-being. A reassuring test occurs over a twenty-minute period and shows evidence of 1) two accelerations of the fetal heart to at least 15 beats above the baseline, lasting at least 15 seconds; 2) no decelerations, which suggests fetal compromise. A reassuring NST is termed "reactive" (Figure 5-4A), and a nonreassuring test is termed "nonreactive" (Figure 5-4B). Unfortunately, the NST has a false-positive rate as high as 90%.

The Contraction Stress Test

The CST is similar to the NST except that the fetal heart rate is evaluated under conditions of stress (i.e., contractions). If the client is not having spontaneous contractions, they are induced by nipple stimulation (warm towels on the breast or nipple rolling) or an IV infusion containing oxytocin. A CST often is the preferred test when uteroplacental insufficiency is suspected, as in preeclampsia or chronic maternal disease. The CST can have a false-positive rate of 65%.

Measurement of Amniotic Fluid Volume: The Amniotic Fluid Index

Amniotic fluid provides protection to the fetus when trauma occurs to the maternal abdomen, maintains the intrauterine environment at a consistent and normal temperature, and shields the umbilical cord against constriction. Its origin in early pregnancy is unknown. As pregnancy advances, fetal urination is the major source, and fetal swallowing removes it. The amount of fluid rises progressively from about 30 mL at 10 weeks' gestation to approximately 800 mL from 32 weeks to term. After 40 weeks the fluid decreases, averaging 400 mL at 42 weeks (Moore, 1997). The amount of amniotic fluid in the uterine cavity is a reflection of fetal well-being.

The AFI is a measurement of amniotic fluid and is obtained by measuring the largest vertical "pocket" of fluid in each of the four quadrants of the pregnant uterus and then adding the four measurements together. Figure 5-5 shows AFI values for normal pregnancies. A second technique to measure amniotic fluid volume, the 2-diameter pocket technique, also measures the largest fluid pocket in each quadrant. But in this technique, the vertical measurement is multiplied by the horizontal measurement. The largest pocket of the four quadrants is the 2-cm pocket measurement. The normal measurement ranges from 15.1 to 50 cm².

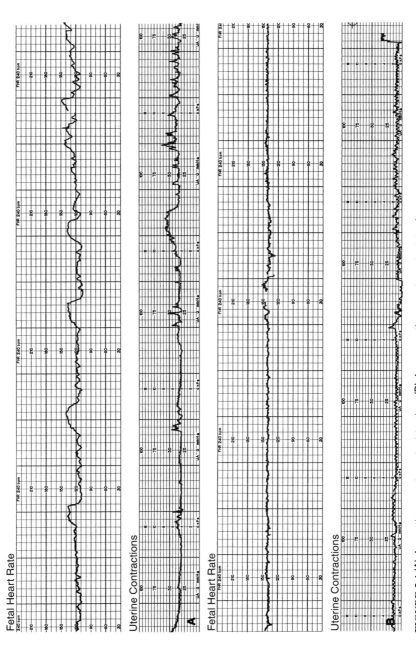

FIGURE 5.4 (A) A reactive nonstress test tracing. **(B)** A nonreactive nonstress test tracing.

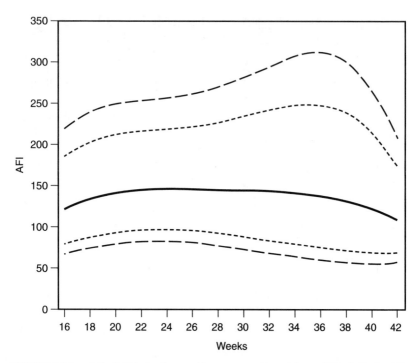

FIGURE 5.5 Amniotic fluid index in normal pregnancy. From Moore, T.K., & Cayle, J.E. (1990). The amniotic fluid index in normal pregnancy. *American Journal of Obstetrics and Gynecology, 162*, 1168.

Unfortunately, amniotic fluid determinations made during ultrasound examination are imprecise, and the measurement that necessitates intervention has not been studied in randomized controlled trials. The influence of maternal hydration on the amount of amniotic fluid is under investigation. Controlled trials to determine the usefulness of oral or intravenous hydration are needed to identify short-term and long-term benefits and risks.

Oligohydramnios

An AFI of 5 cm or less or a 2-diameter pocket measurement of <15 defines oligohydramnios. Prior to term, oligohydramnios is associated with low birth weight and major malformations. At term, oligohydramnios has been associated with meconium-stained amniotic fluid and cesarean delivery for fetal distress. However, this association is not consistent. A recent report of 1001 women with high-risk pregnancies found no difference in intrapartum complications between women diagnosed with oligohydramnios and those found to have a normal amount of amniotic fluid. The authors concluded that while the AFI reliably determines normal amniotic fluid volumes, it can overestimate low volumes by as much as 89%, leaving the usefulness of the test open to question (Magann et al., 1999).

Polyhydramnios

Polyhydramnios is defined as an AFI of 25 cm or greater or a 2-diameter pocket of more than 50 cm². Its cause is usually unknown, but it may be associated with fetal anomalies, insulin-dependent diabetes, gestational diabetes, or Rh isoimmunization. Fluid accumulation usually occurs slowly, but it may also be acute, accruing in as little as 24 hours. It may be great enough to interfere with maternal breathing. A clinical finding in cases of polyhydramnios is an inability to palpate the fetus. Preterm birth will occur in up to one third of the cases, but the underlying cause of polyhydramnios rather than excess fluid may determine whether PTL will occur (Many, Hill, Lazebnik, & Martin, 1995).

Biophysical Profile

A fourth test to evaluate fetal well-being is the BPP. This test uses ultrasound to assess the baby's muscle tone, movement, and breathing, as well as the amount of amniotic fluid. A positive finding in each category is given a score of 2. Negative findings are given a score of 0. The four measurements are combined with results of the NST, 2 points being awarded when the NST shows desired accelerations in the absence of worrisome decelerations. The desired score is 10/10 (Table 5-6).

Unfortunately, there is no agreement on how to obtain the amniotic fluid measurement that makes up one part of the BPP. Three methods have been described. One defines normal volume as a pocket of fluid that is free of umbilical cord and fetal parts and measures at least 2 cm horizontally and 2 cm vertically (2 × 2). Another uses 1 cm by 1 cm in two perpendicular planes (1 × 1)(Cunningham et al., 2001), and a third uses one pocket measuring at least 2 cm in two perpendicular planes (Manning, 1999). A BPP can have a false-positive rate of 60%, usually due to performing the examination while the baby is in a sleep cycle.

Indications for Testing

The American College of Obstetricians and Gynecologists lists the following pregnancy-related conditions as indications for antepartal fetal surveillance (ACOG, 1999a):

- Pregnancy-induced hypertension
- Decreased fetal movement
- Oligohydramnios

TABLE 5.6 Biophysical Profile Scoring: Technique and Interpretation*

Biophysical variable	Normal score	Abnormal (Score = 0)
Fetal breathing movements	At least one episode of FBM of at least 30-sec duration in 30-min observation	Absent FBM or no episode of ≥30 sec in 30 minutes
Gross body movement	At least three discrete body/limb movements in 30 min (episodes of active continuous movement considered as single movement)	2 or fewer episodes of body/limb movements in 30 min
Fetal tone	At least one episode of active extension with return to flexion of fetal limb(s) or trunk. Opening and closing of hand considered normal tone	Either slow extension with return to partial flexion or movement of limb in full extension or absent fetal movement with fetal hand held in complete or partial deflection
Reactive FHR	At least 2 episodes of FHR acceleration of ≥15 beat/min and of at least 15-sec duration associated with fetal movement in 30 min	Less than 2 episodes of acceleration of FHR or acceleration of <15 beats/min in 30 min
Qualitative AFV†	At least 1 pocket of AF that measures at least 2 cm in 2 perpendicular planes	Either no AF pockets or a pocket <2 cm in two perpendicular planes

*FBM = fetal breathing movement; FHR = fetal heart rate; AFV = amniotic fluid volume; AF = amniotic fluid.

†Modification of the criteria for reduced amniotic fluid from <1 cm to <2 cm would seem reasonable.

From Manning, F. (1994). Fetal biophysical assessment by ultrasound. In R. Creasy and R. K. Resnik (Eds.), *Maternal-fetal medicine: Principles and practice* (p. 345). Philadelphia: W.B. Saunders.

- Polyhydramnios
- IUGR
- Postterm pregnancy
- Isoimmunization (moderate to severe)
- Previous fetal demise (unexplained or recurrent risk)
- Multiple gestation (with significant growth discrepancy)

The appropriate time to initiate special studies in women who have had a stillborn baby has not been determined. In practice it is common to begin testing 2 to 3 weeks before the gestational age at which the stillbirth occurred.

Antenatal testing is certainly responsible for a significant number of unnecessary labor inductions. As Cunningham and colleagues state, "How many movements, respirations, or accelerations? In what time period? . . . Abnormal results are seldom reliable, prompting most clinicians to use antenatal testing to forecast fetal wellness rather than illness" (Cunningham et al., 2001, p. 1108).

Despite the shortcomings of antenatal testing, it is widely used and is likely to be the standard of care in most communities.

❖ Conclusion

Midwives must be cognizant not only of routine tests associated with pregnancy, but also of the time frames within which they should be performed. Additional tests may be indicated, and routine tests may need to be repeated. Appendix K identifies normal values for selected laboratory tests.

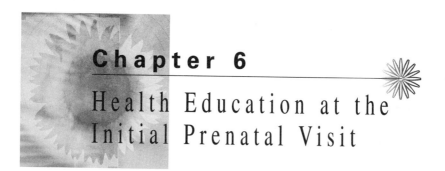

Chapter 6
Health Education at the Initial Prenatal Visit

Health education is an important part of each prenatal visit. Because the initial visit is lengthy, particularly when conducted by a novice practitioner, it is important to choose topics for discussion carefully to avoid "information overload." Many subjects could be discussed, but it is often wise to confine your discussion to questions posed by the client, signs and symptoms that require notification of the health care provider, and information on how to contact someone in the practice to answer questions or resolve an emergency. Put this information in writing and review it with the client. While nutritional counseling is often in order, a diet history can be deferred until a future visit. A brief discussion of weight gain recommendations based on the client's body mass index (BMI) may be appropriate. A written list of what to avoid during the pregnancy and information on behaviors that contribute to a healthy pregnancy can be given to the client to read before the next visit. Ask the client to bring the lists with her so that you can go over them together.

If the client is unfamiliar with midwifery care, an explanation of the role, routines of the practice, and medical backup is in order. In particular, the philosophy of the practice should be explained and might include beliefs about 1) prenatal care, 2) preparation for birth, 3) use of technology, and 4) the general approach to such things as "social" induction and pain relief in labor. When the practice consists of more than one midwife, the "call" schedule should be discussed, and the client should understand the policies of the practice in regard to how midwives are assigned to births.

✳ Danger Signs

A discussion of danger signs should relate to signs and symptoms of potential complications. In the first half of pregnancy, women should know to report vaginal bleeding, cramping, or contractions; fever above 38°C; persistent vomiting; rupture of membranes; and symptoms of a urinary tract infection (UTI).

Danger signs applicable to the first half of pregnancy should also be reported in the second half of pregnancy. Additionally, decreased fetal movement and symptoms of preterm labor (PTL) and preeclampsia should be reported. Although preeclampsia is relatively common and dangerous, clinicians often fail to discuss this disease when talking about the complications of pregnancy. Health care providers need to be diligent about making pregnant women and their families as knowledgeable about preeclamptic symptoms as they are about PTL and fetal movement. Danger signs and symptoms are summarized in Box 6-1. A list of these should be given to clients at the initial prenatal visit.

❖ Communication Between Midwife and Patient

Clients appreciate knowing how to contact the midwife to discuss a minor problem or ask questions that cannot wait until the next visit. They must also know the procedure to follow when an emergency occurs. This information should be provided in writing.

Some practices are experimenting with electronic mail (e-mail) as a means of communicating with clients. E-mail can prevent "telephone tag" and

---

Box 6.1

Danger Signs in Pregnancy

FIRST HALF OF PREGNANCY

- Vaginal bleeding
- Fever ≥101°F
- Rupture of membranes
- Persistent or severe vomiting
- Contractions or cramping
- Abdominal pain or persistent pain anywhere
- Dysuria, urgency, and burning on urination

SECOND HALF OF PREGNANCY

Include previous signs plus the following:
- Decreased fetal movement
- Unusual, generalized edema
- Visual problems: scotoma, blurred vision
- Persistent or severe headaches
- Low-back pain, menstrual-like cramps (either uterine or bowel), increased vaginal discharge, pelvic pressure before term
- General feeling of being unwell
- A rigid abdomen

clarify advice given orally at a prenatal visit. Imagine not having to go to multiple "branches" when calling the clinic or office and then being put on "hold." "Prescription refills, lab results, appointment reminders, insurance questions, and routine follow-up inquiries are well-suited to e-mail. It also provides the patient with a convenient way to report home health measurements, such as blood pressure and glucose determinations" (Kane & Sands, 1998, p. 106).

An additional advantage of e-mail is that links to educational materials can be imbedded in the message. Copies of e-mail communication are easily placed in the client's medical record. Because e-mail communication between client and health care professional is a developing field, guidelines for its use are evolving. Box 6-2 summarizes guidelines for communicating with clients

---

Box 6.2

Guidelines For Communicating With Clients By E-mail

SUMMARY OF COMMUNICATION GUIDELINES

- Establish turnaround time for messages. Do not use e-mail for urgent matters.
- Inform patients about privacy issues. Patients should know:
  Who besides addressee processes messages
    During addressee's usual business hours.
    During addressee's vacation or illness.
  That message is to be included as part of the medical record.
- Establish types of transactions (prescription refill, appointment scheduling, etc.) and sensitivity of subject matter (HIV, mental health, etc.) permitted over e-mail.
- Instruct patients to put category of transaction in subject line of message for filtering: "prescription," "appointment," "medical advice," "billing question."
- Request that patients put their name and patient identification number in the body of the message.
- Configure automatic reply to acknowledge receipt of messages.
- Print all messages, with replies and confirmation of receipt, and place in patient's paper chart.
- Send a new message to inform patient of completion of request.
- Request that patients use autoreply feature to acknowledge reading provider's message.
- Maintain a mailing list of patients, but do not send group mailings where recipients are visible to each other. Use blind copy feature in software.
- Avoid anger, sarcasm, harsh criticism, and libelous references to third parties in messages.

Reprinted with permission from Kane, B., & Sands, D. Z. (1998). Guidelines for the clinical use of electronic mail with patients. *Journal of the American Medical Informatics Association, 5*(1), 106.

by e-mail. Appendix L summarizes medicolegal and administrative guidelines. If you wish to consider using e-mail with clients who identify this method as a communication preference, discuss the issues with administrative personnel. Guidelines are available from the American Medical Informatics Association in Bethesda, Maryland.

❖ What to Avoid

The list of situations to avoid in pregnancy should be reviewed at some point with the mother-to-be. The initial visit is appropriate for this discussion if there is enough time. A handout listing recommendations of situations to avoid (Appendix 6-1) can be given to clients.

❖ Tips for a Healthier Pregnancy

Chapter 2 discusses ways to have a healthy pregnancy and contains a list of activities that can be made into a handout for clients. In addition, suggestions for a client handout summarizing tips for a healthy pregnancy can be found in Appendix 6-2.

Prenatal Vitamins

Clients are often taking a daily prenatal vitamin at the time of their initial prenatal visit. The role of prenatal vitamins in prenatal care is unclear. The Institute of Medicine does not recommend prenatal vitamins for healthy, nonsmoking women whose prepregnancy weight is appropriate for height (National Academy of Sciences, 1992). However, many women will have initiated supplemental vitamins before the initial prenatal visit. It does not seem advantageous for them to stop.

Routine Iron Supplementation

Official recommendations vary on the use of oral iron in pregnancy. Many clinicians feel that the iron in prenatal tablets is a good safeguard against iron deficiency anemia in pregnancy. However, the U.S. Preventive Services Task Force concluded, "There is currently little evidence from published clinical research to suggest that routine iron supplementation during pregnancy is beneficial in improving clinical outcomes for the mother, fetus, or newborn. The evidence is insufficient to recommend for or against routine iron supplementation during pregnancy." (1993, p. 2846). This statement differs from the

Institute of Medicine's recommendation that healthy pregnant women begin iron supplementation with 30 mg of elemental iron at the thirteenth week of pregnancy (National Academy of Sciences, 1992).

Exercise

Women who do not engage in a regular exercise program may wonder if they should start one. Women already engaged in an exercise program may wonder about continuing. While specific health benefits (e.g., shorter labors and fewer operative deliveries) from an exercise routine during pregnancy have not been documented by research studies, the psychological benefits for some women make it important to address the issues. Recent investigations have shown that women who exercised regularly before pregnancy can continue a moderate-intensity exercise for 60 minutes, 5 days a week, throughout the pregnancy (Clapp, 2001). Clients should be told about the benefits of weight-bearing exercise—improving cardiovascular functioning, keeping down weight, decreasing backache, improving sleep, increasing energy, and for some, increasing emotional well-being. The latter can include an increased sense of control and improved self-image (Ezmerli, 2000). Caution clients to avoid exercise with potential for falling and/or trauma to the baby, as well as exercise at high altitudes. (See Chapter 3 for additional information about exercise during pregnancy.)

✱ Frequency of Prenatal Visits

In 1989, the U.S. Public Health Service (PHS) convened an expert panel to evaluate the content and scheduling of prenatal care. The traditional visit schedule—every 4 weeks until 28 weeks, every 2 weeks from 28 to 36 weeks, and weekly thereafter-was designed many years ago in an attempt to identify women with preeclampsia, and it had never been evaluated. Box 6-3 shows the prenatal visit schedule proposed by the expert panel (Public Health Service Expert Panel on Prenatal Care, 1989). Note that the recommendations for nulliparas and multiparas are different.

Clinicians have varying reactions to an alternate schedule. Deleting visits makes health care providers who care for socially or emotionally vulnerable women uneasy because vulnerable women often benefit from more frequent contact. If fewer visits become the norm, these women may be even more at risk. On the other hand, some health care providers like the recommendations because they allow providers to offer fewer visits to women with uncomplicated pregnancies.

Box 6.3

Prenatal Visit Schedule Recommended by the U.S. Public Health Service

NULLIPARAS

First visit: 6–8 weeks
Second visit: Within 4 wks of first
Third visit: 14–16 weeks
Fourth visit: 24–28 weeks
Fifth visit: 32 weeks
Sixth visit: 36 weeks
Seventh visit: 38 weeks
Eighth visit: 40 weeks
Ninth visit: 41 weeks

MULTIPARAS

First visit: 6–8 weeks
Second visit: 14–16 weeks
Third visit: 24–28 weeks
Fourth visit: 32 weeks
Fifth visit: 35 weeks
Sixth visit: 39 weeks
Seventh visit: 41 weeks

From Public Health Service Expert Panel on the Content of Prenatal Care. (1989). *Caring for our future: The content of prenatal care.* (NIH Publication No. 90-3182). Washington, DC: U.S. Department of Health and Human Services.

 HELPFUL HINT

Most pregnant women have not heard about the U.S. Public Health Service recommendations. If they have had a baby before, they may think care is inadequate if you suggest a longer interval between visits than they followed previously. Other women like fewer prenatal visits. Give women with an uncomplicated pregnancy a choice. For example, you could ask a multipara at 30 weeks' gestation, "Would you like to come back in 2 weeks, 3 weeks, or 4 weeks?"

If you are using a fetoscope to detect early fetal heart tones (FHTs) and confirm an estimated date of birth (EDB) established by last menstrual period, be sure that a prenatal visit is scheduled at 20 weeks' gestation, the latest time to initially hear FHTs with a fetoscope. (Note that this may be an exception to both the traditional revisit schedule and the PHS recommendations.) If the client is seen at 18 weeks and FHTs are not heard, schedule the next visit 2 weeks later (20 weeks). If the client is seen at 19 weeks and FHTs are not heard, schedule a visit 1 week later.

❋ Conclusion

The initial prenatal visit is a time to learn about the woman who is seeking prenatal care. It is a time to establish a climate of friendliness and concern that will make her want to return for guidance, encouragement, and monitoring of her well-being and that of her baby.

Appendix 6-1

What to Avoid While You Are Pregnant
(Handout for Clients)

- Cigarettes, which can cause the baby to be born small with weak lungs
- Alcohol, because it can cause mental retardation, learning problems, poor judgment, and aggressive behavior in children
- Recreational or illicit drugs, because they can cause the newborn baby to go through the pain of withdrawal and can later cause personality and learning problems, delayed development, and poor judgment
- Sports in which you are more likely to hit your abdomen if you fall (such as snowboarding, snow skiing, horseback riding, jogging, and waterskiing)
- Biking or hiking vacations at altitudes above 10,000 feet
- Medicines, herbs, and vitamins that might cause harm to the baby (including aspirin; nonsteroidal anti-inflammatory drugs, such as ibuprofen and naproxen; and vitamin A doses above 5000 IU daily). Always check with your midwife before taking over-the-counter medicine, someone else's prescription, extra vitamins, herbs, special teas, and so on.
- Herbicides, pesticides
- Deodorizers and air fresheners
- Kitty litter
- Saunas and warm hot tubs, because they can increase your body temperature to a point where it might be harmful to the baby
- Sick people (to avoid becoming sick and to avoid needing medicine if you become sick)
- Sex in which your partner blows air into your vagina
- A new sex partner who might have a sexually transmitted disease
- Vaginal douching
- More than five caffeine-containing beverages per day

Appendix 6-2

What to Do to Promote a Healthy Pregnancy
(Handout for Clients)

- Use gloves when gardening.
- Open windows to keep fresh air in the house.
- Vacuum carpets frequently.
- Take off your shoes before entering your house to avoid tracking in toxins in dirt. (Merely wiping your feet before entering is not helpful.)
- Wash fruits and vegetables before eating them.
- Cook meat until it is well done.
- Take a prenatal vitamin tablet or iron pill every day.
- Eat a well-balanced diet. Make sure the amount of food eaten is reasonable.
- Get your body moving by walking, swimming, or participating in an exercise program.
- Wash your hands thoroughly after changing diapers and being around young children to minimize the chance of cytomegalovirus infection (ACOG, 2000).
- Shield pelvic structures adequately if x-rays are necessary.
- Wear seat belts.
- Find new homes for pets that might be dangerous to a baby (such as ferrets and some breeds of dogs).
- If there are many pets or animals in your home that strain the boundaries of a clean environment, find new homes for them.
- Keep your prenatal appointments.

PART 3 The Prenatal Revisit

The prenatal revisit is a time to renew the bond established with the client at the initial visit, evaluate the data that has been gathered, and determine whether the pregnancy is progressing normally. Just as important as vigilance for complications are discussions about healthy lifestyle habits and options for labor and birth. Chapter 7 discusses the routine assessments that midwives make at each "return" prenatal visit. Chapter 8 discusses common complications, and Chapter 9 discusses health education at the prenatal revisit.

Chapter 7

Routine Assessments

Preparation for the prenatal revisit should begin with a thorough review of the client's record. As you review the record, have a piece of paper by your side so that you can jot down information that you will need to obtain because it is missing or incomplete. Note all dating information—menstrual history, recent hormonal contraception, date(s) of pregnancy test(s), date of fetal heart tones (FHTs) heard with a Doppler-type instrument, date of FHTs heard with a fetoscope, date of quickening, uterine landmarks, and an ultrasound examination. Then decide whether the data support the estimated date of birth (EDB).

 HELPFUL HINT

Laminate the shorter version of the Chart Review Guide (Appendix N). Carry it in your lab coat pocket, so that it is available for quick reference when seeing clients.

Note findings from the physical examination as well as the results of laboratory tests. Before entering the examining room, refer to Table 7-1, *Important Data and Key Moments in Prenatal Care*, to identify assessments, procedures, and laboratory tests that should be performed at this visit. If you fail to write down the results of your chart review or fail to refer to Table 7-1, it is easy to get involved with the client and forget essential portions of the visit. A Chart Review Guide, such as the one in Appendix M, may be helpful.

 HELPFUL HINT

Laminate Table 7-1, *Important Data and Key Moments in Prenatal Care,* or place it in a plastic sleeve. Keep it where you review charts and refer to it after reviewing the prenatal record to identify tests, procedures, and/or counseling appropriate at this visit.

TABLE 7.1 Important Data and Key Moments in Prenatal Care*

	Objective data	Emotional assessment	Laboratory	Health education
First Visit	Accurate EDB Accurate BP Cervical length and dilatation Size/dates Body mass index	Feelings about this pregnancy, previous birth/losses Stressors Support system Need for referral: mental health counseling, food, shelter, genetic counseling, etc.	Consider: HIV, UDS PPD Sonogram Glucose screen	Danger signs What to avoid Weight gain recommendations Books and classes Provider policies
16 to 19 weeks			Triple screen (15–20 wks) Amniocentesis	Childbirth classes Anticipate body changes and fetal movement Document quickening
20 weeks	Fetal heart tones with fetoscope Weight gain	Stressors Body image	Consider: US for dating and structural anomalies (18–20 wk)	Parenting. Relate own childhood, fears and need for help
24 to 26 weeks	Cervix check if history of preterm labor (PTL) or if first baby	Dreams Fears		Signs/symptoms of PTL Fetal movement parameters
28 weeks	Weight gain Dating review	Body image Stressors	Glucose screen Rh immune globulin	Signs/symptoms of preeclampsia Expectations about labor Family planning
36 weeks	Presentation	Labor fears	Consider repeating: Hematocrit, GBS GC and chlamydia RPR, HIV, HBsAg Schedule version if breech	Preparation for baby Review signs/symptoms of labor and preeclampsia Parenting: own childhood/fears Sibling preparation Birth planning meeting
41 weeks	Presentation		NST, AFI	Offer membrane sweeping Post-dates testing

*In addition to routine assessment (blood pressure, weight, urine evaluation, fetal heart rate, and fundal height).

After reviewing the prenatal record, note any data obtained today by an assistant. This information commonly includes maternal weight and evaluation of urine for protein and glucose. Some clinics or offices also screen for the presence of leukocyte esterase and/or nitrites in the urine specimen. In many practices, a nurse or assistant also measures blood pressure (BP).

After a bit of social "chitchat" with the client, ask about her questions and concerns. Discuss any pertinent information, such as laboratory results, obtained since the last visit. Determine if the client has followed through on any previous plans—such as signing up for the Women, Infants, and Children (WIC) Program or childbirth classes. Follow up on complaints identified at the last visit. If a weight gain goal has not been set in conjunction with the client, do it at this visit and record it next to the body mass index (BMI) information. Finally, ask any questions you jotted down during your review of the client's record.

After evaluating this data, ask the Healthy Pregnancy Questions in Box 7-1 to identify the common discomforts of pregnancy, screen for complications, and evaluate health habits. Measure fundal height, count the fetal heart rate, and determine presentation (after 34 weeks' gestation). Midwives in some settings use a "Revisit Questionnaire" (Appendix N) that incorporates the Healthy Pregnancy Questions. Clients complete the questionnaire while waiting to be seen.

❋ Objective Data

Evaluation of Maternal Weight

Weight gain comparisons from one prenatal visit to another alert the clinician to a variety of problems. BMI, as discussed in Chapter 4, should be used to evaluate weight gain.

Weight Loss

Weight loss in early pregnancy is usually associated with "morning sickness" or hyperemesis gravidarum. Weight loss later in pregnancy may be due lack of appetite, flu syndrome, illness, alcohol or drug use, insufficient resources to buy or find food, an eating disorder, poor fetal growth, or to fetal death.

Low Weight Gain

Women with low pregnancy weight gain have been found to have an increased risk for preterm delivery. In one study, "The risk of preterm delivery was 5.8% among women who had an average BMI before pregnancy and who had an average weight gain during pregnancy. Compared with that group, the risk of

Box 7.1

The Healthy Pregnancy Questions

AT EACH VISIT

At each visit, ask about the following conditions:
1. Headaches
2. Scotoma or blurred vision
3. Nausea and/or vomiting
4. Pain: chest, abdomen, back, or legs
5. Contractions, cramping, or pelvic pressure
6. Burning with urination, urgency, dysuria, or urinary retention
7. Vaginal bleeding
8. Vaginal discharge
9. Skin changes
10. Fever or exposure to infectious disease
11. Edema
12. Numbness or tingling of the hands or wrists
13. Genital lesions, sores, or growths
14. Trauma
15. Fetal movement
16. Over-the-counter or prescribed medications, as well as herbal remedies
17. Emotional well-being, relationships, stress, or abuse

PERIODICALLY

Periodically ask about the following conditions:
1. Appetite, heartburn, constipation, leg cramps, breast tenderness, fatigue, faintness, hemorrhoids, or varicosities
2. Cravings (to eat or to smell)
3. Concerns about sexual activity, desire, or comfort
4. Sleep or dreams
5. Pets

AS INDICATED BY HISTORY

Ask about the following conditions as indicated by the client's history:
1. Use of cigarettes
2. Alcoholic beverages and illicit or recreational drugs

preterm delivery was markedly higher for two groups: women with low prepregnancy BMI and low weight gain (14.0% preterm risk), and women with average prepregnancy BMI and low weight gain (19.6%). Preterm risk was also higher among women with a high prepregnancy BMI and low or average weight gain (9.3% and 9.0%, respectively). Lower risk (2.4%) was noted for women with a high prepregnancy BMI and high weight gain" (Schieve et al., 2000, p. 197).

In an analysis of data from 5931 births occurring at gestational ages ranging from 28 to 43 weeks, these same researchers found "a low rate of pregnancy weight gain between 14 and 28 weeks' gestation increased the risk of subsequent preterm delivery. The magnitude of that risk varied according to prepregnancy BMI. There were high risks for underweight and average-weight women with low weight gain, whereas a moderate increase in risk (OR 1.6) was suggested for overweight or obese women with low weight gain. Although low BMI alone has been implicated as a risk factor for preterm delivery in previous studies, we found that underweight women were at increased risk only if they failed to gain weight at an adequate rate" (Schieve et al., 2000, p. 198).

A helpful guideline for following weight gain in women with a normal BMI is to aim for a gain of at least 10 pounds by 20 weeks' gestation in women who have a low or average BMI. When this gain fails to occur, a thoughtful assessment of fetal growth and a diet assessment should be conducted.

Excessive Weight Gain

Excessive weight gain is defined as a total weight gain greater than 50 pounds or a weekly gain in the last trimester of more than 2 pounds per week. Possible causes of the latter include edema, excessive caloric intake, and preeclampsia. Excessive weight gain associated with preeclampsia often involves increases of 4 or more pounds in 1 week. A meeting with a nutritionist or dietitian can be helpful when one is available. When not available, a diet history can help determine the cause of the increase.

When weight gain is due to excess calories, suggest substituting healthy foods for poor food choices. Possibilities include substituting fresh fruit for fruit juice and baking or broiling foods instead of frying them. Common culprits for excessive weight gain in pregnancy from calories are fruit juice, soda, candy, whole-fat dairy products, and not enough activity.

Pregnant women often think that milk should be an essential component of their diet. In truth, milk should be thought of as a vehicle for obtaining protein and calcium. Skim and 1-percent milk provide about the same amounts of calcium and protein, but they are much lower in fat and calories than 2-percent and whole milk. An 8-ounce glass of 2% milk gets about 35% of total calories from fat, and 1% milk gets 22% of its 100 calories from fat. Skim milk gets only 4% of its total calories from fat. Recognize that it takes a long time for many people to learn to enjoy milk with a lesser fat content. The shift to a lesser fat-containing product should occur one step at a time and often is accomplished only after many months or even years.

Reagent Strip Testing

Random urine samples should be tested for the presence of protein and glucose at each visit. Evaluation for leukocyte esterase and nitrites is also useful.

Proteinuria

Proteinuria may be a sign of preeclampsia and/or a urinary tract infection (UTI). When reagent strip testing demonstrates proteinuria in a random urine sample, repeat the test with a clean-catch specimen as blood or vaginal bacteria may be the source of a positive result. Do not ask the client to drink water so that she can void sooner, as this will dilute the specimen and can give a false-negative result. Obese women who find it hard to reach their vulva for appropriate cleaning can gently insert part of a vaginal tampon into the vagina before cleansing.

While trace amounts of protein in a urine specimen are often considered insignificant, one study found that, "Although proteinuria of ≥5 gm per day is virtually excluded by the presence of negative or trace protein on dipstick, negative or trace values were found in 81 of 243 pregnancies with mild proteinuria (sensitivity of dipstick ≥1+ equals 67%) and should not be used to rule out significant proteinuria." (Meyer, Mercer, Friedman, & Sibai, 1994, p. 139).

When the clean-catch urine specimen tests positive, inquire about symptoms of both a UTI and preeclampsia. Look for a BP elevation, rapid weight gain, and edema. Consider kidney disease if proteinuria is the only finding. A 24-hour urine sample for protein is appropriate for proteinuria (clean-catch specimens) with or without an elevated BP, unless the cause of the proteinuria can be attributed to a UTI.

Glucosuria

The same reagent strip used to test urine for protein usually contains a second reagent that tests for glucose. A clean-catch specimen of urine is not required for accurate results. Be careful about assuming that glucosuria in a pregnant woman can be attributed to a recent diet high in sugar. Because glucosuria in the first two trimesters is associated with a higher incidence of gestational diabetes, request a 1-hour glucose screen whenever glucosuria is identified in the first 26 weeks of pregnancy. Third-trimester glucosuria found after a normal 1-hour glucose screen at 24 to 28 weeks' gestation has not been found to be significant, and no additional testing is indicated (Gribble, Meier, & Berg, 1995).

Leukocyte Esterase and Nitrites

Use a reagent strip that tests for leukocyte esterase and nitrites to test for a UTI, as bacteria in the urine may cause proteinuria. See Chapter 5 for a discussion of a positive result.

HELPFUL HINT

Teach pregnant women to test their own urine with the reagent test strip and have them note the results in their record.

Blood Pressure

Diastolic blood pressure decreases a maximum of 10 mm Hg at 28 weeks, after which it rises toward prepregnant levels by term (Monga, 1999). An elevated BP during pregnancy is one with a systolic reading at or greater than 140 mm Hg or a diastolic reading at or greater than 90 mm Hg. For many years, an increase in BP of 30 mm Hg systolic or 15 mm Hg diastolic from early values was also considered diagnostic if proteinuria and/or edema were also present. Current guidelines from the American College of Obstetricians and Gynecologists (ACOG) state, "This concept is no longer considered valid" (1996a, p.2). (See Chapter 8 for a discussion of elevated blood pressure in pregnancy.)

Fetal Heart Tones

The normal fetal heart rate ranges between 120 and 160 beats per minute (bpm). Listen for at least 30 seconds to increase your chances of detecting any slowing of the heart rate. Accelerations and short bursts of tachycardia are often associated with fetal activity and are normal. An acceleration returning to baseline can be mistaken for a deceleration. Listen to the fetal heart for at least a full minute in these situations.

A fetal heart rate below 100 bpm is extremely rare. It may indicate a congenital heart block and requires medical consultation. Rates between 100 and 110 bpm also require consultation. Persistent rates above 160 bpm, as can occur in fetal hydrops, are always serious and require medical consultation. Irregular fetal heart rates are almost always benign but do require consultation.

Finding FHTs in the first half of pregnancy is discussed in Chapter 4. FHTs are easier to find after 26 weeks' gestation (Figure 7-1). When FHTs are found in one of the upper quadrants, the baby may be in a breech presentation.

Some clinicians determine fetal position before listening to FHTs, knowing that it is easiest to hear them through the fetal back. This technique works well except that babies in utero frequently assume posterior positions, making the back unavailable. Clinicians are notoriously wrong in identifying fetal position from abdominal palpation.

Fundal Height

Fundal height (described in Chapter 4) is used in early pregnancy to identify a multiple gestation or an error in dating and in later pregnancy to determine fetal growth. Remember that, while these measurements are useful, they are imprecise.

Guidelines for Growth

Of the many studies that have tried to determine parameters for distinguishing between normal and abnormal growth, the only conclusion that can be drawn

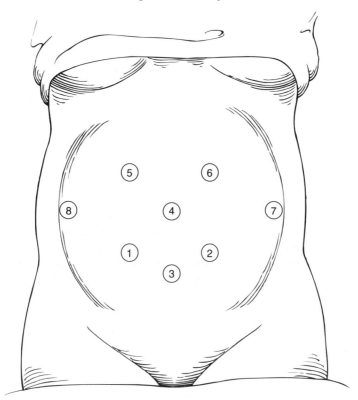

FIGURE 7.1 Finding fetal heart tones after the 26th week of pregnancy.
1 and 2: Listen first in the middle of either of the lower quadrants of the abdomen.
3. If heart tones are not found, listen in the middle of an imaginary line drawn from the umbilicus to the middle of the top of the pubic hair.
4. If not found, listen directly over the umbilicus.
5 and 6. If not yet found, listen in the middle of either of the upper quadrants of the abdomen.
7 and 8. If still not found, listen about 4 inches away from the umbilicus toward the flank.

is that the fundal height measurement is inexact. And of the many studies that have looked at fundal height determinations throughout pregnancy, none agree on the gestational ages at which the measurement is most useful.

This is not to say that the measurement should be discarded. Rather it should be a starting point for evaluating fetal growth. Clinicians in a given practice setting should agree on guidelines for requesting an ultrasound to evaluate fetal growth when the fundal height measurement in centimeters is outside of the guidelines. One guideline is this: Between 26 and 36 weeks' gestation, the fundal height measurement in centimeters should equal the current weeks of gestation, plus or minus 2 cm. For example, if a woman is 28 weeks pregnant, the fundal height should measure between 26 cm and 30 cm.

Accurate measurement of fundal height depends on identifying the top of the symphysis and the top of the uterine fundus. Start at the top of the symphysis or at the top of the fundus; do whatever is comfortable for you. Feel *carefully* for the top of the symphysis, as it can be tender. Its location varies. Differences in measurements between practitioners usually come from differences in identification of the top of the fundus. Ideally, the same examiner will measure the fundal height at each visit.

 HELPFUL HINT

To measure the fundus in centimeters, think of the uterus as a lightbulb. You want your measurement to extend to that part of the lightbulb where the wattage and brand name would be printed. This means that you will have to go over the top of the uterus and push down a bit.

When there is a discrepancy between fundal height and gestational age, the first action should be to carefully review dating parameters. If the due date is correct, examine all the data available. Estimate the baby's weight. While these estimates are particularly inaccurate when precision is most important (i.e., when a baby is thought to be larger or smaller than expected for the gestational age), the estimate of fetal weight may be useful when added to other available information.

 HELPFUL HINT

Always turn the measuring tape so that you cannot see the centimeter markings. After measuring, turn the tape over, and read the corresponding centimeter marking. This way you won't be tempted to make the centimeters agree with the gestational age.

Request an ultrasound for fetal growth when there is a 4-cm discrepancy between fundal height and gestational age prior to 36 weeks' gestation. Some clinicians feel that a sonogram is appropriate when a 3-cm discrepancy exists. Occasionally, a 2-cm discrepancy requires follow-up, as when slower growth is accompanied by poor maternal weight gain or weight loss.

Size Less Than Dates

When the fundal height is 3 to 4 cm less than the gestational age in weeks, the uterus is said to be "small for dates" (not small for gestational age [SGA]). Possible explanations include a dating error, intrauterine growth restriction (IUGR), transverse presentation, fetal infection, a chromosomal or genetic abnormality, a constitutionally small but healthy baby, descent of the presenting part into the pelvis, oligohydramnios (a small amount of amniotic fluid), or fetal death. Oligohydramnios, particularly during the second trimester, is associated with increased perinatal morbidity and mortality. It may be caused by rupture of membranes, maternal dehydration, or lack of fetal urine as a result of fetal renal agenesis or urinary tract obstruction. Intrauterine growth restriction is often categorized as symmetric or asymmetric. Symmetric growth restriction is thought to be caused by early insults such as infection, exposure to some drugs, chromosomal abnormalities, and congenital malformations. Asymmetric growth restriction is thought to be caused primarily by the hypertensive disorders of pregnancy (Creasy & Resnik, 1999). These causes are listed in Boxes 7-2A and 7-2B.

Size Greater Than Dates

When the fundal height is 3 to 4 cm or more than the gestational age in weeks in the second and third trimesters, the uterus is said to be "large for dates" (not LGA). Possible explanations include a dating error, a baby that is macrosomic because of maternal diabetes, a multiple gestation, a constitutionally large baby, and polyhydramnios (excess amniotic fluid).

After 36 weeks' gestation, a fundal height that continues to increase by 1 cm each week beyond 36 weeks is reassuring (unless, of course, it is way too high). If the fundal height does *not* increase after 36 weeks, always consider the possibility of fetal growth restriction. Another possibility is descent of the presenting part into the pelvis. An abdominal or vaginal examination to determine descent may confirm this possibility.

A third possibility is that the mother-to-be is carrying her baby in a way that does not allow accurate evaluation by the fundal height measurement. If the client has had a baby before, ask her how much she thinks her baby

---

Box 7.2A

Causes of Symmetric IUGR

Genetic
  Low growth potential
  Genetic abnormalities
Congenital abnormalities
  Congenital heart disease
  Central nervous system
  Gastrointestinal
  Musculoskeletal
Intrauterine infection
  Rubella
  Toxoplasmosis
  Cytomegalovirus
Severe malnutrition
  Famine
  Gastric bypass surgery

Maternal habits
  Tobacco
  Drug addiction
  Alcohol
Maternal medications
  Coumadin
  Steroids
Maternal hypoxic disease
  Severe asthma
  Cyanotic congenital heart disease
  High altitudes
  Severe anemia

From Burlbaw, J. (1996). Intrauterine growth restriction. *OB-GYN Ultrasound Today, 3*(1), 30.

---

weighs. Mothers are remarkably good at knowing whether the baby they are carrying is smaller, about the same as, or larger than previous babies. Ask also if the fundal height measurement followed a similar pattern previously.

Macrosomia is variously defined as a baby weighing more than 4000 or 4500 grams. Evaluate the client for risk factors for macrosomia (previous large baby, gestational diabetes, diabetes mellitus, obesity, prolonged gestation). Estimate the weight of the baby by abdominal palpation and request an ultra-

---

Box 7.2B

Causes of Asymmetric IUGR

Maternal vascular disease
  Toxemia
  Chronic hypertension
  Advanced stage diabetes
Multiple gestation
  Discordant twins

Transfusion syndrome
Placental malformation
  Abnormal insertion
  Hemangioma
  Multiple infarcts

From Burlbaw, J. (1996). Intrauterine growth restriction. *OB-GYN Ultrasound Today, 3*(1), 32.

sound for fetal size. At term, ultrasound determinations of fetal weight are accurate to $+/-15\%$.

Management of births involving macrosomia varies from scheduled cesarean section to induction at 38 to 40 weeks to awaiting spontaneous labor. If the person providing prenatal care will not be the birth attendant, the prenatal care provider should alert the birth attendant when macrosomia is suspected. Factors that may influence the decision of how to manage care include 1) the dimensions of the maternal pelvis, 2) the size of previous infants delivered vaginally without delivery-related problems, 3) previous cesarean delivery for excessive fetal size, or 4) failure to progress in second stage (Nahum, 2000). Studies of induction for macrosomia have not conclusively demonstrated a benefit.

HELPFUL HINT

When discussing fetal size with mothers, avoid use of the word "big" whenever you can. Is there any woman who can respond enthusiastically to the thought of a big baby coming through her vagina? If a pregnant woman has a baby that you think is big and the client asks you how much you think the baby weighs, you can recall how inaccurate estimates of fetal weight can be when babies are either small or large. Give this information to the client, and ask her how much she thinks the baby weighs.

Fundal height measurements may be difficult to determine when the client is obese. If you are unable to assess fetal growth in an obese woman, order ultrasound examinations at 28 to 30 weeks' gestation and at 34 to 36 weeks' gestation to verify that growth is appropriate.

HELPFUL HINT

When using disposable measuring tapes to measure the height of the fundus, note the fundal height on the tape at each visit. Keep the tape in the client's record, and give the tape to the new mother at the time of delivery or when she comes for her postpartum examination. Then it can be added to her mementos of the pregnancy.

Presentation

At 34 weeks' gestation and beyond, the abdominal examination should include identification of the presentation (the part of the fetus that lies over the pelvic inlet). Presentation may be cephalic, breech, face, or shoulder (Figure 7-2). (Use of the term "vertex presentation" should be saved for the intrapartal period when both the anterior and posterior fontanelles can be palpated on vaginal examination, as technically speaking, the vertex is the area between the fontanelles.) Any presentation other than cephalic at delivery increases the risk for poor perinatal outcome.

Use Leopold maneuvers to determine presentation. Grasp the uterine fundus between the thumb and middle finger of one hand. When something soft is felt, it is usually the fetal buttocks; when something is round, firm, and easily moved, it is usually the fetal head. Next feel the maternal pelvis (Figure 7-3). Then feel on the sides of the maternal abdomen for the baby's back and "small parts." Some clinicians may feel certain that they feel the baby's head in the pelvis and omit examining the fundus. The baby's buttocks can feel quite firm at times and can easily trick you into thinking you have found the head!

 HELPFUL HINT

Babies are often in a posterior position prenatally. This has nothing to do with the position the baby will decide to use during labor, as most babies in a cephalic presentation enter the pelvis in a transverse position regardless of the position they favored earlier in pregnancy. (The widest diameter of the pelvic inlet is the transverse diameter.) Because women who attend childbirth classes are often taught that posterior labors are long and difficult, hearing that her baby is in a posterior position late in pregnancy can cause the mother unnecessary worry. If a mother asks about the position of her baby and you think it is posterior, respond by saying, "I think it's posterior now, but we don't know what position the baby will choose for labor."

When uncertain of fetal presentation late in pregnancy, a vaginal examination may help. If suture lines on the fetal head can be felt with the examining fingers, the presentation is cephalic. Be careful, however, because sometimes the crease in the baby's buttocks can be mistaken for a suture line. Feeling a fontanelle makes you certain that the baby's head is "down." When-

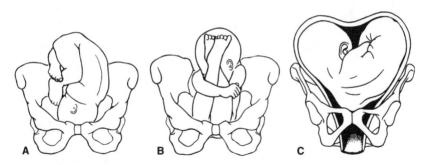

FIGURE 7.2 The fetus in various presentations. (**A**) Vertex. (**B**) Frank breech. (**C**) Transverse lie.

ever you are uncertain about presentation and the gestation is 36 weeks or more, request an ultrasound examination to avoid the client going into labor with the baby in a breech presentation.

If the presentation is not cephalic at 36 weeks' and beyond, refer the client to a clinician experienced in external cephalic version, the procedure used to try to turn the baby so that the presentation is cephalic. This procedure should be done only with ultrasound monitoring of the fetal heart rate and availability of a cesarean operation, as fetal distress could occur. A short cord or a tight

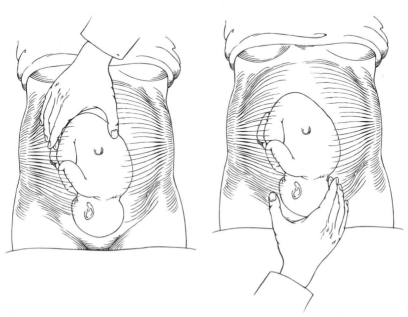

FIGURE 7.3 Procedure for determining fetal presentation.

nuchal cord may cause placental abruptions. Performing external version under epidural anesthesia has been used in some instances to increase the success rate (Mancuso, Yancey, Murphy, & Markenson, 2000). You might first recommend moxibustion or acupuncture, because these procedures have been helpful in "turning" babies.

 HELPFUL HINT

Women usually enjoy hearing your explanation of how the baby is positioned. Offer to draw a picture of the baby on your client's abdomen if she is at or greater than 32 weeks (or earlier if you are artistically inclined). While those of us who do not consider ourselves artists may panic, anyone can do a drawing that a pregnant mother will like. If you follow the lines shown in Appendix O, you cannot go wrong.

You may wish to keep the drawings from Appendix O taped to a wall in the examining room to use as a guide. Practice on a piece of paper first. Follow the numbers, unless you can do better on your own. Draw with a permanent marker (a "Sharpie" laundry marker works well and dries in a few seconds). As you become proficient, try drawing five fingers and toes, an ear, and hair. The drawing will last about 3 days. Most women will be delighted with your artwork. For many, this visual image helps to make the baby real, and some women have reported that the drawing facilitated attachment to the baby. Some women take a picture of their bellies and put the pictures in a baby book.

Of course, some women will not want you to draw on their abdomens, and their wishes should be respected. However, most women appreciate at least one drawing, and some want it done at each visit.

❊ The Healthy Pregnancy Questions

The Healthy Pregnancy Questions presented in the following sections and Box 7-1 can identify potential complications, as well as the common discomforts of pregnancy. Some questions should be asked at each prenatal visit, and some should be asked periodically. Some questions depend on the client's history to determine whether they should be asked and at what intervals. The common discomforts of pregnancy are frequently trivialized because they are "normal" happenings during pregnancy, yet they can cause great distress and can disrupt family life. Unfortunately, few of the commonly advised measures have been studied to determine their effectiveness.

 HELPFUL HINT

Laminate the Healthy Pregnancy Questions presented in Box 7-1. You will find it easier to refer to a readily available list than to attempt to recall each question. Ask the questions in groups to save time. You might use this approach: "I am going to ask you that long list of questions I asked you at your last visit. Since you were here last, have you had any headaches, spots before your eyes, nausea, or vomiting?" Then proceed with the rest of the questions.

Questions to Ask at Each Visit

Headaches

Most headaches during pregnancy are benign and respond to rest or acetaminophen. (Neither aspirin nor ibuprofen are recommended during pregnancy. Aspirin's effect on platelets can cause bleeding problems. Ibuprofen may cause premature closure of the ductus arteriosus in the fetus and persistent pulmonary hypertension in the newborn.) Box 7-3 lists questions that may help distinguish among the more common headaches—tension, migraine, cluster, sinus, and benign vascular headache of pregnancy—and a headache requiring immediate evaluation.

While many women who have experienced migraine headaches in the past find that they occur less frequently when they are pregnant, some women experience their first migraine headache at this time. The clinical issue with migraines is how to treat them. The safest approach is to avoid "triggers" and treat with acetaminophen. However, acetaminophen may not relieve the pain, and consultation with a physician may be necessary.

A very small number of pregnant women with headaches and a normal physical examination will have intracranial pathology. Only if the headache is severe, constant, unusual, or associated with neurologic signs (stiff neck and/or neurologic deficits) is there likely to be a problem—subarachnoid and other brain hemorrhages, hematomas, cerebral aneurysm, or tumors.

Remember to think of the possibility of preeclampsia when pregnant women complain of a headache. The headache of preeclampsia is usually severe, unremitting, and unresponsive to acetaminophen. It requires immediate evaluation.

Box 7.3

Questions to Ask Pregnant Women About Headaches

1. Is this a new type of headache?
2. Did it begin precipitously?
3. How often do the headaches occur?
4. How long do they last?
5. Have they changed significantly?
6. Does anything trigger them, such as lights, sounds, or smells?
7. Do they come on suddenly or gradually?
8. What do they feel like?
9. Where is the pain?
10. Does anything make them worse?
11. Do you have any other symptoms when they occur, such as neck pain, vomiting, fever, or change in the level of consciousness?
12. Does anything happen right before you get them?
13. What do you do to relieve the pain? Does it work?
14. What medicines have you taken?
15. Do the headaches interfere with any of your activities?
16. Do you have a history of migraines?
17. What do you think causes them?

Scotoma and Blurred Vision

Visual changes, particularly spots or flashing lights in front of the eyes or blurred vision, can also be signs of preeclampsia or even a brain tumor. These "sparkly" spots always must be taken seriously. They should not be confused with "floaters."

Nausea and/or Vomiting

Between 50% and 80% of pregnant women experience nausea or vomiting (morning sickness) in early pregnancy. Why this phenomenon exists is unknown. Attempts to attribute a psychological cause, such as wanting to get rid of the baby, are not valid. While morning sickness is the usual cause of nausea and vomiting, other causes include hyperemesis gravidarum, multiple gestation, molar pregnancy, hepatitis, gallbladder disease, gastroenteritis, pyelonephritis, migraine, flu syndrome, food poisoning, appendicitis, bowel obstruction, increased intracranial pressure, malaria, migraines, medication effect or toxicity, drug or alcohol effect, pancreatitis, and intestinal parasites. Box 7-4 summarizes the differential diagnosis for vomiting in pregnancy.

Recent research involving 160 pregnant women who kept diaries of the frequency, duration, and severity of nausea and vomiting found that traditional

---

Box 7.4

Differential Diagnosis for Vomiting During Pregnancy

1. Appendicitis
2. Bowel obstruction
3. Bulimia
4. Drug or alcohol effect
5. Flu syndrome
6. Food poisoning
7. Gallbladder disease
8. Gastroenteritis
9. Gestational trophoblastic disease
10. Hepatitis
11. Hyperemesis gravidarum
12. Hyperthyroid
13. Increased intracranial pressure
14. Intestinal parasites
15. Malaria
16. Medication effect or toxicity
17. Migraines
18. Multifetal pregnancy
19. Pancreatitis
20. Pyelonephritis

---

notions of "morning sickness" should be revised. Findings of the study included the following:

- Nausea was reported as early as the first week of conception.
- The mean gestational age for the onset of nausea was 5.7 weeks.
- Vomiting began as early as the 4th gestational week.
- While 90% of women who experienced nausea in pregnancy developed it by the 8th week of gestation, a few women noted the onset during or after the 10th week.
- Peak severity occurred at 11 and 13 weeks.
- Fifty percent of women were through with nausea by 14 weeks, but it took until the 22nd week for the nausea to disappear in 90%.
- Eighty percent experienced nausea all day long.
- Women who reported nausea in a previous pregnancy were more likely to experience nausea and vomiting in the following pregnancy.
- Symptom relief was most likely to occur when ingesting dry foods and carbonated beverages, spending time outside in fresh air, or lying down (Lacroix, Eason, & Melzack, 2000).

Supportive measures that are often recommended to treat morning sickness, alone or in conjunction with antiemetic medication, include lying down, changing diet, drinking teas, and using acupressure, acupuncture, or hypnosis. Dietary recommendations are numerous and include eating small amounts of food frequently, eating potato chips and dry crackers, restricting fat, drinking lemonade and eating potato chips, drinking various teas, avoiding spicy foods, taking vitamin B_6, and delaying vitamin/iron therapy. A review of 20 studies in the Cochrane Pregnancy and Childbirth Group Trials Register and the

Cochrane Controlled Trials Register concluded that antiemetic medication appears to reduce the incidence of nausea in early pregnancy, and pyridoxine (vitamin B_6) may decrease the severity of nausea. Studies using acupressure show equivocal results (Green, 2000). Hypnosis can be helpful (Simon & Schwartz, 1999). Gingerroot has not been shown to be effective.

Prenatal vitamins and iron may cause or worsen morning sickness and should be eliminated temporarily if either is identified as a contributing factor. Folic acid should be continued through the 7th gestational week. Some practitioners attempt to replicate the ingredients in Bendectin, a drug used in the past to treat morning sickness. It was very effective but was removed from the market because of litigation expenses from claims that the drug was teratogenic. Bendectin contained 10 mg of doxylamine succinate and 10 mg of pyridoxine (vitamin B_6). Midwives often recommend that clients take vitamin B_6 (25 to 50 mg) and half of a doxylamine (Unisom) tablet at night. Doxylamine is a nonprescription hypnotic drug.

Antiemetics can be useful for controlling morning sickness that is somewhat incapacitating. Promethazine (Phenergan), 12.5 to 25.0 mg every 6 hours rectally or orally, and prochlorperazine (Compazine), 5 to 10 mg orally every 6 hours or 25 mg rectally twice a day, are commonly prescribed for pregnant women with morning sickness. These medications are summarized in Box 7-5. While considered safe and effective, prochlorperazine can precipitate adverse reactions in certain individuals. One side effect is severe muscle spasm, requiring 10 to 100 mg of IV or IM diphenhydramine (Benadryl), followed by oral diphenhydramine for 72 hours to relieve the spasm (Given, 2000).

Box 7.5

Drugs Used to Treat Morning Sickness

1. Pyridoxine (Vitamin B_6): 10 to 25 mg three to four times a day
2. Pyridoxine (as above) + Doxylamine (the active ingredient in Unisom Sleep tabs): 12.5 mg three to four times a day (use one half of a scored 25 mg tablet)
3. Diphenhydramine (Benadryl): 25 mg three or four times a day
4. Promethazine (Phenergan): 12.5 to 25.0 mg orally or rectally every 4 hours
5. Prochlorperazine (Compazine): 5 to 10 mg orally every 3 to 4 hours or 25 mg rectally twice a day
6. Metoclopramide (Reglan): 10 mg orally 4 times daily 30 minutes before meals and at bedtime
7. Ondasetron (Zofran): 8 mg orally every 12 hours

Pressure bands are also suggested to treat morning sickness, although their effectiveness is not well documented. These stretch bracelets, originally marketed for tourists who go deep-sea fishing, are placed over an acupressure point above the wrist. They can be bought at pharmacies, maternity stores, and some AAA travel stores. ReliefBand is a battery-powered, watchlike wristband with five patient-controlled power settings, which uses electric impulses to prevent nausea. The mechanism of action is unknown. ReliefBand is relatively expensive and currently available only by prescription.

Chest, Abdominal, Back, or Leg Pain

Various aches and pains occur throughout the body during pregnancy. Occasionally, pain may signal a serious problem. Chest pain, for example, may be indicative of a pulmonary embolus, heart attack, or preeclampsia. During pregnancy, abdominal pain may be caused by an aneurysm, appendicitis, bowel obstruction, cholecystitis, colitis, constipation, Crohn disease, cystitis, diverticulitis, gastritis, gastroenteritis, hepatitis, hernia, inflammatory bowel disease (including ulcerative colitis), neoplasm, ovarian cyst or torsion, pancreatitis, peritonitis, pyelonephritis, renal colic, splenic rupture, trauma, or an ulcer. Obstetric causes include preeclampsia, premature labor, abruption, degenerating myoma, ectopic pregnancy, round ligament pain, or a ruptured corpus luteum cyst.

Table 7-2 summarizes the differential diagnosis for abdominal pain in pregnancy based on location of the pain. Traditional belief has been that right upper quadrant (RUQ) rather than right lower quadrant (RLQ) pain is the common finding when appendicitis occurs in the last trimester of pregnancy. However, a recent study has found RUQ pain to be rare. Although subjects in the study reported pain in the left lower quadrant, mid-abdomen, epigastric region, and a combination of locations, RLQ pain remained the most common symptom of appendicitis in all trimesters (Mourad, Elliott, Erickson, & Lisboa, 2000). When evaluating abdominal pain, use the mnemonic OLDCART (onset, location, duration, characteristics, associated symptoms, relieving factors, timing/treatments tried), to remember questions to ask about the pain. Also ask about worsening symptoms, and precipitating factors (such as fatty food ingestion or position change).

Nephrolithiasis often begins as a severe, dull pain in the flank that radiates down to the lower quadrant of the abdomen. Nausea and dysuria (in about one third of cases) and bacteriuria and hematuria (in about 75% of cases) have been noted (Butler, Cox, Eberts, & Cunningham, 2000). Ultrasound remains the initial tool for diagnosis, despite the fact that 40% of renal calculi can be missed with this method. Treatment includes analgesia, intravenous hydration, and antimicrobial therapy for concomitant infection. When ultrasound examination fails to find renal calculi, persistent symptoms should lead to single-shot intravenous pyelography. With an ultrasound diagnosis of calculi, per-

TABLE 7.2 Differential Diagnosis for Abdominal Pain in Pregnancy

Obstetric Possibilities: Spontaneous abortion (SAB), threatened abortion (AB), ectopic pregnancy, degenerating myoma, round ligament pain, abruption, preeclampsia/HELLP, ruptured corpus luteum cyst

Other Possibilities: aneurysm, appendicitis, bowel obstruction, cholecystitis, colitis, constipation, Crohn disease, cystitis, diverticulitis, gastritis, gastroenteritis, hepatitis, hernia, inflammatory bowel disease (including ulcerative colitis), neoplasm, ovarian cyst/torsion, pancreatitis, peritonitis, pyelonephritis, renal colic, splenic rupture, trauma, ulcer

Data to gather: OLDCART (onset, location, duration, characteristics, associated symptoms, relieving factors, timing/treatments tried), worsening symptoms, precipitating factors (e.g., fatty food or position change)

Obstetric causes First trimester	Second trimester	Third trimester
Ectopic pregnancy	PTL	Labor
SAB/threatened AB	Abruption	Abruption
Degenerating fibroid	Fibroid	Fibroid
Ruptured corpus luteum cyst	Round ligament pain	Round ligament pain
	Preeclampsia/HELLP	Preeclampsia/HELLP

Other causes based on location Location	Cause
Diffuse	Gastroenteritis
	Constipation
	Trauma
	Peritonitis
	Intestinal obstruction
	Abruption
	Dissecting aortic aneurysm
	Sickle cell crisis
Periumbilical	Gastroenteritis
Epigastric	Liver swelling/rupture (preeclampsia)
	Esophagitis
	Pancreatitis
	Cancer (pancreatic/gastric)

table continues on page 206

TABLE 7.2 Differential Diagnosis for Abdominal Pain
in Pregnancy continued

Location	Cause
RUQ	Pyelonephritis (R)
	Pneumonia
	Pancreatitis
	Kidney stone
	Cholecystitis
	Hepatitis
	Appendicitis
	Peptic ulcer
LUQ	Pyelonephritis (L)
	Pneumonia
	Pancreatitis
	Kidney stone
	Gastritis
	Splenic abscess/rupture
	Diverticulitis
	Aneurysm
	Constipation
RLQ	SAB/threatened AB
	Appendicitis
	Intestinal obstruction
	Ectopic pregnancy
	Ovarian cyst
	Twisted ovary
	Diverticulitis
	Kidney stone
	Degenerating fibroid
	Round ligament pain
	UTI (cystitis)
	Inguinal hernia
LLQ	SAB/threatened AB
	Appendicitis
	Intestinal obstruction
	Ectopic pregnancy
	Ovarian cyst

TABLE 7.2 Differential Diagnosis for Abdominal Pain
in Pregnancy continued

Location	Cause
	Twisted ovary
	Diverticulitis
	Kidney stone
	Degenerating fibroid
	Round ligament pain
	UTI (cystitis)

sistent symptoms suggest renal obstruction, which may occur in 25% to 50% of symptomatic pregnant women with kidney stones (Butler, Cox, Eberts, & Cunningham, 2000).

A "degenerating" fibroid may cause severe abdominal pain. It occurs most often between the twelfth and eighteenth week of pregnancy and can be accompanied by vomiting. The condition is self-limiting. Analgesia is required.

Leg pain may be caused by thrombophlebitis, sciatica, or displacement of the sacroiliac joint. Pain in the lumbar area with or without radiation to the legs that is caused by a shifting center of gravity should be differentiated from posterior pelvic pain (also called sacroiliac pain, sacroiliac joint syndrome, and pelvic girdle relaxation) and pyelonephritis. Careful questioning of the client can help identify situations requiring consultation with or referral to a physician.

Contractions, Cramping, and Pelvic Pressure

Reports of contractions, cramping, and pelvic pressure pose a challenge to clinicians as these may be normal pregnancy occurrences or signs of preterm labor (PTL). Identifying women with these signs and symptoms who will actually give birth prematurely is difficult. How many contractions within a given time period can be considered normal? What patterns precede PTL? Unfortunately, there is no normative data to answer these questions. But two recent developments can help with diagnosis and management: 1) measurement of the length of the cervical canal by ultrasound and 2) detection of fetal fibronectin, a gluelike substance in the lower uterine segment that leaks out of the cervix in the second half of pregnancy prior to some cases of preterm birth (see Chapter 5).

Reports of premature contractions, cramping, and pelvic pressure, whether associated with discomfort, should always be taken seriously. Ask about the frequency of the contractions, as well as additional subtle, associated symptoms: continuous backache, increased vaginal discharge, and blood-stained vaginal discharge.

While the exact number of contractions in a given time period that predicts PTL is unknown, most women will not give birth prematurely if they have fewer than 4 to 6 contractions per hour.

 HELPFUL HINT

Teach clients a "magic number"—four to six contractions per hour before 36 weeks' gestation—that requires notification of the clinician. Begin referring to this number at 24 weeks' gestation, and periodically ask the client if she remembers the "magic number" for contractions.

Burning with Urination, Urgency, Dysuria, and Urinary Retention

Urinary tract infections (UTIs) are described in terms of their location: cystitis, inflammation in the bladder or urethra (lower urinary tract), or pyelonephritis, inflammation of the kidney (upper urinary tract). The most common symptoms of cystitis are dysuria, frequent voidings of small amounts of urine, and urgency. Lower abdominal pain, particularly when the bladder is palpated; hematuria; and nocturia may be present. Pyelonephritis presents with flank pain, costovertebral angle tenderness, fever, chills, nausea, vomiting, headache, and malaise with or without symptoms of lower tract infection. The differential diagnosis should include vaginitis, urethritis, and an allergic/chemical reaction to soap or a feminine hygiene product.

Inquire at each visit about urgency, dysuria, and burning with urination. Urinary frequency can be a difficult symptom to evaluate in pregnant women. Traditional teaching states that urinary frequency is common in the first trimester, when the enlarging uterus sits on the bladder, and in the third trimester for the same reason. However, "Urinary frequency in early pregnancy is unlikely to be related to increasing uterine size because frequent urination begins while the uterus is still far too small to exert any significant pressure on the bladder. Lower urinary tract symptoms in early pregnancy are far more likely to be caused by dramatic changes in hormone levels, plasma volume expansion, and increases in renal blood flow and glomerular filtration than they are to be caused by mechanical factors. The notion that urinary frequency should improve as the uterus gets dramatically larger but 'rises up out of the pelvis' also seems incongruous. Why should a uterus at 22 weeks' gestation cause less pressure on the bladder than a uterus at 6 or 8 weeks' gestation?" (Thorp et al., 1999, p. 270).

Occasionally, an enlarging retroverted uterus will impinge on the urethra and not allow urine to pass. An indwelling catheter may be necessary for awhile. At times it is possible to "flip" the retroverted uterus into an anterior position during a bimanual examination.

Episodes of urinary incontinence and cough-induced stress incontinence may worsen as pregnancy progresses (Thorp et al., 1999).

Vaginal Bleeding

Vaginal bleeding or spotting can occur at any time in pregnancy. Bleeding and spotting can be caused by benign conditions, such as implantation, cervicitis, cervical polyps, or coitus, or by serious, even life-threatening conditions, such as ectopic pregnancy, placenta previa, abruptio placentae, and miscarriage. The cause of bleeding or spotting may remain unknown in as many as 38% of cases. When the cause is unknown, PTL and congenital anomalies occur at higher rates. All reports of vaginal bleeding should be taken seriously. A differential diagnosis for vaginal bleeding in pregnancy can be found in Table 7-3.

Vaginal Bleeding in the First Half of Pregnancy.

In the first trimester of pregnancy, pregnancy-related vaginal bleeding or spotting can be a sign of an ectopic pregnancy; threatened, impending or missed

TABLE 7.3 Differential Diagnosis for Vaginal Bleeding in Pregnancy

First trimester	Second trimester	Third trimester
Ectopic Pregnancy	GTN	Placenta previa
Implantation bleeding	Incompetent cervix	Abruptio placentae
Miscarriage	Cervical cancer	Bloody show
Cervical polyp	Cervical polyp	Trauma
Cervicitis	Cervicitis	Coitus
STI	Coitus	STI
Cervical cancer	STI	Cervical polyp
Trauma	Abruptio placentae	Cervical cancer
Hemorrhoids	Trauma	Marginal sinus rupture
Hemorrhagic cystitis	Bloody show	Cervicitis
Foreign object	Marginal sinus rupture	Hemorrhoids
	Hemorrhoids	Hemorrhagic cystitis
	Hemorrhagic cystitis	Foreign object
	Foreign object	Bleeding disorder

abortion; or trophoblastic disease. Speculum and digital examinations can be performed in the presence of vaginal bleeding in the first trimester. There is no danger of disturbing the placenta. Inquire about the most recent episode of coitus as the penis thrusting against fragile cervical epithelium may cause bleeding or spotting.

Ectopic Pregnancy. As many as 25% of women with ectopic pregnancies do not know they are pregnant, mistaking their bleeding for menses. Suspect ectopic pregnancy whenever a woman in the reproductive years complains of unusual menses, amenorrhea, vaginal bleeding, or pelvic pain. When a diagnosis of pregnancy has been made, ectopic pregnancy must be a consideration whenever vaginal bleeding or spotting is reported in the first 12 weeks of pregnancy, unless ultrasound examination has determined that the pregnancy is in the uterus.

The presenting complaint in ectopic pregnancy is usually vaginal bleeding or spotting with cramping or abdominal pain, although classic symptoms may be absent. Gastrointestinal symptoms as well as dizziness are often present. A history of a previous ectopic pregnancy, pelvic inflammatory disease, or a bilateral tubal ligation should increase one's suspicion of an ectopic pregnancy, although absence of these risk factors must not delay an assessment. An ectopic pregnancy is potentially fatal.

Ectopic pregnancy is best diagnosed with a combination of transvaginal ultrasound and serum human chorionic gonadotropin (hCG) levels. A positive assay for serum beta-hCG can be found 8 days after fertilization. A transvaginal ultrasound can identify an intrauterine gestational sac 28 days after fertilization. With a beta-hCG level greater than 6000 mIU/mL and an intrauterine gestational sac noted with abdominal ultrasonography, normal pregnancy is almost certain. A vaginal ultrasound examination is useful when the hCG level is 1000 to 2000 mIU/mL.

When a beta-hCG level is greater than 6000 mIU/mL (1000 to 2000 mIU/mL with vaginal ultrasonography) and the uterine cavity is empty, ectopic pregnancy is likely. A beta-hCG level less than 6000 mIU/mL (1000 to 2000 mIU/mL with vaginal ultrasonography) and a definite intrauterine ring of pregnancy means that spontaneous abortion is likely. A beta-hCG level less than 6000 mIU/mL (1000 to 2000 mIU/mL with vaginal ultrasonography) and an empty uterus result in an uncertain diagnosis (Cunningham et al., 2001).

Miscarriage. The medical term "abortion" (also called blighted ovum) is used to refer to pregnancies that never develop that cause vaginal bleeding or bloody discharge in the first half of pregnancy (threatened abortion), present with the cervical os open and tissue seen (inevitable abortion), and end with all or part of the "products of conception" being "expelled" (spontaneous abortion), in addition to situations in which the fetus dies but is not expelled (missed abortion). The lay public refers to these conditions as miscarriages. It is appropriate to use this term when referring to first-trimester losses that are not induced (as elective or therapeutic terminations of pregnancy). Most miscarriages occur in the first 12 weeks of pregnancy. At least half are probably caused by chromosomal anomalies.

The first sign of a spontaneous abortion is usually bleeding, with or without pain/cramping. The picture is inconsistent from one woman to another in regard to both. Some will bleed heavily, and others will merely spot. Some have bleeding daily; others bleed intermittently. For some women the color will be pink, while others note brown or red. Pain can be absent or severe and anywhere in between. It can be in the back as well as in the lower abdomen, and it may be rhythmic or constant (Thorstensen, 2000).

When a woman reports vaginal bleeding early in pregnancy, perform a speculum examination to determine the source and amount of bleeding. If tissue is seen at or coming from the cervical os, loss of the baby is inevitable. If no tissue has been passed or can be seen at the os, and the gestational age of the fetus is at least 6 weeks, an ultrasound examination will be able to determine if the pregnancy is intact.

If a client reports vaginal bleeding before the 6th gestational week, order a *quantitative* hCG level (as opposed to a *qualitative* hCG level, which usually will only state that the level is less or more than 25 IU/L). Human chorionic gonadotropin levels rise rapidly after implantation, doubling about every 31 hours until 9 weeks' gestation, when levels peak at 100,000 IU/L. Repeat the test in 48 to 72 hours, when the hCG level should have doubled if the baby is still alive.

It may be appropriate to order an ultrasound when a previous ultrasound examination showed that the fetal heart was beating. Despite the fact that the vast majority of babies demonstrating a beating heart at an early ultrasound examination do well, women with autoantibodies are known to miscarry after documented fetal heart tones.

Women who experience vaginal bleeding may call to report that they have passed tissue at home. If bleeding is not heavy, the client usually does not need to come to the clinic or office to be seen. Women who have miscarried should be counseled to report fever, severe cramps, or heavy bleeding. If a missed abortion has occurred, many women request a surgical procedure to remove the tissue from the uterus. Some women prefer to avoid surgery and await spontaneous expulsion of the fetus. The chances of blood coagulation problems (from retention of a dead fetus for a long period of time—about 4 weeks) or of infection are slight.

Whether or not the pregnancy was planned is not helpful in predicting a woman's reaction to her baby's death. Family and friends may minimize the loss or remain silent, fearing to inflict emotional pain. Be helpful to the grieving mother by discussing the grieving process and comments she is likely to hear. Tell the mother that the sadness may last a year or two or even longer.

Her partner is likely to experience resolution of the grief before she does. Encourage her to talk about her experience with others. Acknowledgment of the pain experienced may prompt other women to share stories of their own losses, helping a woman feel that she is not alone. Also important is the provider's continuing expression of concern as evidenced by periodic phone calls.

Gestational Trophoblastic Neoplasia. Gestational trophoblastic neoplasia (GTN) is a term that includes three diagnoses: hydatidiform mole, invasive mole, and choriocarcinoma. Most women with GTN experience first-trimester bleeding. Other symptoms include excessive nausea and vomiting and a discrepancy between uterine size and gestational age. The discrepancy can be either larger or smaller than expected. GTN requires referral to a physician. Follow-up depends on the diagnosis

Vaginal Bleeding in Later Pregnancy

Bleeding in the second half of pregnancy can be caused by polyps, cervicitis, trauma, cancer, and coitus, as in the first half of pregnancy. Additionally, bloody show, placenta previa, and abruptio placentae can cause it.

When bleeding occurs in the second half of pregnancy, a speculum examination should be performed if an ultrasound examination has determined there is no placenta previa. Both speculum and digital examinations can cause a fatal hemorrhage if the placenta is disrupted. When a speculum examination is unable to determine the cause of vaginal bleeding or spotting, a detailed second-trimester ultrasound scan should be requested, if it has not been previously performed (Chan & To, 1999).

Placenta Previa. Placenta previa, a major cause of third-trimester bleeding, is a condition in which the placenta implants in varying degrees in the lower uterine segment, below the presenting part of the baby. A total or complete previa covers the entire internal cervical os; a partial previa covers part of the internal os; and a marginal previa means that the edge of the placenta has reached the internal os. The classic presentation of placenta previa is painless, vaginal bleeding. The initial bleeding episode usually stops spontaneously, but bleeding recurs.

A placenta previa identified incidentally on ultrasound examination in the first 20 weeks of gestation is likely to "migrate" away from the cervix toward the uterine fundus as the uterus grows and the placenta is pulled up farther into the uterus. In 90% of cases, the previa disappears (Baron & Hill, 1998). When an early sonogram identifies a placenta previa, a repeat sonogram for placental localization is recommended at 26 to 28 weeks' gestation. Women with a placenta previa who have any vaginal bleeding should be referred for physician care. These women should also observe "pelvic rest," that is, nothing in the vagina, including intercourse, a tampon, and douching. Masturbation should also be avoided to avoid provoking uterine contractions that may arise with orgasm.

Low-Lying Placenta. A low-lying placenta is one in which an ultrasound examination locates a placental edge within 2 cm of the internal os. This condition is found in approximately 1% of normal pregnancies when ultrasound examination is performed between 15 and 20 weeks' gestation. Fourteen percent of these low-lying placentas are present at delivery (Lauria et al., 1996). Studies report an association between low-lying placentas and vasa previa and velamentous cord insertion. In a study of 18 women with antepartum bleeding, both vasa previa and velamentous cord insertion were found in six of 18 women (Lee et al, 2000).

Abruptio Placentae. An abruptio placentae is one in which all or part of the placenta separates from the uterine wall before the baby is born. The separation may be abrupt or occur over a period of weeks. It can occur in the second or third trimester. In addition to vaginal bleeding, the mother usually reports abdominal pain, contractions, and back pain if the placenta is implanted posteriorly, although vaginal bleeding and uterine tenderness are absent in 25% of cases. Preterm labor may be the initial diagnosis (Baron & Hill, 1998). A "boardlike" abdomen, uterine irritability, and tetanic contractions may be present. Hypotension, shock, fetal bradycardia, and fetal death may occur. Any indication of abruption requires immediate hospitalization for the well-being of both mother and baby.

Vaginal Discharge

An increase in vaginal discharge is common in pregnancy, especially in the last few weeks when the cervical glands are particularly active. However, increased vaginal discharge may also be a symptom of a sexually transmitted disease, cervicitis, vaginitis, or PTL and may be confused with ruptured membranes. Many women are unaware of the characteristics of normal vaginal discharge. A discussion about symptoms of vaginal infection should be part of prenatal health education. Be sure to include unusual discharge; malodor, including a fishy odor after intercourse; and itching, burning, or dysuria. Instruct women to report an increase or change in vaginal discharge. An office or clinic visit to differentiate between normal increase in vaginal discharge, infection, and PTL is indicated. Microscopic examination of vaginal discharge to rule out vaginitis is always appropriate, as is a cervical examination to rule out premature effacement or dilatation (unless membranes are ruptured). Remember to perform the cervical examination after obtaining the fFN specimen when this test is indicated.

Ruptured Membranes Whenever rupture of the membranes is a possibility, a sterile speculum examination should be performed to confirm or refute the suspicion. If no obvious "pool" of fluid is noted in the vagina, asking the client to cough sometimes results in fluid visible at the cervical opening if the membranes are truly ruptured. Three positive findings substantiate a diagnosis of ruptured membranes: pooling of fluid in the vagina, "ferning" of the fluid when examined under a microscope, and a basic pH (identified when amniotic fluid touches pH paper and the color changes from yellow to blue). Dip a sterile cotton swab into the pool of amniotic fluid and touch it to the pH paper. Dip another sterile swab into the pool, roll it across a microscope slide, let it dry, and examine it for "ferning." Blood can affect the nitrazine paper used to identify pH.

Rupture of membranes in a preterm pregnancy is associated with infection and malpresentation as well as low-birth-weight babies. Clients should be especially vigilant about leaking of amniotic fluid before the 37th week of pregnancy. Under no circumstances should a digital examination of the cervix be performed in the clinic or office when membranes are ruptured unless delivery is imminent. The chance of uterine infection greatly increases once a digital examination is performed.

Skin Changes

Pregnancy can precipitate a number of skin changes. Those unique to pregnancy that may be bothersome include pruritus gravidarum, pruritic urticarial papules and plaques of pregnancy (PUPPP), and herpes gestationis (HG). Additional diagnoses with either rash or itching include erythema multiforme, viral exanthem, scabies, contact urticaria, and an adverse drug reaction.

The initial symptom of pruritus gravidarum, also known as intrahepatic cholestasis of pregnancy, is general body itching. "Anorexia, malaise, epigastric discomfort, steatorrhea, and dark urine are common" (Fagan, 1999). Intrauterine death can occur unexpectedly despite close fetal monitoring.

When a client reports pruritus and no rash can be found (except for those caused by scratching), liver function tests should be ordered, and medical consultation should be obtained to diagnose cholestasis. When this occurs, the client is at increased risk for PTL and poor pregnancy outcome; induction of labor may be appropriate as soon as the pregnancy reaches 36 weeks.

Pruritic urticarial papules and plaques of pregnancy (PUPPP) is a condition in which a pruritic, macular, papular rash appears on the abdomen and sometimes the extremities, buttocks, and lower chest in the third trimester. The lesions begin on the abdomen and usually involve the striae, sometimes developing within the striae first. The rash usually occurs only in first pregnancies. It resolves by the end of the first postpartum week. No vesicles are present, and pruritus (severe in 80% of the cases) is the only systemic symptom. While topical corticosteroids and oral antihistamines may give relief, referral to a physician for oral corticosteroid therapy may be necessary. Induction of labor at term to relieve symptoms can be appropriate.

The HG erythematous eruption is followed by papules, vesicles, and bullae over the abdomen, buttocks, back, and upper extremities. Malaise, fever, and anorexia may also be present. HG commonly occurs in multiparas, while PUPPP is more common in women having their first baby. HG also is likely to recur, while PUPPP recurs infrequently. Consultation with a dermatologist is usually necessary.

Fever and Exposure to Infectious Disease

Fever in pregnancy is usually caused by flu, sinusitis, or a respiratory infection. While low-grade fevers usually are not significant, a fever above 38°C (100.4°F) poses the possibility of damage to the fetus, particularly if it occurs in the first 16 to 18 weeks. Clients should be advised to notify the provider when a temperature is elevated and to take acetaminophen (Tylenol) for fever reduction. "Data from animal studies and fever during pregnancy indicate that core temperature elevations of 38.9°C or higher may increase the rate of spontaneous abortion or birth defects, most notably neural tube defects" (Colie, 1997, p. 16).

Varicella. One of the most significant infectious diseases in pregnant women is varicella (See Chapter 5). Fortunately, the risk of congenital varicella syndrome (cutaneous scars, limb hypoplasia, and eye and central nervous system abnormalities) is small, particularly if maternal infection occurs in the first 4 months of pregnancy. Varicella pneumonia in pregnancy can be fatal. Any pulmonary symptoms (cough, chest pain, dyspnea, hemoptysis) require immediate notification of the clinician. If hemoptysis occurs, the maternal death rate can be as high as 50%.

If a pregnant woman reports that she has been exposed to a child with chickenpox and has no history of varicella infection, determine susceptibility by requesting an immunoglobulin G (IgG) titer. Testing should be completed within 48 hours of exposure. The presence of IgG antibodies reflects immunity. Absence of IgG antibodies reflects susceptibility. In cases of susceptibility, varicella zoster immune globulin (VZIG) should be administered as soon as possible. "It may be effective up to 96 hours after exposure" (Chapman, 1998).

Cytomegalovirus. Cytomegalovirus (CMV) is a herpes virus commonly found among women who work in daycare centers, newborn nurseries, renal dialysis centers, and mental institutions. CMV infection is the most common congenital viral infection in the United States. Approximately 9% of women who develop a primary CMV infection during pregnancy will have an affected infant. Intrauterine growth restriction, microcephaly, hydrocephaly, and spleen or liver enlargement accompany fetal infection. While most infected newborns are asymptomatic, by the age of 2 years, between 5% and 17% develop symptoms that include deafness, learning disabilities, and mental retardation.

Transmission rates are thought to be higher in the third trimester, but primary infection in the first half of pregnancy seems to cause more severe effects (Leguizamon & Reece, 1997; Liesnard et al., 2000). Women who are seronegative for CMV before pregnancy and who develop a primary infection while pregnant have intrauterine transmission rates of 14% to 50% compared with seropositive women who have a transmission rate of 1% (Leguizamon & Reece, 1997).

Pregnant women with a primary CMV infection rarely have symptoms. Occasionally, fever, headache, swollen glands, a mild sore throat, and sore muscles may be present. Routine prenatal screening is not recommended because screening is not cost-effective, no vaccine is available, testing is unreliable, and seropositivity does not prevent recurrence. Primary infection is diagnosed when IgG seroconversion is demonstrated or a fourfold increase in titers is identified. A negative result may require follow-up because of a delay of up to 4 weeks in the rise of the titer (Leguizamon & Reece, 1997).

Parvovirus B19. Another potentially dangerous virus associated with a low-grade maternal fever is parvovirus B19 (erythema infectiosum). It is also known as fifth disease "as it was the fifth exanthem identified. The other exanthems, in order of discovery, are measles (first disease), scarlet fever (second disease), rubella or German measles (third disease), Duke's disease (fourth disease), and roseola infantum (sixth disease)" (Turnquest & Brown, 1999, p. 75). Treatment for parvovirus B19 is not available.

Parvovirus B19 is spread primarily by respiratory droplets, hand-to-mouth contact, and blood transfusions. It does not cause birth defects, but second-trimester fetal loss has been noted (Mead, 1997). Parvovirus infection can cause nonimmune fetal hydrops, an accumulation of serous fluid in body cavities and subcutaneous tissue, 4 to 6 weeks after maternal infection. When hydrops is identified on ultrasound, the mother should be tested for parvovirus infection whether or not she is aware of exposure.

"Acute arthralgias and arthritis of the hands, knees, and wrists may occur as the only manifestation of infection in adults. A flu-like illness is also common as are numbness and tingling of the peripheral extremities. Approximately one quarter of adults infected with B19 will have a nonrash illness, and another quarter of them will be asymptomatic" (Mead, 1997, p. 21). Some individuals have a mild anemia. A brief period of low-grade fever may be followed by a "lacy, reticular" rash on the trunk and extremities. The "slapped cheek" rash characteristic of fifth disease in children is not as common in adults.

Parvovirus B19 is diagnosed by screening for IgG and IgM antibodies against parvovirus. The absence of B19 IgG and IgM antibodies means the woman is susceptible to infection. A positive IgG screen denotes previous infection and immunity against the disease. The presence of B19 IgM antibodies alone is indicative of a very recent infection (probably within the last 7 days). The presence of both B19 IgG and IgM antibodies suggests exposure from 7 days to 6 months previously (Turnquest & Brown, 1999).

When a pregnant woman has been exposed to parvovirus B19 or has symptoms of the disease, obtain B19 IgG and IgM determinations between 4 days and 4 weeks after onset of symptoms or 2 weeks after exposure if no symptoms are present. If maternal infection is diagnosed, physician referral is indicated for identification and follow-up of fetal hydrops, which may occur in up to 30% of cases of maternal infection. It frequently resolves spontaneously over a 6-week period.

Table 7-4 summarizes the signs and symptoms, diagnosis, and management of selected infections during pregnancy.

Edema
Swelling in both normal and preeclamptic pregnancies is caused by movement of fluid from the bloodstream to the interstitial spaces. Almost all pregnant women have edema at some time during their pregnancies. While it occurs primarily in hands and feet, facial edema is also common. Worrisome edema in pregnancy is the kind that comes on suddenly or is excessive. Preeclampsia may be the cause, although edema is no longer considered necessary for a diagnosis of preeclampsia (National Institutes of Health, 2000). Still, it is prudent to consider preeclampsia when significant edema is noted.

The definition of excessive or significant edema is elusive. Weight gain is often used as a marker for edema.

Numbness and Tingling of the Hands and Wrists
Prickly sensations, tingling, numbness, weakness, swelling, stiffness, burning, and pain are common symptoms of carpal tunnel syndrome. The median nerve and nine flexor tendons of the hand pass through the carpal tunnel (Figure 7-4). In pregnancy, swollen soft tissue decreases the space available for the median nerve, causing the classic triad of symptoms—numbness, tingling, and pain—at night, often in both hands. Nocturnal symptoms are probably due to fluid shifts from the lower to the upper extremities when the client lies down (Lublin, Rojer, & Barron, 1998).

Carpal tunnel syndrome usually develops in the second and third trimesters and resolves within 2 weeks' postpartum. Symptoms can be mild or severe. In severe cases, the client may not be able to write or hold a cup.

Wrist splints worn at night and during activities that increase symptoms may provide some relief. The splint has a metal slat that prevents flexion of the wrist yet permits movement of the thumb and fingers. Without flexion and extension of the wrist, nerve compression is avoided. Prolonged immobilization by full-time use of the splint is discouraged. Women who work with keyboards should adjust the level of the keyboard to keep the wrist in a neutral position. Induction of labor after 37 weeks is occasionally necessary because of extreme discomfort, distress, and disability.

Genital Lesions, Sores, and Growths
The herpes virus, syphilis, or chancroid may cause genital lesions. Because neither herpes nor syphilis always present in the classic textbook manner, as

text continues on page 221

TABLE 7.4 Selected Viral Infections in Pregnancy

Disease	Signs & symptoms	Effects on fetus	Diagnosis	Prevention	Transmission	Remarks
Parvovirus	Bright red macular rash Erythroderma of face (slapped cheek) Flulike symptoms Arthralgias Low-grade fever May be none in >50% of adults	Not teratogenic but causes fetal death due to hydrops from anemia caused by erythroid aplasia (RBC fail to mature) Abortion	IgM-specific antibody IgG antibody titers, with acute and convalescent sera		Horizontally by droplet infection	Risk of fetal death = 9% Infants who survive the severe anemia appear to develop normally Prophylactic immune globulin not recommended
Cytomegalo-virus	15% have monolike syndrome, fever, sore throat, lymph-adenopathy, polyarthritis	At birth, symptomatic: low birth weight(LBW), microcephaly chorioretinitis, developmental delay, mental retardation, sensorineural deficits, hepa-tosplenomegaly, jaundice, anemia, purpura At birth, asymp-tomatic: 5–15% with long-term neurologic sequelae later in childhood (usually hearing loss)	Primary infection: 4× IgG titers in paired acute and convalescent sera measured at the same times		Horizontally by droplet infection and contact with saliva and urine STD Vertically from mother to fetus	30–40% of women with primary infections transmit virus to fetus with 10% symptomatic at birth Acquisition in early pregnancy ↑ severity of infection Recurrent infections = 0.5% to 1% with ↓ severity Seroconversion should be followed by amniocentesis for viral identification

	Signs/Symptoms		Diagnosis	Treatment/Prevention	Comments
Rubeola	Fever, malaise Koplik spots Cough Photophobia Periorbital edema Rash	↑ Abortion and LBW if maternal measles shortly before birth; ↑ risk of death especially if preterm Not teratogenic	Visual inspection Titers	Passive immunity: Immune serum globulin, 5 mL IM, within 3 days of exposure No vaccine during pregnancy	
Listeria (L. *Monocytogenes*: Gram-positive bacillus)	Febrile illness—may be mild	50% mortality	Blood culture Amniocentesis	Found in soil, water, sewage, manure, cabbage, pasteurized milk and cheese	Infection similar to group B strep Treat with ampicillin and gentamicin or TMP-SMZ
Rubella	¼–½ of cases are subclinical Viremia precedes signs/symptoms by 1 week Only ½ of women with affected infants give history of rash Termination of pregnancy after 10 wks not recommended as rate of infection and birth defects is lower	If rash appears 12–21 days from LMP, 31% fetal infection; if 3–6 wks from LMP, 100% infection; if 13–14 wks, 54%; if >17 wks, no severe damage but no long-term studies Congenital rubella syndrome: cataracts, glaucoma, patent ductus; microphthalmia, septal defects; deafness; CNS defects; IUGR; TCP and anemia; hepatitis; pneumonitis; bone changes; chromosomal abnormalities ↑ abortion	Visual inspection Titers	Vaccination (MMR)	No fetal damage reported after inadvertent vaccination in pregnancy

table continues on page 220

TABLE 7.4 Selected Viral Infections in Pregnancy continued

Disease	Signs & symptoms	Effects on fetus	Diagnosis	Prevention	Transmission	Remarks
Varicella	Vesicular rash on trunk, hands, feet, face Fever May develop pneumonia	Early chorioretinitis, cerebral cortical atrophy, hydronephrosis, cutaneous and bony leg defects If delivery occurs while mother has varicella, disseminated visceral and CNS disease ⅓ of infants with congenital varicella syndrome die in neonatal period and most survivors have serious problems	Visual inspection Titers	VZIG (varicella zoster immune globulin) within 96 hours–125U/10kg IM VZIG to neonate when onset of maternal clinical discharge is within 5 days before delivery or 2 days postpartum	Transplacental	Risk of congenital varicella syndrome 1.8% if maternal infection in Δ and less than 1% after Δ
Toxoplasmosis	Few if any	Chorioretinitis with 50% having severe visual impairment if no treatment	Seroconversion from a negative to a positive titer or IgM antibodies or four-fold ↑ in specific IgG titer when done at 3-week intervals with no treatment Amniocentesis US (hydrocephalus, intracranial calcifications)	Avoid poorly cooked meat, unwashed vegetables and fruit Avoid cat feces in garden, litter boxes	Transplacental	4 out of 1000 susceptible pregnant women will get toxoplasmosis; if not treated 40% will have an infected baby Fetal infection ↑ with gestational age (17% at 17–20 wks and 29% after 20 wks) but severity ↓ with gestational age Treat with antibiotics

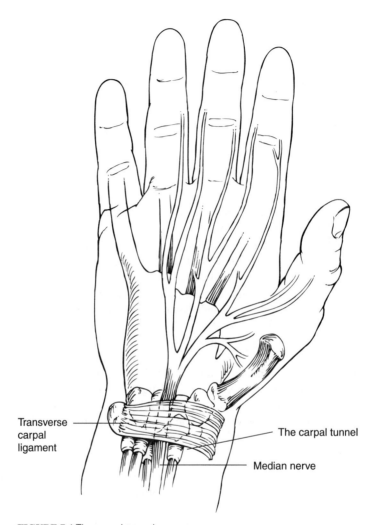

Transverse carpal ligament

The carpal tunnel

Median nerve

FIGURE 7.4 The carpal tunnel.

many as 50% of lesions may be misdiagnosed (Hoffman & Schmitz, 1995). Accordingly, a serologic test for syphilis and a culture or other lesion test or type-specific serologic testing for herpes simplex virus should be performed regardless of the appearance of the lesion.

Herpes. Herpes simplex virus (HSV) type 1 commonly causes fever blisters on the mouth or face, while type 2 causes lesions to develop in the genital area and buttocks. However, both types can cause oral *and* genital infections. Both types are transmitted through kissing, skin-to-skin contact, or vaginal, oral, or anal sex. A primary outbreak of HSV type 2 (HSV-2) in the first trimester may increase the risk of spontaneous abortion (ACOG, 1999d). Later, primary infection increases the incidence of PTL. Women who do have symptoms with an initial outbreak are likely to experience fever, dysuria, and enlarged, painful lymph glands. A second crop of lesions may arise. Recurrence varies and is usually preceded by vulvar irritation, itching, burning, and erythema, as well as perianal and vulvar fissures (Corey & Handsfield, 2000).

A diagnosis of HSV is made by isolating the virus with a cell culture. "Early primary and non-primary first-episode ulcers yield the virus in 80% of patients, whereas ulcers from recurrent infections are less likely to be culture-positive; only 40% of crusted lesions contain recoverable virus. When testing for HSV, overt lesions that are not in the ulcerated state should be unroofed and the fluid sampled" (ACOG, 1999d, p.4).

Women who may be having their initial HSV-2 infection while pregnant should have a herpes antibody titer done as soon as there is suspicion of a herpes lesion. If the IgG screen is positive, immunity is present. If the IgM screen is positive but the IgG is negative, the test has identified an initial outbreak. A second titer should be drawn 2 to 3 weeks after the first. The presence of a titer in the first specimen "strongly suggests non-primary first episode or recurrent infection" (ACOG, 1999d, p. 4) and should not be cause for alarm.

Chapter 3 discusses the use of antiviral agents to prevent herpes outbreaks in late pregnancy. The Acyclovir Registry of 1246 women who used acyclovir during pregnancy found no neonatal outcomes likely to be drug related. However, noting that the prophylactic dose of acyclovir involves long exposure to the fetus with a dose significantly higher than that given to nonpregnant women, the small sample of women in the Acyclovir Registry, and the fact that no long-term follow-up is involved in the registry study, Brown concluded, "it is presumptuous to say that the drug has no adverse effects on the developing human fetus" (2000, p. 68).

Syphilis. Primary syphilis usually presents with a small macule that turns into a single, painless ulcer (chancre) with well-defined edges on the vulva or anus or, more commonly, on the cervix or vagina, where the lesion goes unnoticed. The inguinal lymph glands will be enlarged, reflecting the systemic nature of the disease. Symptoms of secondary syphilis include condylomata lata (a flat, papular growth on the genitalia), sore throat, musculoskeletal pain, generalized lymphadenopathy, and a generalized maculopapular body rash that can even be seen on the palms of the hands and the soles of the feet. Syphilis rates tend to be high in urban areas, where crack cocaine is used and money or drugs are exchanged for sex (CDC, 1996).

Trauma

Trauma may result from many activities, including assault, physical or sexual abuse, a motor vehicle accident, falls, and stab or gunshot wounds. Uterine trauma may be lethal to both mother and baby, as the large amount of blood in the uterus means that uterine injury can lead to exsanguination. Injuries can also damage the fetal skull and brain, particularly if the fetal head is engaged (Pearlman & Cunningham, 1996), and can cause premature separation of the placenta (abruptio placentae). This condition often leads to fetal death and, depending on blood loss, maternal death as well. Abruptio placentae may occur in 1% to 5% of minor injuries and 20% to 50% of major injuries (Bowen, 1994).

Any woman who has had trauma to her abdomen after 20 weeks' gestation should be seen in an obstetrics unit to monitor fetal well-being. Large, prospective studies have not validated the length of monitoring needed. However, 2 to 6 hours are recommended in the literature. "Monitoring should be continued and further evaluation carried out if uterine contractions, a nonreassuring fetal heart rate pattern, vaginal bleeding, significant uterine tenderness or irritability, serious maternal injury, or rupture of the amniotic membranes is present" (ACOG, 1998b, pp. 4-5).

Fetal Movement

Quickening, the first movement of the baby in utero perceived by the mother, occurs between 18 and 20 weeks' gestation in most women having a first baby and between 16 and 18 weeks' gestation in most women having a subsequent baby. In the early 1970s, researchers in Israel and England studying fetal movement hoped to establish a minimum number of movements in a selected time period that would differentiate a fetus in danger of dying from one that was healthy. The researchers found that most babies moved hundreds of times each day, although there was tremendous variation from one fetus to another. The researchers also found that decreased fetal movement could be a sign of fetal jeopardy.

Studies looking at fetal movement have been unable to pinpoint a precise number of movements in a specific time period that identify either the healthy or unhealthy baby in utero. "Consistent evidence that a formal program of fetal movement assessment will result in a reduction in fetal deaths is lacking" (ACOG, 1999a, p. 934). Still, many practices ask pregnant women to count fetal movements if a subjective decrease in movement is noted. Without evidence-based guidelines, the clinician should individualize directions for counting the movements and the form for recording movements and then expect that the client's lifestyle will vary. Methods that require counting for extended time periods may not be reasonable for women who are employed or distracted by other children. Forms that initiate counting in the morning may not be appropriate for women who work nights. Many charts and forms may not work well for women with low literacy skills, particularly if the chart requires use of a graph.

One guideline for fetal movement is 10 movements in a 10- or a 12-hour period. If the baby does not move 10 times within the specified time period, a movement alarm signal has occurred, and the client should notify the health care provider immediately so that a nonstress test can be arranged.

On rare occasions a baby moves so little that the mother describes fetal movement as absent. While lack of maternal awareness may explain failure to perceive movement at times, reports of absent or decreased movement should always be taken seriously and special testing ordered. Because some women still think it is normal for the baby's movements in utero to slow down before labor begins, be certain that every mother knows this is not so.

Prescription, Over-the-Counter, and Herbal Medicine

Most medicines used appropriately contribute significantly to quality of life, but during pregnancy, practitioners must be aware of the FDA category of all medicine prescribed. The clinician is responsible for knowing what medicine, if any, the client is taking; the dosage and the frequency; any side effects the client may be experiencing; and whether the client wants to discontinue the medicine.

 HELPFUL HINT

Both beginning and experienced practitioners would do well to maintain a system of information that provides pertinent information about the use of drugs in pregnancy and lactation. Any commercially available set of drug cards can serve as a starting point. Discard the cards you are not likely to use, punch holes in the upper left-hand corner of those remaining, and insert them onto a large metal key ring. When you prescribe a drug, read about it extensively, note the FDA category, call a pharmacy for the price, look in the *Physicians' Desk Reference* to see how it is supplied, and add this information to your card. Each practice should also have a recent edition of a "drugs in pregnancy" book.

Remember that herbal products, including vitamins, minerals, and amino acids, are classified as dietary supplements. As such, they are not subject to FDA procedures that require testing for adverse effects before they are marketed. Nor are there manufacturing standards that would address harvesting, handling, packaging, and storing the products. Herbal products are not regulated for purity or potency; therefore, the amount of an active ingredient from one product to another may vary (Ramsey, Ross, & Fischer, 2000). While Dietary Supplements Research Centers that emphasize botanicals (medicinal plants) have recently been established by NIH's Office of Dietary Supplements, questions about the efficacy, safety, and reliability of herbal products remain. Unfortunately, much of the past research on herbal products involved anecdotal data, small sample sizes, problems with quality control of the product, short duration of therapy, differing end points, and failure to report side effects. Pending the results of a systematic evaluation of health benefits, practitioners must carefully review what is known about herbal products before recommending them to clients.

Prenatal Vitamins. For decades women have been told that a daily prenatal vitamin is important. However, routine use of prenatal vitamins is not recommended by the Institute of Medicine. These vitamins are big and powerful, and there is no proof that they help fetuses of women who 1) are at a weight appropriate for their height, 2) eat a well-balanced diet, 3) carry one fetus, and 4) are not abusing drugs, alcohol, or cigarettes. A multivitamin and mineral preparation is recommended by the Institute of Medicine (1992) when the client

- Has iron deficiency anemia
- Is a complete vegetarian
- Is carrying more than one baby
- Resists improving a poor-quality diet
- Is a heavy cigarette smoker
- Abuses alcohol
- Is under age 25
- Is not able to or interested in consuming calcium-rich milk products

In regard to the institute's recommendations for the content of prenatal vitamins, a review of the 1996 *Physicians' Desk Reference* (PDR) for prescription drugs showed that neither "the prescription or the non-prescription supplements reviewed in the PDR conform to these recommendations and almost none come close. Perhaps it is time to reconsider the formulation of prenatal supplements and to assess the safety and effectiveness of their use" (Brown & Kahn, 1997).

Many pregnant women come to their first prenatal visit already taking prenatal vitamins. These women usually feel uncomfortable not taking them, and they probably should not be asked to stop, even when they do not fall into the Institute of Medicine groups for whom supplementation is recommended. It is easy to understand why most women feel that prenatal vitamins are essential in pregnancy. The prenatal vitamin-and-iron ritual has a long tradition. Clinicians themselves find it difficult not to prescribe these vitamins routinely. However, the potential effect of high doses of vitamins is unknown, and large doses can mask a vitamin B_{12} deficiency. Megadoses of vitamin A can cause birth defects.

The price of prenatal vitamins varies greatly. There is no evidence that any one brand is more effective than any other.

Emotional Well-being, Stress, and Abuse

Emotional lability is common during pregnancy. Mood swings may be related to hormones, physical discomfort, changes in body image, or anxiety about the profound way that a baby may affect relationships, lifestyle, and responsibilities. To initiate a discussion of this topic, you might say to the client, "Most women note some mood swings or changes in their emotions when they are pregnant. I'm wondering if you have noticed anything."

Because stressors and their intensity in a person's life often change during pregnancy, it is also appropriate to ask how things are going. You might ask, "What is the biggest stress in your life right now?" or "How much stress are you under?" You can use the "1-to-10 scale" and ask, "On a scale of 1 to 10, with 1 being awful and 10 being great, how are things going for you right now?" Women who report high stress, unexplained somatic symptoms, or irritability, alone or in combination, should be screened for depression.

Do not hesitate to ask about abuse if it seems appropriate. "In general, safety is the dominant concern in women's decisions to disclose or reveal abuse. As a woman's sense of safety changes, so do her disclosure decisions. For this reason, it is essential for women to be screened for abuse at multiple points of contact with the health care system" (Fishwick, 1998, p. 663).

Questions to Ask Periodically

Information about some symptoms, problems, and practices during pregnancy needs to be obtained only at intervals or as appropriate given the client's history.

Appetite, Heartburn, Constipation, Leg Cramps, Breast Tenderness, Fatigue, Faintness, Hemorrhoids, and Varicosities

It is easy to forget to ask about heartburn, constipation, leg cramps, fatigue, and so on because they are common and seem so "ordinary." Yet pregnant women often appreciate the clinician's awareness that these seemingly small things can make aspects of pregnancy unpleasant, if not difficult. Asking about these common discomforts of pregnancy also allows the midwife to ask about remedies the client is using and provides an opportunity to suggest safe relief measures.

Cravings

Consumption of nonfoods and excessive consumption of some food staples during pregnancy is known as pica, a poorly studied phenomenon that can occur in both pregnant and nonpregnant women. Some practitioners know of a special type of clay from the southern part of the United States that is often shipped to other parts of the country to be baked and eaten by pregnant women who have a craving for it. Pregnant women may also crave the smell of certain substances. Pica suggests iron deficiency (Blackwell & Hendrix, 2001) and can cause medical complications as well as pain, nausea, and vomiting (Adler & Olscamp, 1995).

Pregnant women seldom volunteer information about cravings because of feelings of guilt or fear that they have harmed their baby. Ask at intervals, "Do you ever crave to put something in your mouth or to smell anything? What about cravings for clay, ice, dirt, starch, cornstarch, or anything else?"

Sexual Activity, Desire, and Comfort

Information about sexual response, concerns, and/or questions that was obtained at the initial prenatal visit can be appropriate to bring up at subsequent prenatal visits. Women (and their partners) often appreciate knowing that a decrease in desire for sex, particularly in the first and third trimesters, is common. In early pregnancy, lack of interest is often due to breast tenderness, fatigue, morning sickness, and urinary frequency. Later in pregnancy, physical aches and a large abdomen may make coitus low on a woman's priority list. Alternate forms of showing affection may be helpful, as well as alternate coital positions late in pregnancy, particularly ones that allow the woman to control the depth and angle of penile thrusting, such as the woman astride.

At times, "desire discrepancies" may be a continuation of a situation existing before conception. In such cases, it may be helpful to determine whether the differences in desire for sex fall within the wide range considered normal or whether other factors play a role. Be sure to explore differences in how couples define such topics as frequency of intercourse. Statements such as, "We have sex all the time" and "We never have sex," can have very different meanings to different individuals. Factors that can affect libido include anxiety, depression, pain, fatigue, alcohol, a history of sexual abuse, and the quality of the couple's relationship. Sexual aversion is occasionally present. Invite women to talk about sex by asking, "Is there anything you wonder about in regard to having sex in general or having it when you are pregnant?"

Pregnant women should know that some men experience anxiety about having sexual relations with a woman who is pregnant, especially once the pregnancy begins to show. These men may be fearful of injuring the baby, or they may have personal or culturally derived concerns about having sex at this time. Men have also reported fearing that intercourse may be too noisy for the baby. They may be reassured to know that the baby is accustomed to hearing loud noises in the mother's body—liquids entering her stomach, air entering and leaving her lungs, her heartbeat, food moving through the intestines, and urination. A pregnant woman may be frustrated or confused about a man's reluctance to have intercourse and may attribute his reticence to her being unattractive because of weight gain, edema, and increased discharge. Couples should be alerted to the fact that fetal movement may occur during sexual activity.

Many women wonder about the safety of intercourse as the pregnancy advances. They should know that there are generally four reasons to avoid intercourse during pregnancy: vaginal bleeding, ruptured membranes, labor, and lack of desire. Additionally, women with a history of PTL are usually asked to avoid intercourse and orgasm from a few weeks before their earliest gestation at delivery until 37 weeks' gestation. Orgasm, associated with the release of oxytocin, can induce uterine contractions. Although these contractions usually subside about 30 minutes after orgasm, women who are predisposed to PTL may find that the contractions persist, and they may go into labor.

Sleep and Dreams

Getting to sleep and staying asleep can be problems during pregnancy. Nausea, vomiting, urinary frequency, and breast tenderness often explain why sleep is difficult in early pregnancy. Physical discomfort from fetal movement, a pendulous abdomen, leg cramps, joint pain, heartburn, backache, nonlabor contractions, and urinary frequency can make it difficult to get to sleep and stay asleep later in pregnancy. A small study of 33 pregnant women showed that significant changes in sleep occur as early as 11 weeks' gestation. In this study, a decrease in restorative, deep sleep did not improve until after the baby was born (Lee, Zaffke, & McAnany, 2000). Problems with sleep can also be a sign of depression, a possibility that should not be ignored.

Pregnant women also experience the same sleep problems encountered by the non-pregnant population. Strategies for limiting the amount of time spent awake include earplugs or a fan for background noise when external noise from co-sleepers causes wakefulness, requests for help from a partner in caring for children who get up at night, extra pillows to facilitate comfortable sleep positions, and daytime naps (Baratte-Beebe & Lee, 1999). These suggestions may be particularly appreciated at the end of pregnancy when the quality of sleep is at its lowest. Many women appreciate acknowledgment of their sleep problems and associated fatigue.

Unusual dreams and nightmares are occasional occurrences for some pregnant women and may be another source of sleep disturbance. Common themes include having an abnormal baby and not being a good mother. Women also seem to have recurring vivid images. Ask clients if they are aware of their dreams. Reassure them that dreaming about having an abnormal baby or of placing the baby in jeopardy by poor parenting does not mean that these will occur.

Pets

Because of the potential danger that the presence of some animals pose for babies or children, ask periodically if the family has a new pet. If a client indicated at the initial visit that there are potentially dangerous animals in the house or indicated that there were many animals that could pose hygiene problems, follow up on these reports.

Questions to Ask as Indicated by History

Use of Cigarettes

At each visit ask women who smoke about the number of cigarettes smoked per day. Consistent, repeated attention to cigarette smoking is critical to success. Be sure that the record of each client is flagged with a special sticker to indicate whether the client has never smoked, is a past smoker, or smokes currently. Assess smokers with the five A's at each visit (see Chapter 3).

Be sure to ask women who have quit smoking because of the pregnancy how they are doing. Heap on praise and support for the cessation. Determine whether smokers in the home have made efforts to quit. Begin or continue discussions of the high incidence of postpartum relapse and help the client think of ways to decrease her risk.

Ingestion of Alcoholic Beverages and Use of Illicit and Recreational Drugs

At each visit, women who have used alcohol or illicit drugs in the recent past (the last 2 years) or during the pregnancy should be asked about continued use. If a special program exists for women abusing these substances, transfer of care may be appropriate. However, women may not want to change their health care provider, and it may be best to ensure ongoing care in a nonspecialized program rather than have the client give up prenatal care altogether or participate inconsistently by changing.

❊ Conclusion

Beginning practitioners will find that a considerable amount of time is required to not only prepare for a return prenatal visit, but also to conduct a thorough visit. Do not compare yourself with experienced practitioners who may be able to review charts quickly or even walk into a client's room without having reviewed the chart at all. It is more important to develop a habit of systematically reviewing information and establishing a complete database than to work rapidly.

Novice practitioners should get in the habit of thoroughly documenting subjective and objective findings, the meaning of the findings, and the plan of care that evolved. Midwives in busy practices often omit this kind of charting. However, not only the legal climate in which we practice, but also the quality of care the expectant mother deserves depend on everyone involved in her care understanding the thinking that guided care to date.

By paying close attention to the significance of the objective data gathered at each prenatal visit and by asking the Healthy Pregnancy Questions to identify potential complications, you will be working toward ensuring a healthy outcome for both mother and baby.

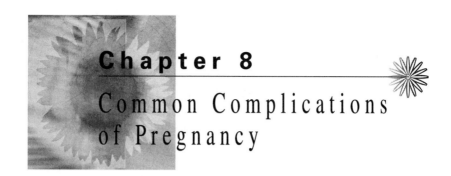

Chapter 8

Common Complications of Pregnancy

Nurse-midwives often manage or comanage a number of common complications of pregnancy. This chapter discusses tests of fetal well-being, as well as the following complications: hyperemesis gravidarum, iron deficiency anemia, preterm labor (PTL), lower urinary tract infection, size-date discrepancies, gestational diabetes mellitus (GDM), selected blood pressure (BP) elevations, and postdate pregnancies.

❋ Hyperemesis Gravidarum

Intractable vomiting in pregnancy is known as hyperemesis gravidarum and is associated with significant weight loss (more than 5% of body weight), dehydration, acidosis, alkalosis, and hypokalemia. Intravenous fluids and antiemetics are usually required for both outpatient and inpatient treatment. A diagnosis is based on a rapid maternal pulse (greater than 100 beats per minute [bpm]), poor skin turgor, moderate to heavy ketonuria, and weight loss. Helpful laboratory tests include a urinalysis to measure specific gravity and blood chemistries to identify electrolyte imbalance.

When moderate to heavy ketonuria is present, intravenous fluids are needed. "This requires appropriate amounts of sodium, potassium, chloride, lactate or bicarbonate, glucose, and water." (Cunningham et al., 2001, p. 1275). Whether to administer intravenous fluids in the outpatient or inpatient setting depends on how sick the client appears. In addition to the antiemetic drugs prochlorperazine (Compazine) and promethazine (Phenergan), oral diphenhydramine (Benadryl) and oral or intramuscular hydroxyzine (Vistaril) can be useful. Reglan, 10 mg orally given 30 minutes before eating, may also be used, as can Zofran, although the latter is still very expensive. Hyperalimentation may be necessary. Drugs frequently used to treat hyperemesis are listed in Box 8-1.

Intravenous hydration and/or hospitalization may need to be repeated as hyperemesis may persist for either brief or extended periods of time. Rapid treatment of hyperemesis with "moderately aggressive" intravenous hydration

---

Box 8.1

Drugs Used to Treat Nausea and Vomiting in Pregnancy

1. Diphenhydramine (Benadryl) 50 mg IV over 30 minutes every 6 hours
2. Promethazine (Phenergan): 12.5 to 25.0 mg orally or rectally every 4 hours
   or
   12.5 to 25 mg IV every 4 hours
3. Metoclopramide (Reglan): 10 mg orally 4 times daily 30 minutes before meals and at bedtime
   or
   5 to 10 mg IV every 8 hours
4. Hydroxyzine (Vistaril): 50 mg 30 minutes before meals and at bedtime with metoclopramide
5. Ondasetron (Zofran): 8 mg every 12 hours orally
   or
   8 mg IV over 15 minutes

---

and a progressive diet may be the best approach to breaking the cycle of vomiting. Since 1989, women with hyperemesis at Women's Hospital in Long Beach, California, have been treated with the approach described in Box 8-2. The rehospitalization rate with this approach has been reported as about 15% (Briggs, 1997a). In rare cases, women choose an abortion to control intractable vomiting.

"With persistent vomiting, appropriate steps should be taken to diagnose other diseases, such as gastroenteritis, cholecystitis, pancreatitis, hepatitis, peptic ulcer, pyelonephritis, and fatty liver of pregnancy" (Cunningham et al., 1997, p. 1147).

❋ Iron Deficiency Anemia

Complete blood count (CBC) values that fall outside the range of normal require accurate interpretation to distinguish iron deficiency anemia in pregnant women from other anemias and hemoglobinopathies. Here are some guidelines:

- If either the hemoglobin or the hematocrit is low, as well as the mean corpuscular volume (MCV) and mean corpuscular hemoglobin (MCH), treating for iron deficiency anemia is reasonable.
- If the MCV is not low, do not assume iron deficiency.
- If a low MCV does not respond to iron, look for hidden sources of bleeding. Request ferritin and transferrin saturation levels.

Box 8.2

Drug therapy for patients hospitalized with hyperemesis gravidarum

DROPERIDOL

Solution: 25 mg in 500 mL D5W (or NS) (0.05 mg/mL)
Start at 1 mg (20 mL) per hour (use infusion pump)
Give 1- to 2.5-mg bolus dose over 30 minutes if vomiting is present; if no vomiting, start without bolus dose
Dose adjustments: 0.25-mg (5 mL) increments every 4 hours (see text)

DIPHENHYDRAMINE

50 mg IV over 30 minutes every 6 hours (not prn)
First dose immediately prior to starting droperidol
Give extra dose at anytime if required (see text)

BENZTROPINE

Use if patient unresponsive to diphenhydramine (rare)
1 mg IV (or IM) initially, then 1 mg IV/IM every 12 hours

METOCLOPRAMIDE

10 mg po 1/2 hour before meals and at bedtime (4 × daily) (Give with hydroxyzine)

HYDROXYZINE

50 mg po 1/2 hour before meals and at bedtime (4 × daily) (Give with metoclopramide)

From Briggs, G. G. (1997). A guideline for testing hyperemesis gravidarum. *Contemporary OB/GYN, 42*(4), p. 74.
Reprinted with permission.

- If microcytic anemia is present without iron deficiency, consider thalassemia carrier status (Himes, 1998).
- If the client has African, Greek, Italian, Middle Eastern, Southern and Southeast Asian, or Pacific Island ancestry, offer carrier testing for thalassemia. ("Ethnic background is often impossible to determine by sight; patients must be asked" [Himes, 1998, p. 4.])

The treatment of iron deficiency anemia varies in regard to the amount of iron to take, whether supplements should also be taken, whether a slow-release preparation is acceptable, and how long to continue therapy. Recommendations include:

- Sixty to 120 mg of elemental iron per day, plus a multivitamin and mineral supplement containing 15 mg of zinc and 2 mg of copper—but no more than 250 mg of calcium and no more than 25 mg of magnesium per dose, considering both can interfere with iron absorption (Institute of Medicine, 1992)
- Two-hundred milligrams of elemental iron (Cunningham et al., 1997)
- Ferrous sulfate, 320 mg, one to three times a day with 500 mg of ascorbic acid with each dose (Kilpatrick & Laros, 1999)

The Institute of Medicine recommends a slow-release iron preparation with meals if persistent gastrointestinal symptoms are present. Other experts find no advantage in slow-release products (Cunningham et al., 2001). When anemia is identified, therapy should be continued after delivery for 3 (National Academy of Sciences, Institute of Medicine, 1992) to 6 months (Kilpatrick & Laros, 1999) to ensure that iron stores have been replenished.

The amount of elemental iron in iron tablets varies and is usually different than the dose of iron indicated on the label. Generally, iron deficiency anemia during pregnancy can be treated with 60 mg/dL of elemental iron, the amount contained in one ferrous sulfate tablet. While absorption is best on an empty stomach, gastrointestinal effects (mainly nausea and constipation) are less likely when the tablet is taken with meals. Liquid and chewable preparations can be prescribed for those who cannot take pills. Some liquid preparations contain alcohol and can stain teeth unless the client places it in the back of her mouth, dilutes it with juice, or brushes her teeth right after ingesting it. To increase absorption, iron tablets should be taken separately from prenatal vitamins

A response to iron therapy should be seen in 2 to 4 weeks. If no response is seen (an increase in the hemoglobin level of at least 1 g/dL or an increase in hematocrit of 3%), a ferritin level should be obtained, if not done previously, to be certain that the anemia is truly caused by iron deficiency. "The most useful single test for diagnosing iron deficiency anemia is the serum ferritin assay. Levels of this iron-storing glycoprotein reflect total body iron stores. Ferritin levels between 30 μg/L and 300 μg/L are considered normal; levels below 12 μg/L are typical of iron deficiency anemia" (Blackwell & Hendrix, 2001, p. 61).

Ferritin levels are rather expensive to obtain. Accordingly, it is reasonable to await a response from iron therapy before requesting this laboratory evaluation.

Hematocrit may not improve despite iron therapy when acute or chronic blood loss, parasites, a multiple pregnancy, a folate deficiency, pica, or chronic disease are factors. When no rise in hematocrit occurs, think of these possibilities as well as whether the client is taking the medication as prescribed.

Intrauterine growth restriction (IUGR) is not associated with maternal anemia until the maternal hematocrit reaches 24%. In fact, strange as it seems, women with mild anemia have bigger babies than nonanemic women. Why? Perhaps it is because less viscous blood perfuses the placenta better.

❈ Preterm Labor

Clients who report uterine contractions, abdominal cramping, continuous low back pain, pelvic pressure, or a change in vaginal discharge may be in premature labor. While benign contractions before 37 weeks are relatively common, it may be difficult to distinguish between true and false labor. If there are fewer than four to six contractions in an hour, the contractions will usually disappear with time. Often drinking two to four glasses of water will cause them to cease. When contractions continue despite hydration, or when other symptoms persist, the client should be evaluated for PTL. In gestations at or beyond 34 weeks, most institutions will not try to delay labor. Still, women with symptoms of PTL should be evaluated, because malpresentation occurs more frequently in earlier gestations.

Evaluation of a woman who reports signs and symptoms of PTL after 24 weeks' gestation and before 34 weeks can include a wet smear, to rule out vaginitis, and a fetal fibronectin (fFN) test (see Chapter 5) if the client has not had intercourse in the last 24 hours and there is no bleeding. Be sure to review previous ultrasound results to identify cervical length, remembering that a length shorter than 2.5 to 3 cm predisposes the client to PTL. If an ultrasound reporting cervical length findings has not been obtained and resources permit, order this examination.

After obtaining the fFN specimen, evaluate cervical dilatation (the internal cervical os) and effacement as well as the consistency of the cervix and its location (posterior/mid/anterior). Any woman with a dilated cervix prior to 28 weeks or a cervix dilated more than 2 cm between 28 and 34 weeks should be referred for further evaluation. A firm and posterior cervix is less likely to mean PTL.

A recent review of randomized controlled trials of tocolytics for women in PTL showed that although these drugs prolong pregnancy, they have not improved perinatal or neonatal outcomes, and they have significant side effects. Among those reported are maternal palpitations, nausea, chorioamnionitis, hyperglycemia, hypokalemia, dyspnea, vomiting, endometritis, and hypotension. At this time, it appears that the benefits to the infants are not enough to justify the risk to the mother, except to delay labor for 48 hours to allow administration of corticosteroids to speed up fetal lung maturity (Gyetvai, Hannah, Hodnett, & Ohlsson, 1999).

❈ Lower Urinary Tract Infection

Urinary tract infections (UTIs) during pregnancy are diagnosed based on a positive reagent strip test or a urine culture. Women without symptoms are said to have asymptomatic bacteriuria. Symptomatic infections are either cystitis (lower tract UTI) or pyelonephritis (upper tract UTI). Both asymptomatic bacteriuria (ASB) and cystitis can lead to pyelonephritis, with its potential for serious maternal morbidity. Whether ASB leads to anemia, preeclampsia, prematurity, or low birth weight is unproven (Gibbs & Sweet, 1999).

Drugs commonly used to treat lower tract UTIs in pregnant women include nitrofurantoin (Macrodantin) and trimethoprim/sulfamethoxazole (TMP/SMX). The usual dose of the former is 100 mg, orally, every 12 hours for 3 days. ACOG recommends a 3-day course of antibiotics to treat uncomplicated cystitis in an otherwise healthy woman, provided a follow-up culture is obtained approximately 10 days after completion of therapy. A positive repeat culture with the same organism "will necessitate a longer subsequent course of antibiotics and possibly long-term suppressive therapy" (ACOG, 1998a, p. 8). In practice, many clinicians commonly prefer a 7- to 10-day course of treatment.

Some clinicians avoid prescribing nitrofurantoin for African American women, as it can cause acute hemolytic anemia in people with glucose-6-phosphate dehydrogenase (G6PD) deficiency, a problem present in approximately 10% of the African American population. This occurrence, however, is rare (Mikhail & Anyaegbunam, 1995). No case of neonatal hemolytic anemia from in utero exposure to nitrofurantoin has been reported (ACOG, 1998a). Nitrofurantoin is a pregnancy class C drug.

Most clinicians refrain from using TMP/SMX (Bactrim, Cotrim, Septra) during the first trimester, because trimethoprim is a folate antagonist in bacteria (not in humans). Clinicians may also refrain from late third-trimester use (after 38 weeks' gestation), because theoretically, the sulfonamides can displace bilirubin, leading to newborn jaundice and, potentially, kernicterus. However, "despite many years of use of sulfonamides, there are no reported cases of neonatal kernicterus resulting from prenatal exposure at any gestational age" (ACOG, 1998a, p. 234). Trimethoprim is a pregnancy class C drug.

Amoxicillin, 500 mg orally, 3 times daily for 7 to 10 days, is a cheap and reasonable alternative to nitrofurantoin. However, it is not as good for resistant *Escherichia coli*, the most common urinary pathogen during pregnancy. A 3-day course is thought to be appropriate for an acute, uncomplicated UTI in pregnancy. This therapy also avoids potential fetal and neonatal side effects, and most patients tolerate the drug well.

Combination therapy with amoxicillin and clavulanate potassium (Augmentin) is an option, but it is expensive and has gastrointestinal side effects (Carson, Boggess, Colgan, Hooton, & Kerr, 2000). The American College of Obstetricians and Gynecologists recommends that ampicillin/amoxicillin not be used empirically, because up to one third of organisms isolated in UTIs are resistant to these drugs (ACOG, 1998a).

Group B streptococcus (GBS) in urine is a marker for GBS colonization of the genital tract and requires intravenous penicillin during labor to prevent GBS neonatal sepsis (Hager, Schuchat, Gibbs, Sweet, Mead, and Larsen, 2000). Not all clinicians consider GBS a urinary pathogen, and consequently, some physicians, choose not to treat GBS in urine during pregnancy.

If a pregnant woman has two lower tract UTIs during pregnancy, she should take a daily dose of a urinary antiseptic such as nitrofurantoin to prevent another UTI. The dosage in this case is 50 to 100 mg per day.

The standard of care in most communities is hospitalization of pregnant women with pyelonephritis to prevent the serious complications of respiratory insufficiency, PTL and birth, or septic shock. These recommendations were not based on clinical trials. Some evidence is available that outpatient treatment of selected women may be appropriate, that is if they can be observed while being hydrated, receiving initial parenteral doses of antibiotics, and awaiting results of laboratory testing. Subsequent close outpatient follow-up is essential (Wing, 1998).

❊ Size-Date Discrepancies

Fundal height that deviates from normal parameters requires an ultrasound examination to confirm or refute the clinical suspicion of a large or a small baby. The cause of aberrations in fetal growth should be identified as soon as possible, so that intervention to decrease the likelihood of perinatal morbidity or mortality can be initiated. However, the first action to be taken when a size-date discrepancy is noted is a thorough review of dating parameters. Remember that birth weight depends on uterine and genetic factors. Both low and high birth weights tend to recur in families, but the paternal side has little to do with birth weight (Creasy & Resnik, 1999).

Size Less Than Dates

Reliable clinical guidelines do not exist for identifying babies whose growth in utero does not conform to standard norms. Fundal height measurements and estimates of fetal weight based on abdominal palpation are known to be imprecise. Nevertheless, practitioners have developed rules of thumb found to be clinically useful.

Measurement Guidelines

A helpful rule of thumb states that the fundal height between 26 and 36 weeks' gestation should be within 2 cm of the gestational age in weeks. When the difference is 3 cm, clinicians can look at other parameters (such as maternal weight gain and fundal height measurements in previous pregnancies, when records are available) to determine whether an ultrasound examination is warranted. When the discrepancy between fundal height and gestational age is 4 cm, an ultrasound examination should be ordered. Reasons for fetal size being less than it should be given the gestational date include IUGR, transverse lie, a constitutionally small baby, and fetal death.

Creasy & Resnik note that repeated fundal height measurements by the same observer help document fetal growth but often lack sensitivity to pick up most cases of IUGR. Looking at data from a 1967 study, they also note that experienced obstetricians are able to estimate fetal weight to within 450 g (1 lb) only 40% of the time when babies weighed less than 2270 g (Creasy & Resnik, 1999).

Intrauterine Growth Restriction

IUGR is a significant cause of neonatal mortality and morbidity, as well as long-term neurologic and intellectual disabilities. It is associated with increased stillbirths, meconium aspiration syndrome, hypoglycemia, and asphyxia. Known causes of IUGR include congenital anomalies, congenital malformations, intrauterine infection with rubella or cytomegalovirus (and possibly varicella-zoster virus and HIV), multiple gestation, inadequate maternal nutrition, antiphospholipid syndrome, maternal vascular disease, and cigarette smoking (Creasy & Resnik, 1999).

IUGR is diagnosed when the ultrasound measurements are less than either the 10th percentile or the third percentile (two standard deviations from the mean). Institutions vary in the percentiles selected for diagnosis. Findings should be plotted on a fetal growth grid. Repeat ultrasound examinations to measure growth are often requested at 2- to 3-week intervals. A diagnosis of IUGR requires tests to determine fetal well-being.

Decisions about inducing labor should be made in consultation with a physician. The possibility of neonatal death from respiratory distress syndrome in preterm birth must be balanced with maternal health, tests of fetal well-being, and tests of fetal lung maturity.

Intrauterine growth restriction is one of the situations in which babies may benefit from mothers lying in the left lateral recumbent position as much as possible. This position increases blood flow to the uterus and, thereby, improves fetal oxygenation and nutrition. Clients should be asked to drink large quantities of liquids to ensure an adequate amount of amniotic fluid. Women who smoke should stop.

Size Greater Than Dates

Fundal height measurements are also used to detect fetal size that is greater than the gestational age, with discrepancies of more than 3 to 4 cm between 26 and 36 weeks' gestation again being significant, but this time the measurement is greater than the gestational age. Causes of size greater than dates include macrosomia, polyhydramnios, and a multiple gestation. Polyhydramnios is discussed in Chapter 5.

Macrosomia

Macrosomia is a result of fetal hyperinsulinemia, the baby's response to maternal hyperglycemia in which fetal insulin serves as a growth hormone. It is variously defined as a baby weighing more than 4000 g, more than 4500 g, or greater than the 90th percentile for age and gender. Although the risk for maternal and fetal morbidity increases between 4000 and 4500 g, the risk sharply increases beyond 4500 g (ACOG, 2000a). Mothers have an increased chance of cesarean birth or, if the birth is vaginal, an increased chance of trauma to maternal tissue. Macrosomic babies are more likely to have birth trauma and hypoglycemia. "Altered fetal body shape" may cause the higher incidence of shoulder dystocia with macrosomic babies of diabetic women. "These macrosomic infants tend to have greater total body fat, greater shoulder and upper-extremity circumferences, greater upper-extremity skin-fold measurements, and smaller head-to-abdominal circumference ratios than macrosomic infants of mothers without diabetes" (ACOG, 2000a, p. 3). Risk factors for macrosomia include a previous macrosomic baby, high prepregnancy weight, excessive pregnancy weight gain, multiparity, abnormal maternal glucose metabolism, and advanced gestational age. Maternal birth weight over 8 pounds (3600 g) has also been shown to increase the risk of giving birth to an infant weighing more than 4000 g (ACOG, 2000a).

Predicting Fetal Weight

As with small babies, clinical examinations to estimate fetal weight are not reliable predictors of fetal weight, particularly in macrosomic babies. Combining Leopold maneuvers and fundal height measurements results in better prediction of macrosomia than either assessment alone. Ultrasound examinations using biparietal diameter and abdominal circumference or biparietal diameter, abdominal circumference, and femur length can improve precision of fetal weight estimates of babies with birth weights ranging from 2080 to 4430 g (Chien, Owen, & Khan, 2000). However, "the superiority of ultrasound-derived estimates of fetal weight over clinical estimates has not been established. Indeed, parous women are able to predict the weight of their newborns as well as clinicians who use ultrasound measurements or Leopold's maneuvers" (ACOG, 2000a, p. 3).

Unfortunately, risk factors are likely to be absent when the baby is macrosomic. When macrosomia is suspected, consultation with a physician is appropriate. Induction of labor has not been found to decrease morbidity or mortality. The risk of cesarean delivery increases with induction, and the incidence of shoulder dystocia is not lowered. Prophylactic cesarean section may be con-sidered when fetal weight is estimated to be >5000 g, despite the fact that published reports do not support such a policy (ACOG, 2000a).

 HELPFUL HINT

Research has shown that between 37 and 40 weeks' gestation, babies gain approximately 25 g per day in utero (Owen, Donnet, Ogston, Christie, Howie, & Patel, 1996). Therefore, when an ultrasound is obtained late in pregnancy because of suspected macrosomia, add 25 g to the ultrasound-estimated fetal weight for every day between 37 and 40 weeks.

❖ Gestational Diabetes Mellitus

The management of women with GDM varies greatly. It usually involves 1) instituting a special diet, 2) identifying women who need insulin, and 3) watching for preeclampsia, the incidence of which may be as high as 10% in women with GDM. While diet therapy is recognized as an important facet of GDM management, optimal components of the diet are unknown.

GDM is monitored by measuring fasting and/or postprandial blood sugar levels at intervals. The norms for these tests and the frequency at which they should be performed are subjects of debate. In some practices, fasting blood sugars are measured at each clinic visit as long as the value is below 105 mg/dL. Some practitioners even choose to measure glucose levels only every 3 to 4 weeks if the fasting values are low (below 85 mg/dL). In other practices, women with GDM monitor blood glucose at home three or four times each day. Some practitioners prefer to follow glucose levels with a 2-hour post-prandial test, administered either alone or in addition to a fasting blood sugar. Norms for the 2-hour postprandial test vary between 120 mg/dL and 140 mg/dL. The American College of Obstetricians and Gynecologists recom-mends weekly glucose evaluations to identify women who will require insulin, that is women with persistent fasting blood sugar above 105 mg/dL or 2-hour plasma glucose levels above 120 mg/dL (ACOG, 1994). The term "persistent" can be defined as occurring on two or more occasions after 2 weeks of fol-lowing a diabetic diet.

When, or if, to begin tests of fetal well-being in women with GDM is also controversial. Some practices initiate twice-a-week nonstress testing at 40 weeks based on the knowledge that the placentas of women with GDM may deteriorate prematurely. (Remember that diabetes is a vascular disease.) The American College of Obstetricians and Gynecologists recommends that gestational diabetics requiring insulin, those with hypertension, and those with a history of delivering a stillborn baby have more intensive monitoring. However, "In most cases, women with GDM can be managed expectantly as long as fasting and postprandial glucose values remain normal" (ACOG, 1994, p. 6).

❊ Blood Pressure Elevations

Hypertension in pregnancy predisposes women to a variety of complications. Mothers may develop abruptio placentae, renal failure, liver failure, disseminated intravascular coagulation, cerebral hemorrhage, and blindness. Babies may have restricted growth from compromised placental function. Classification of hypertensive diseases of pregnancy, criteria for diagnosis, and guidelines for treatment have varied over time. The most recent guidelines (2000) are from the National High Blood Pressure Education Program Working Group on High Blood Pressure in Pregnancy. New recommendations include

- Classifying the hypertensive disorders in pregnancy as chronic hypertension, preeclampsia or eclampsia, preeclampsia superimposed upon chronic hypertension, and gestational hypertension. Transient hypertension, previously used interchangeably with gestational hypertension, is now reserved for BP elevations noted for the first time in pregnancy and not associated with preeclampsia. Normal BP should be found by 12 weeks postpartum.
- Ignoring BP increases of 30 mm Hg systolic and 15 mm Hg diastolic as diagnostic criteria (as did ACOG in 1996), although the working group did suggest vigilance in this group of women "especially if proteinuria and hyperuricemia (uric acid [UA] greater than or equal to 6 mg/dL) are also present" (National High Blood Pressure Education Program Working Group on High Blood Pressure in Pregnancy, 2000, p. 4)
- Eliminating edema as a criterion for diagnosis. Even rapid weight gain and facial edema, often regarded as ominous features of preeclampsia, were downgraded. "Although rapid weight increase and facial edema may indicate the fluid and sodium retention of preeclampsia, they are neither universally present nor uniquely characteristic of preeclampsia. These signs are, at most, a reason for closer monitoring of blood pressure and urinary protein" (National High Blood Pressure Education Program Working Group on High Blood Pressure in Pregnancy, 2000, pp. 17 to 18).
- Using Korotkoff 5, disappearance of sound, rather than Korotkoff 4, muffling of sound, for diastolic BP determinations.
- Basing a diagnosis of proteinuria on a 24-hour urine test "because of the discrepancy between random protein determinations and 24-hour urine protein in preeclampsia (which may be either higher or lower)" (National High

Blood Pressure Education Program Working Group on High Blood Pressure in Pregnancy, 2000, p. 4)
• Using 2.0 g or more of protein in 24 hours (2+ or 3+ on qualitative examination) to diagnose what has traditionally been called severe preeclampsia

Chronic Hypertension

Chronic hypertension is defined as a BP of 140/90 before pregnancy or before the twentieth week of pregnancy *or* a BP of 140/90 identified for the first time in pregnancy and persisting beyond 6 weeks postpartum. Obviously, the latter definition is not helpful during pregnancy, as it is not possible to wait until the postpartum period ends to decide about the significance of the elevation. Women who enter prenatal care after the 20th week of pregnancy can pose a diagnostic problem, because the physiologic fall in blood pressure that occurs in the first two trimesters can be exaggerated in women with chronic hypertension, thereby "masking" the diagnosis. Mild to moderate chronic hypertension (systolic BP of 140 to 179 mm Hg or diastolic BP of 90 to 109 mm Hg) in women with normal renal function is not likely to pose problems for pregnant women or their babies (National High Blood Pressure Education Program Working Group on High Blood Pressure in Pregnancy, 2000).

Baseline data that should be obtained when a pregnant woman with known or suspected chronic hypertension is seen for an initial prenatal visit include serum creatinine and serum uric acid levels to evaluate kidney function and a 24-hour urine protein measurement to determine if excessive protein is being excreted by the kidneys. Creatinine levels above 1.4 mg/dL increase the risk of fetal loss as well as the worsening of maternal disease (National High Blood Pressure Education Program Working Group on High Blood Pressure in Pregnancy, 2000).

Care of pregnant women with chronic hypertension requires vigilance for superimposed preeclampsia and poor fetal growth. Fetal growth should be determined by sonographic evaluation and fundal height measurements. The initial sonographic examination should be performed at 18 to 20 weeks' gestation. If subsequent fundal height measurements indicate appropriate growth and preeclampsia can be excluded, tests of fetal well-being are not indicated (National High Blood Pressure Education Program Working Group on High Blood Pressure in Pregnancy, 2000). However, if factors such as obesity or multiple examiners interfere with determination of fundal height, additional sonographic evaluations of growth should be performed at 28 to 32 weeks' gestation and monthly thereafter. Any diagnosis of IUGR requires tests of fetal well-being. Box 8-3 summarizes the recommendations for fetal monitoring in cases of mild to moderate chronic hypertension in pregnancy and normal renal function.

Box 8.3

Guidelines for the Evaluation and Management of Fetal Growth in Pregnant Women With Mild to Moderate Chronic Hypertension and Normal Renal Function

Management should include

1. Ultrasound for fetal size at 18 to 20 weeks
2. Fundal height assessment for fetal growth in the second half of pregnancy
3. Ultrasound examinations for growth at 28 to 32 weeks and then monthly until delivery if fetal growth cannot be determined with fundal height measurements (as in obese women or multiple examiners)
4. Test(s) of fetal well-being for IUGR

From NIH National High Blood Pressure Education Program Working Group on High Blood Pressure in Pregnancy (2000).

Gestational and Transient Hypertension

In the new classification of hypertensive disorders of pregnancy, gestational hypertension is defined as hypertension that develops for the first time after midpregnancy without the presence of proteinuria. If the preeclamptic laboratory test results (blood and 24-hour urine) are normal, the baby is growing well, and the amount of amniotic fluid is within the normal range, prenatal visits and checking of urine with a reagent strip for protein should occur twice weekly. Evaluation of amniotic fluid and nonstress testing should occur at diagnosis. If both tests are normal, repeat testing is needed only if there is "significant change in maternal condition" (National High Blood Pressure Education Program Working Group on High Blood Pressure in Pregnancy, 2000, p. 18). Box 8-4 contains guidelines for fetal monitoring in gestational hypertension.

Preeclampsia

Preeclampsia is a complex disease. The fundamental cause is unknown, and progression is poorly understood. Research points to some kind of placental trigger that causes endovascular damage and results in a systemic maternal reaction of various forms. "The endovascular damage leads to a loss of vascular autoregulation, significant vascular spasm, and vascular leakage (Katz, Farmer, & Kuller, 2000, p. 1392).

In its extreme form, preeclampsia affects the liver, kidneys, central nervous system, and blood coagulation mechanism. It may cause maternal convul-

Box 8.4

Fetal Monitoring in Gestational Hypertension

Gestational Hypertension (hypertension only without proteinuria with normal laboratory test results, and without symptoms)

- Estimation of fetal growth and amniotic fluid status should be performed at diagnosis. If results are normal, repeat testing only if there is significant change in maternal condition.
- Nonstress test (NST) should be performed at diagnosis. If NST is nonreactive, perform biophysical profile (BPP). If BPP value is eight or if NST is reactive, repeat testing only if there is significant change in maternal condition.

From NIH National High Blood Pressure Education Program Working Group on High Blood Pressure in Pregnancy. (2000). *Working Group Report on High Blood Pressure in Pregnancy.* Washington, DC: U.S. Department of Health and Human Services, p. 18.

sions (eclampsia), intracranial hemorrhage, pulmonary edema, and clotting disorders. Long thought to progress linearly from mild preeclampsia to severe preeclampsia and, finally, to eclampsia, this thinking may be a "flawed paradigm." In a retrospective analysis of 53 pregnancies complicated by eclampsia, 60% of the women had seizures as the first sign of preeclampsia (Katz, Farmer, & Kuller, 2000). Two decades ago, reviewing data from 67 cases of eclampsia, researchers noted that prior to convulsing, 21% of the women had a diastolic BP below 90 mm Hg, and 21% had no proteinuria (Sibai, McCubbin, Anderson, Lipshitz, & Dilts, 1981).

Preeclampsia occurs most frequently in women with one of the following circumstances:

A first pregnancy
More than one fetus
Pregnancy by a new sexual partner
Chronic hypertension
Diabetes
Obesity
Maternal autoimmune disorders
Renal disease
Family history of severe preeclampsia
Primipaternity
High BP before 34 weeks in a previous pregnancy
A mother or sister who has been eclamptic or severely preeclamptic
Age younger or older than usual. (The age curve for risk is J-shaped.)

Attempts to prevent preeclampsia have been ineffective. Results of at least 15 randomized trials using antihypertensives or diuretics, seven placebo-controlled trials using calcium supplementation, seven multicenter trials using low-dose aspirin, as well as reports describing the use of magnesium, fish oil, and zinc indicate that neither dietary supplementation nor pharmacologic therapy is effective in the prevention of preeclampsia (Sibai, 1998). Increasing protein intake, a practice common among some midwives, is not helpful.

Elevated BP is the usual signpost for special care. The further development of proteinuria and symptoms of systemic involvement (headache, visual disturbances, disorientation, nausea and vomiting, liver involvement [epigastric pain, right upper quadrant abdominal pain from swelling of the liver capsule, hepatic hemorrhage, or liver rupture], and general malaise) require immediate attention. Some clinicians feel that hyperreflexia contributes to the diagnosis. However, the presence, absence, and degree of hyperreflexia have not been shown to contribute to the diagnosis (ACOG, 1996a; Roberts, 1999).

An elevated BP or proteinuria must always raise the question of preeclampsia. Blood and urine tests should be performed to distinguish between preeclampsia and chronic or gestational hypertension and, if preeclampsia is present, to assess the severity of the disease. Unfortunately, the use of these tests varies widely, as do the norms used to define abnormality. Serum creatinine and uric acid assess kidney involvement, aspartate aminotransferase (AST) assesses kidney and liver involvement, hematocrit identifies the extent of hemoconcentration, and a platelet count identifies potential clotting problems. As in chronic hypertension, a 24-hour urine test should be performed to determine the amount of protein being excreted. Additional tests should be ordered in the case of severe disease. These tests and the rationale for performing them are summarized in Table 8-1. Table 8-2 contains normal pregnancy values for selected tests requested in the evaluation of a woman who develops hypertension during the second half of pregnancy. "It is important to recognize that in women with preeclampsia, one or more abnormalities may be present even when blood pressure deviation may be minimal" (National High Blood Pressure Education Program Working Group on High Blood Pressure in Pregnancy, 2000).

Unfortunately, laboratory tests to either confirm a diagnosis of preeclampsia or identify severity have poor sensitivity (the number of true positives identified by a test) and poor positive predictive value (the likelihood that a patient with a positive test will actually have the disease), and therefore, they have limited value in clinical practice. A recent study of 445 women with severe preeclampsia and eclampsia found no laboratory values that would predict either placental abruption or eclampsia (Witlin, Saade, Mattar, & Sibai, 1999).

TABLE 8.1 Laboratory Tests and the Rationale for Performing Them in Women Who Develop Hypertension After Midpregnancy

Test	Rationale
Hemoglobin and hematocrit	Hemoconcentration supports diagnosis of preeclampsia and is an indicator of severity. Values may be decreased, however, if hemolysis accompanies the disease.
Platelet count	Thrombocytopenia suggests severe preeclampsia.
Quantification of protein excretion	Pregnancy hypertension with proteinuria should be considered preeclampsia (pure or superimposed) until it is proved otherwise.
Serum creatinine level	Abnormal or rising serum creatinine levels, especially in association with oliguria, suggest severe preeclampsia.
Serum uric acid level	Increased serum uric acid levels suggest the diagnosis of preeclampsia.
Serum transaminase levels	Rising serum transaminase levels suggest severe preeclampsia with hepatic involvement.
Serum albumin, lactic acid dehydrogenase, blood smear, and coagulation profile	For women with severe disease, these values indicate the extent of endothelial leak (hypoalbuminemia), presence of hemolysis (lactic acid dehydrogenase level increase, schizocytosis, spherocytosis), and possible coagulopathy, including thrombocytopenia.

Adapted from NIH National High Blood Pressure Education Program Working Group on High Blood Pressure in Pregnancy. (2000). *Working Group Report on High Blood Pressure in Pregnancy.* Washington, DC: U.S. Department of Health and Human Services, p. 10.

Women with mild preeclampsia are managed either at home or in the hospital, although an initial in-hospital assessment may be made. At-home management usually includes daily fetal movement counts, daily monitoring of BP, and daily protein testing of a clean-catch urine specimen with a reagent strip (despite the random nature of protein excretion). Decreased activity can be advised instead. The purported benefits of bed rest include the reduction of

TABLE 8.2 Normal Laboratory Values for Selected Tests Used in the Evaluation of Clients Who Develop Hypertension in the Second Half of Pregnancy

Test	Values
Uric acid	<5.0 mg/dL at 28 weeks, <5.4 mg/dL at term
AST	<40 IU/mL, (Mild elevation = 50–200 IU/mL)
Creatinine	<0.8 mg/dL
Platelets	>150,000/cc or 100,000/cc to 150,000/cc if a value obtained before the development of signs and symptoms was in the same range
Hematocrit	<38%

edema, improved fetal growth, and prevention of progression to severe preeclampsia. However, randomized trials to support these outcomes are lacking. In addition, maintaining a side-lying position for extended periods of time can be stressful to the expectant mother and does not make a significant difference in perinatal outcome when *normal fetal growth* is present. The left-lateral position is probably most useful when the baby is not growing well.

The client should be instructed to immediately report 1+ or greater proteinuria on a clean-catch urine specimen, as well as any headaches not relieved with rest or acetaminophen, persistent scotoma, epigastric pain, right upper quadrant pain, disorientation, abdominal pain, nausea or vomiting, and "not feeling right." Blood tests should be repeated twice weekly.

Ultrasound examinations to measure fetal growth should be ordered when fundal height measurements and estimates of fetal weight are either outside accepted norms or are difficult to assess (as in maternal obesity). Birth size decreases with 1) increasing severity of preeclampsia, 2) early-onset disease (at or before 32 weeks), and 3) recurrent disease. A recent study from Norway reported a 12% reduction in expected birth weight when severe preeclampsia was diagnosed and a 23% reduction with early-onset disease. No correlation was found in mild preeclampsia (Odegard, Vatten, Nilsen, Salvesen, & Austgulen, 2000). Recommendations for tests of fetal well-being include evaluation of amniotic fluid status every 3 weeks and weekly non-stress test (NST), biophysical profile (BPP), or both as long as the results are normal and the maternal condition is unchanged (National High Blood Pressure Education Program Working Group on High Blood Pressure in Pregnancy, 2000). Box 8-5 summarizes fetal monitoring recommendations in preeclampsia.

Box 8.5

Fetal Monitoring in Preeclampsia

Mild preeclampsia (mild hypertension, normal platelet count, normal liver enzyme values, and no maternal symptoms)

- Estimation of fetal growth and amniotic fluid status should be performed at diagnosis. If results are normal, repeat testing every 3 weeks.
- NST, BPP, or both should be performed at diagnosis. If NST is reactive or if BPP value is eight, repeat weekly. Testing should be repeated immediately if there is abrupt change in maternal condition.
- If estimated fetal weight by ultrasound is <10th percentile for gestational age or if there is oligohydramnios (amniotic fluid index ≤5 cm), then testing should be performed at least twice weekly.

From NIH National High Blood Pressure Education Program Working Group on High Blood Pressure in Pregnancy. (2000). *Working Group Report on High Blood Pressure in Pregnancy.* Washington, DC: U.S. Department of Health and Human Services, p. 18.

When mild preeclampsia is diagnosed at term, induction of labor usually is recommended because only delivery of the baby permits resolution of the disease process. Women with severe preeclampsia should always be hospitalized with comanagement by or referral to a physician. Severe preeclampsia is distinguished from mild by the severity of the BP (systolic BP of 160 or more; a diastolic BP of 110 or more), the amount of proteinuria (2.0 g or more in 24 hours or 2+ or greater on dipstick evaluation), serum creatinine >1.2 mg/dL, platelet count less than 100,000 cells/mm³, elevated hepatic enzymes (alanine aminotransferase [ALT] or AST), and/or the presence of subjective symptoms (persistent headaches, visual disturbances, epigastric pain, right upper quadrant abdominal pain, nausea and vomiting, or "not feeling well"). These findings necessitate hospitalization. These indications for hospitalization are summarized in Box 8-6.

"Disease severity varies not only from patient to patient but also from organ system to organ system within an individual. One woman may have oliguria but no change in liver functions, whereas another may have severe hypertension and minimal proteinuria" (Katz, Farmer, & Kuller, 2000, p. 1392).

Because preeclampsia is not preventable at the present time, proper respect for signs and symptoms of the disease is essential. Common diagnostic mistakes include:

- Ignoring a BP elevation
- Not testing for proteinuria or not taking it seriously when it is found

Box 8.6

Indications for Hospitalization for Women with Elevated Blood Pressure in the Second Half of Pregnancy

1. Systolic blood pressure of 160 or more
2. Diastolic blood pressure of 110 or more
3. Proteinuria of 2.0 g or more in 24 hours or 2+ or greater on dipstick evaluation
4. Serum creatinine >1.2 mg/dL
5. Platelet count less than 100,000 cells/mm^3
6. Elevated hepatic enzymes (ALT or AST)
7. Persistent headaches, visual disturbances, epigastric pain, right upper quadrant abdominal pain, nausea and vomiting, or "not feeling well"

From NIH National High Blood Pressure Education Program Working Group on High Blood Pressure in Pregnancy. (2000). *Working Group Report on High Blood Pressure in Pregnancy.* Washington, DC: U.S. Department of Health and Human Services.

- Misinterpreting the cause of abdominal pain, nausea, vomiting (which are symptoms of gallbladder disease and gastroenteritis as well as preeclampsia), and "just not feeling well"
- Failing to look for clotting derangements (Redman & Walker, 1992)

Remember four things about preeclampsia: it is largely silent, it gets progressively worse, it can become fulminating overnight, and it is easy to miss because the symptoms can be so variable.

The HELLP Syndrome

The hemolysis, elevated liver enzymes, and low platelets (HELLP) syndrome is a form of severe preeclampsia or eclampsia most often seen in a partial form (i.e., hemolysis and/or low platelets, and/or elevated liver enzymes). BP is not always elevated, and proteinuria may be minimal. Any woman in the third trimester who reports epigastric or right upper quadrant pain should be seen immediately, as this condition is very serious and requires hospitalization and physician management. The diagnosis of HELLP is based on laboratory findings.

Chronic Hypertension With Superimposed Preeclampsia

Women with chronic hypertension may also develop preeclampsia. Because of increased danger for both mother and baby when it occurs, clinicians must be watchful for indicators. These include the following (National High Blood Pressure Education Program Working Group on High Blood Pressure in Pregnancy [2000]):

- Proteinuria (0.3 g [300 mg] or greater) in a hypertensive woman who did not demonstrate proteinuria before 20 weeks' gestation
- Hypertension and proteinuria before 20 weeks' gestation
- Sudden increase in proteinuria
- Sudden increase in BP
- Platelet count below 100,000 cells/mm³
- An increase in ALT or AST to abnormal levels

Eclampsia

Eclampsia is "the new onset of convulsions during pregnancy or postpartum, unrelated to other cerebral pathologic conditions, in a woman with preeclampsia" (Mattar & Sibai, 2000, p. 307). Traditionally, seizures before 20 weeks' gestation or after the 10th postpartum day have been attributed to causes other than preeclampsia. However, in a recent review of 399 eclamptic patients, the authors found six women who convulsed before 20 weeks' gestation. Of 110 women with postpartum eclampsia, 62% convulsed more than 48 hours after delivery (within 3 to 23 days). Women with postpartum eclampsia had "significantly higher incidences of neurologic deficits" than women with prenatal or intrapartal eclampsia. The authors concluded that women with severe preeclampsia at less than 32 weeks' gestation should be cared for in tertiary care facilities. They also noted that "the development of cerebral complaints (headaches, visual changes, confusion), right upper-quadrant pain, or epigastric pain should be considered an indication for delivery, because these symptoms may herald the development of incipient convulsions" (Mattar and Sibai, 2000, p. 311).

❋ Postdates

As pregnancy progresses beyond 40 weeks' gestation, the ability of the placenta to function optimally in support of the baby's needs declines. Tests for fetal well-being are usually initiated at 41 or 41½ weeks and may include an NST, an amniotic fluid index (AFI), and a BPP. In the management of babies considered to be postdates, opinion varies regarding the optimum frequency of AFI evaluations. While determinations are often made in association with twice-weekly nonstress testing, Moore suggests that the measurement needs to be repeated only weekly when the AFI is greater than 8 cm (Moore, 1997).

Because of data that conclude that pregnancies carried beyond 42 completed weeks of gestation put babies at risk, labor is often induced at this time. However, the optimum time for recommending induction of labor is unclear. The Cochrane database concluded that offering induction to women who have reached 41 weeks' gestation is "reasonable." "A policy of induction of labor after 41+ weeks' gestation slightly reduces the risk of perinatal death, in the range of one death saved for each 500 inductions" (Enkin et al., 2000, p. 238).

However, data from a study that examined pregnancy outcomes at 40, 41, and 42 weeks' gestation in a large sample of low-risk women concluded, "interventions at 41 weeks' gestation are unwarranted because of a lack of proven benefit ... Larger randomized studies must be done before labor induction is done routinely in pregnancies that reach 41 weeks" (Alexander, McIntire, & Leveno, 2000, p. 293). The American College of Obstetricians and Gynecologists recommends induction of labor at 42 weeks' gestation (ACOG, 1997c).

Midwives must evaluate each situation individually when faced with needing to deliver a baby. Induction of labor works best when the cervix is "ripe" (soft, anterior, effaced, and dilated) and the presenting part is low in the pelvis. The Bishop score uses these four cervical characteristics and the station of the presenting part to predict the likelihood of a successful induction (Tables 8-3A and 8-3B). A Bishop score of 9 or 10 means that induction will probably be successful. With a score of 5 or less, induction with oxytocin is often ineffective.

Induction carries with it the possibility of a cesarean birth when the induction "fails." Both cervical condition and parity influence this failure rate. "Nulliparous women with Bishop scores 0 to 3 have a 23-fold increased cesarean rate as compared to nulliparous women with higher Bishop scores, whereas multiparous women with low Bishop scores have a sixfold increased

TABLE 8.3A The Bishop Score

	0	1	2	3
Dilatation	0	1–2	3–4	5–6
Effacement	0–30%	40–50%	60–70%	80%
Station	−3	−2	−1	+1
Consistency of cervix	Firm	Medium	Soft	
Position	Posterior	Midline	Anterior	

TABLE 8.3B Modified Bishop's Score

	Centimeters	Score
Station	−3	0
	−2	1
	−1 or 0	2
	+1 or +2	3
Dilatation	0	0
	1–2	2
	3–4	4
	>4	6
Length of cervix	3	0
	2	1
	1	2
	0	3

failure rate and a twofold increased cesarean rate as compared to multiparous women with higher Bishop scores" (Poma, 1999, p. 658).

When the Bishop score is low, it is prudent to try to "ripen the cervix" to increase the chances of the induction working and to avoid an increased risk of cesarean birth. The cervix may be ripened by a variety of medical methods, some of which are also used for induction. Midwives usually prefer to try other approaches to inducing labor. Recommendations include penis-in-vagina intercourse, nipple stimulation, an orgasm, castor oil, an enema, or acupuncture. The effectiveness of these methods is not well documented, and randomized controlled trials are generally absent. However, experienced clinicians often report some success with each approach.

Vaginal intercourse may effect cervical ripening because of the deposit of prostaglandins from the seminal vesicles into the vagina. Orgasm may be effective because uterine contractions frequently occur following climax. The combination of intercourse, orgasm, and nipple stimulation that may be part of lovemaking may be more effective than either approach by itself. Some clinicians prefer to avoid nipple stimulation when fetal monitoring cannot occur, because of the possibility of strong and frequent contractions that may be dangerous to the baby.

Castor oil alone or in combination with an enema has long been used to induce labor. The mechanism of action is unknown. In the 1950s and 1960s, a common hospital protocol called for castor oil followed by 1000 cc's of a soap solution enema. A recent study of 52 women at 40 to 42 weeks' gestation with a Bishop score of 4 or less and no uterine contractions showed that 30 women who took 2 oz of castor oil went into labor within 24 hours, while only two women in the no-castor-oil group went into labor within this time (Garry, Figueroa, Guillame, & Cucco, 2000).

Anecdotally, castor oil is more effective once the due date has passed, contractions are present, and/or the cervix is "somewhat" favorable. It is rarely effective before the due date unless the cervix is well dilated (3 or more cm). Clients should be told that they might experience abdominal cramps and diarrhea rather than labor. It is best to instruct the expectant mother to take the castor oil concoction early in the morning. If she takes it at night, she is likely to lose a night's sleep because of frequent trips to the bathroom. Castor oil "recipes" are numerous. Four common recommendations can be found in Box 8-7.

In addition to activities that can be recommended to initiate labor, clinicians may "sweep" the membranes to induce cervical change. Sweeping the membranes is also called "stripping" the membranes, but sweeping seems to be a better descriptor because of the negative connotation of the word "stripping." The point of the procedure is to stimulate the release of prostaglandins, the mechanism thought to be the vehicle by which cervical change occurs.

Various techniques to sweep the membranes have been described, but all require some degree of dilatation of the internal cervical os. One technique is to insert a gloved finger as far into the os as possible, encircling the interior portion as if dialing a phone number with a rotary telephone. Two studies reporting the effect of membrane sweeping showed a statistically significant increase in spontaneous labor when performed at 38 weeks (Gupta, Vasishta, Swahney, & Ray, 1998) and between 41 and 42 weeks' gestation (El-Torkey & Grant, 1992). A recent study from Singapore reported that membrane

---

Box 8.7

Castor Oil Recipes

1. Four ounces of castor oil, followed by another 2 ounces 4 hours later. The castor oil can be mixed with a milkshake if the emulsified form is not available. Or put the castor oil in orange juice and place a straw at the separation line. Let the straw mix the castor oil and orange juice as it is sipped (from Elizabeth Gabzdyl, CNM, Seattle).
2. Four ounces of castor oil in 4 ounces of orange juice. Add ½ teaspoon of baking soda immediately before swallowing to reduce the oily feel of the liquid.
3. Two ounces of castor oil in 2 ounces of orange juice every 2 hours and repeat three times
4. Two ounces of castor oil in a root beer float

sweeping in conjunction with labor induction resulted in shorter induction-to-labor intervals (Foong, Vanaja, Tan, & Chua, 2000). Directions vary for the number of "sweeps" (one to two in the literature but many more in actual practice) and depth of insertion of the finger(s) into the lower uterine segment (up to 2 to 3 cm in the literature). Sweeping may be performed according to a variety of frequency schedules that range from daily to weekly. The frequency most likely to be effective is unknown and probably depends on gestational age and the Bishop score at the start of sweeping.

Theoretically, risks to the procedure include infection, accidental rupture of membranes, and bleeding from a low-lying placenta or placenta previa whose existence was unknown before the procedure was initiated. Many clients have a small amount of bloody show after the procedure and should be warned in advance that this might occur. No increases in maternal or neonatal morbidity have been reported.

Herbal preparations and homeopathic solutions for inducing labor appeal to some midwives, as they are believed to be safe, and effective. Additionally, they are cheap, available for home use, and less interventionist (McFarlin, Gibson, O'Rear, & Harman, 1999). Blue and black cohosh are commonly recommended for induction of labor (Allaire, Moos, & Wells, 2000). The lack of studies documenting either safety or effectiveness of herbal products, the lack of standardization, and the possibility of product contamination make recommendation of these products ill advised. For example, increased incidence of meconium-stained amniotic fluid and transient fetal tachycardia has been noted with blue cohosh (McFarlin, Gibson, O'Rear, & Harman, 1999), as has one instance of acute myocardial infarction in a newborn (Jones & Lawson, 1998). A case of severe neurologic damage has been found in the infant of a mother who took a combination of blue and black cohosh to induce labor (Gunn & Wright, 1996). Until prospective studies document both the safety and efficacy of products recommended in herbal therapy and homeopathy, these products should be considered contraindicated.

Prior to any elective induction, data documenting a gestational age of at least 39 weeks must be present. Acceptable criteria for documentation are in Box 8-8.

Box 8.8

Criteria for Documentation of Gestational Age

1. FHTs heard by fetoscope for 20 weeks or by Doppler for 30 weeks
2. Positive pregnancy test for 36 weeks
3. Ultrasound: crown-rump at 6 to 12 weeks or other measurements at 13 to 20 weeks supporting 39 weeks (ACOG, 1999h)

✳ Conclusion

Midwifery management of some complications of pregnancy will depend on the protocols or guidelines established by each practice. Some midwifery practices will be more comfortable with complications than others.

Chapter 9
Health Education at the Prenatal Revisit

Health education is an essential part of each prenatal revisit. What is important to discuss varies according to gestational age and the circumstances of the client and her family. Certainly, danger signs (see Chapter 6) are important, as are recommendations specific to a common discomfort of pregnancy or a complication. Other topics for discussion are breastfeeding, family planning, circumcision, planning for pediatric care, preparation for labor and birth, preparation of other children in the family for the new baby, and ceremonies to honor the pregnant woman. This chapter addresses these topics and concludes with a discussion of appropriate use of health education material.

❋ Breastfeeding

There should be no doubt that breast milk is best for most babies. Research has consistently shown that human milk has health, developmental, psychological, social, economic, and environmental benefits for human babies—a lower incidence of diarrhea, respiratory infections, otitis media, bacterial meningitis, urinary tract infections, sudden infant death syndrome (SIDS), allergic diseases, and digestive diseases (American Academy of Pediatrics, 1997). Mothers who breastfeed experience less postpartum bleeding, faster involution of the uterus, less loss of blood during lactation amenorrhea, delayed return of ovulation, and less risk of ovarian and premenopausal breast cancer.

In the United States, the only situations in which breastfeeding is not in the baby's best interest are in the cases of 1) an infant with galactosemia; 2) an infant whose mother uses illegal drugs; 3) an infant whose mother has untreated, active tuberculosis; 4) an infant whose mother is infected with HIV (American Academy of Pediatrics, 1997); and 5) maternal use of a prescribed drug that contraindicates breastfeeding. These contraindications are listed in Box 9-1.

Most women who give birth in hospitals leave the hospital breastfeeding their newborns. However, few are breastfeeding 6 months later. The exact reasons are unknown. We do know however, that for many women, breastfeeding

Box 9.1

Contraindications to Breastfeeding in the United States

1. An infant with galactosemia*
2. An infant whose mother uses illegal drugs*
3. An infant whose mother has untreated, active tuberculosis*
4. An infant whose mother is infected with HIV*
5. Maternal use of a prescribed drug that contraindicates breastfeeding

*American Academy of Pediatrics, 1997.

is neither automatic nor natural. It can be difficult, particularly when the baby is irritable and hungry. Prenatal education can help women prepare realistically for the breastfeeding experience. Preparation might include discussions of

- The benefits of breastfeeding for infants and mothers
- Common, early problems (engorgement and sore nipples)
- Variability in infant temperament
- Variability in sucking patterns
- The need for help with household chores after giving birth
- The impact of sleepless nights
- The possibility of inconsistent advice from professionals
- The importance of avoiding bottles initially
- The mother's feelings should a professional need to touch the mother's breasts
- Feelings about nursing in front of others
- Leaking breasts
- Community resources for information and support
- Books that may be helpful

While several factors may be associated with early discontinuation of breastfeeding, three variables are of particular significance: maternal age less than 20 years, lack of confidence about continuing breastfeeding, and the mother's perception that the baby enjoys the bottle (Ertem, Votto, & Leventhal, 2001). While the latter issue is not likely to arise until the baby starts to feed, midwives can take advantage of this knowledge to spend extra time with younger clients and help all expectant mothers feel confident about their abilities to nurse their babies.

Fortunately, most women know there are compelling reasons to breastfeed, and they plan to nurse their babies. Those who choose to bottle-feed do so for a variety of reasons. Some women are uncomfortable with the idea of breastfeeding, perceiving it to be embarrassing, painful, inconvenient, energy draining, and time consuming. Some women believe they will never have a chance to get away from the baby or that their partner will be deprived of an opportunity to participate in a meaningful way in the baby's care. Some women see bottle-feeding as a status symbol or, because they will be returning to work, feel they should just start with the bottle. Some women don't like the feel of a baby nursing, and some may have had friends who tried to breastfeed with cracked and bleeding nipples. Some have had a bad experience trying to nurse a previous baby or may be living a chaotic life that allows no time to sit and feed a baby.

What should clinicians do when confronted with a woman who is reluctant or unwilling to try breastfeeding? First determine the mother's reason for preferring bottle-feeding. Ask the client, "Can you share with me how you came to the decision to bottle-feed?" If a previous breastfeeding experience was unsuccessful, be sympathetic with her reluctance to try again. Her lack of success may be directly related to the support and help she received in the initial days of nursing. Ask the client if she would be willing to try again if support and encouragement were likely to be available after the birth of the baby.

Correcting misinformation about breastfeeding will help some women give breastfeeding a try. After that, acknowledging that the client is best equipped to make the best decision for herself and her baby in regard to breastfeeding—and accepting this decision—is the best action to take. Pushing a woman to breastfeed when she does not wish to do so rarely results in a successful breastfeeding experience. Emphasizing the benefits of breastfeeding while devaluing a woman's personal reasons for not wanting to nurse her baby can cause the client to have feelings of guilt that are neither fitting nor helpful. A supportive, considerate response to a woman's desire to bottle-feed her baby, combined with thoughtful and attentive care, may make the client willing to try breastfeeding. Ask the client again later in pregnancy if she would like to reconsider her decision.

❋ Family Planning

Discussions about family planning should be initiated prenatally to allow families to discuss the many facets of decision making in regard to this topic. Good decision making involves an understanding of contraceptive effectiveness, side effects, contraindications, cost, noncontraceptive benefits, and, for those wishing a subsequent pregnancy, the return of fertility. These discussions are best spread out across the prenatal period and can be accompanied by appropriate printed material that has been personally evaluated by the midwife for content and literacy level. Insight into the client's preferences can be gained by asking her about her previous experience with any family planning method, as well as what she has heard from her partner, family, and friends.

HELPFUL HINT

Ask the pharmaceutical representative of the company that sells the intrauterine device (IUD) for a nonsterile sample. Keep the IUD in your lab coat pocket. When discussing family planning methods with clients, pull the IUD out of your pocket as you say, "Have you ever thought about an IUD?" (This approach assumes, of course, that an IUD is not contraindicated.) Most women who have not seen one before will comment, "I didn't know it was so small!"

Differentiate between women who wish to conceive in the future and women who do not wish another pregnancy. Women who state that they do not wish to give birth to more children should be asked if they have considered a permanent method of birth control. If a permanent method is being contemplated, information should be provided about both bilateral tubal ligation (BTL) and vasectomy. BTL is commonly performed within 24 hours of delivery. However, some families delay this procedure for a time because of the concern for neonatal problems and the slight risk of SIDS.

Sterilization regret is an important topic to discuss when women express a desire for permanent sterilization. A prospective, multicenter cohort study involving 11,232 women between the ages of 18 and 44 found poststerilization regret most common when tubal sterilization was performed postpartally in women under 30 years of age or within 1 year of a birth (Hillis, Marchbanks, Tylor, & Peterson, 1999). Certainly, most women who choose permanent sterilization are happy with their decisions. Still, a discussion about the possibility of regret is always appropriate. Further discussion of family planning methods can be found in Chapter 13.

❋ Circumcision

Both parents and midwives often have strong opinions about circumcision. While some feel the practice is barbaric, unnecessary, and unnatural, all clinicians have an obligation to provide unbiased and accurate information to parents so that their decision is an informed one. Most circumcision procedures are performed for social, cultural, or religious reasons.

The frequency of penile problems with and without circumcision is unknown. The main medical benefit lies in the decreased risk of urinary tract infection in the first year of life, a 1 in 1000 chance when a baby has been circumcised versus a 1 in 100 chance for the uncircumcised baby. Circumcision also prevents phimosis (tight foreskin), which occurs only in uncircumcised males and decreases the incidence of penile cancer. Complications of this circumcision, thought to be between 0.2% and 0.6% (American Academy of Pediatrics, 1999), are usually minor and consist primarily of slight bleeding and infection, although the potential for serious bleeding and infection exists. Removal of too much foreskin as well as other trauma to the penis has been reported.

While recognizing the potential medical benefits of circumcision, the American Academy of Pediatrics feels that available data do not support a recommendation to routinely circumcise newborns. The academy recommends that parents "determine what is in the best interest of the child" (American Academy of Pediatrics, 1999, p. 1).

❋ A Visit to the Baby's Health Care Provider

When clients have a choice about pediatric care, encourage the parents to schedule an appointment with potential health care providers. The American Academy of Pediatrics encourages its members to support a variety of visits during the prenatal period. Topics for discussion with a pediatrician include "office hours, telephone hours, fees, hospital affiliations, coverage for night, weekend, and emergency care, and what arrangements can be made if the infant is born at a hospital where the pediatrician is not on staff" (American Academy of Pediatrics, 1996, p. 142).

❋ Planning for Labor and Birth

Every woman deserves an opportunity to talk about her hopes, fears, and plans for the birth of the baby. The role of the midwife is to work with each pregnant woman to help her determine what she feels is most appropriate for her. Expectations and intentions about a particular kind of birth experience will vary based on many factors. Among these are 1) ideas and attitudes acquired from family, especially the client's mother and sister(s), 2) previous labors and births, 3) experiences attending other women's births, 4) individual beliefs about the pain of labor, 5) notions about the spiritual or emotional meaning of labor and birth, 6) cultural norms, 7) a history of trauma (sexual abuse, perinatal loss), and 8) a history of obstetric complications.

A woman anticipating her first child may not know what she wants. Stimulate her thinking with questions such as, "What is important for you when you are in labor and giving birth? Is it important to go through labor without any medicine? Have you thought about how you would like the birth to go? Do you think you will have a vaginal birth or a cesarean birth? Is there anything about giving birth that frightens you? What do you worry about? What have your friends or relatives told you about labor or birth? Is there anything special you would like to do to welcome your baby?"

Midwives come from a long tradition of helping women labor without pain medicine. In the past, women who sought midwifery care did so primarily because they knew that a midwife would support them in their unmedicated journey through labor. Today, however, while some women still seek midwifery care for this support, others seek it because they know a midwife approaches birth from a different perspective than a medical doctor, emphasizing the emotional and spiritual components of birth and valuing client education. Still, these women want analgesia or anesthesia. Another group of women in this country have no choice about the person who attends them in birth. This new group of women in midwifery care may or may not want analgesia in labor.

A discussion about the client's preferences for addressing pain in labor should begin early in prenatal care. The complex nature of pain and its interpretation make any discussion of pain relief in labor challenging for midwives. The midwife must consider the woman's beliefs and preferences, as well as her or his own beliefs about the nature and purpose of labor and the potential value of birthing without analgesia. Many midwives have personally experienced the power and satisfaction that can come from that experience. Others have experienced the relief or satisfaction and sense of control that emerges from the use of pain medication. Inevitably, these personal experiences and beliefs influence care.

Among the dilemmas we face are these:

How can we know when to encourage women to consider a birth without analgesia or anesthesia and when to know that it truly is in her best interest to support her decision to use pharmacologic relief measures?

How should we respond when clients wanting no "intervention" feel that any discussion of possible complications predisposes them to develop the very thing they wish to avoid? Should the midwife insist on a discussion of complications, knowing that failure to discuss them might lead to trauma symptoms if emergency intervention occurs? Or should the midwife refrain from such discussions to avoid generating so much anxiety that the client becomes vulnerable to what she fears most?

How do we decide what recommendations to make about preparation for childbirth (when options are available)? How do we know which classes to suggest, and should they be hospital classes or community-based classes? When should acupuncture, yoga, or hypnosis be suggested? Which books

should we recommend? When do we acknowledge that formal classes might not be appropriate or possible because of client preference, culture, accessibility, cost, content, or availability?
How can we tell when labor pain will be interpreted as trauma, and when it will be interpreted as purposeful and fulfilling?

Simkin suggests that unresolved earlier traumas ("such as unresolved physical, emotional, or sexual trauma, family dysfunction, loss of one or both parents, chronic illness, or others") contribute to posttraumatic stress after childbirth (Simkin, 2000, p. 254). Women with a history of sexual abuse seem to be especially vulnerable in labor. Evolving data suggest that a history of sexual abuse may influence a woman's ability to deliver vaginally. Powerful emotional forces may make women able to "shut labor down" so that they do not have to deal with many people looking at their genitalia or feel the baby emerge from a place that is associated with pain, embarrassment, guilt, and humiliation.

The issue of "control" during labor is a difficult one. Some professionals believe that being "in control" is essential. Others believe that giving up control is key. Green points out that rather than being an objective state, a woman's feeling of being in control depends on her perception of a situation. Some women will even feel in control by transferring decision-making responsibility to family members or the professional staff; the feeling is enhanced by her knowledge that she could have made a different choice (Green, 1999).

The art of midwifery is finding a path through the multiple dilemmas and complexities that each woman's personal situation provides. There is no one answer about what (if any) childbirth classes to take, when to encourage a particular approach to pain management, or what topics or level of discussion can help or hinder a woman's preparation and readiness for birth. Perhaps the best rule is to always try to determine what works for a particular client. To that end you might inquire:

• Is it helpful for you to hear many details or just basic explanations?
• What is the best way to raise a concern or give you information about a potential or actual problem?
• What kind of support works best for you?
• When you are under stress, what kind of communication is most helpful?
• In the past, what have you done to manage pain, fear, or uncertainty?

One of the most effective ways to honor a woman's needs and preferences is to ask her how to proceed if you encounter a dilemma. Suppose, for example, that a client does not want to hear about potential problems because such talk makes her nervous. You might respond by saying, "I understand you want to focus on your body working well. But if I notice something that might interfere with your body working its best, how can you and I, together, find a way to make your nervousness manageable and still help your body do its best job?"

Clinicians need to have an open mind about labor and birth. They must ask about and respect a woman's desires. Because these wishes will cover a wide range of possibilities, the midwife must know about resources to help women prepare for labor in a variety of ways. This requires keeping up-to-date with new books, talking with childbirth educators, and attending their classes when possible. When the midwifery practice serves women from a nondominant culture, particularly a culture in which childbirth classes are not the norm, she should meet with the "wise women" of the cultural group and visit traditional healers in the community to determine culturally sensitive and appropriate approaches to pregnancy and birth.

Women who plan to attend childbirth classes will appreciate a list of classes describing the goals, philosophy, and teaching approach of the instructor; the cost; location; and timing. Some communities offer classes during both the day and evening, including sunrise classes for those who find it best to attend before work or school. Weekend classes allow parents-to-be to have a concentrated period of time to think about labor and birth. Some classes emphasize patterned breathing. Some use techniques of hypnosis or visualization. Others stress "finding your own way through labor" and present a variety of tools that may be helpful. The more the clinician knows about the various classes offered in the community, the more likely it will be for the client to find a group that fits her interests, personality, learning style, and most importantly, her goals.

The Role of Partners

The role of partners in the U.S. childbirth process is evolving. In many instances, the partner is expected to act as coach. However, not all partners are comfortable in that role. A small, exploratory study has shown that some men readily assume the role of coach or teammate, but more are likely to be "witnesses" or "companions" (Chapman, 1992). Men may appreciate a suggestion that they have a support person of their own during labor and birth, someone who can provide food, encouragement, and support, particularly if progress is slow or the mother-to-be is in much pain (Jordan, 2000).

Midwives in the United States must be careful not to assume that American cultural values about the role of the husband, even when it is only his physical presence, serve all women well. A study of 432 Somali women who gave birth in the United States reported, "At least one-half of the women felt pressured to have their partner with them in labor and delivery, when, in fact, a female companion would be far more culturally acceptable than a male companion" (Chalmers & Hashi, 2000, p. 233).

Midwives should discuss the client's preferences as to who will be present at the labor and during the birth and what their role will be.

The Birth Plan

It is common in some midwifery practices to ask the expectant mother to put her desires for labor and birth in writing. This document is called a birth plan. Some birth plans are brief, while others are long and detailed. Some health care providers find them helpful, and others wish they had never been in-vented. Whether a written birth plan is encouraged, take time to help the client consider what she wants to happen during labor, who she wants with her, and how she thinks she will react to the practices and procedures she is likely to encounter. Suggest that she choose people with whom she can be comfortable, as well as people she trusts with her sounds, pain, body exposure, and intimacy.

When possible, request a meeting between you, the client, and all the people she hopes will be present during her labor or at the birth. Reviewing the expectant mother's desires out loud and hearing each person's questions, expectations, hopes, and fears can clear the air and set the stage for a support-ive birth experience. The health care provider may want to review the process of labor with the group, emphasizing how different it is for each person. Talk about long labors and short labors, membranes rupturing before contractions begin, and membranes rupturing just before the birth. Allow those who have given or witnessed birth to express some of their thoughts and feelings. Be sure to ask the expectant mother if there is anything about her that those who attend the birth should know or would find helpful.

 HELPFUL HINT

Use the last month of the pregnancy to help clients understand the policies and procedures at the place of birth. This applies whether the birth will occur at home, in a birth center, or at a hospital. A check-off list can help ensure that all topics are covered that are considered important by the midwives in the practice.

Doulas

Some women appreciate knowing about doulas, specially trained individuals who provide continuous support during labor. Doulas may also accompany the mother to a prenatal visit, take pictures of the birth, and write an account of the birth. They may charge a one-time fee or may charge according to the amount of time spent with the family. They usually are with their clients in early labor at home and are able to focus exclusively on supporting the labor-ing woman. In most instances, a doula will complement the care of the midwife and will not interfere with the support provided by the woman's partner, family, or friends. Postpartum doulas provide support after birth and may do cooking, laundry, and light housekeeping and help with older children.

❊ Preparing Other Children

Take some time to help parents anticipate likely reactions from older children to the baby's birth. No matter how well parents have prepared their other children for the new baby, the initial encounter may be difficult—or the initial encounter may be fine, only to be followed later by the calm announcement, "Let's give the baby back!" If parents are not taken by surprise by these reactions, they will be in a better position to help the children adjust to the new sibling. Sometimes a young child reacts directly toward the baby by hitting or grabbing the bottle. More often it is indirect, often by rough "loves," or more demanding behavior or whining. Children who were toilet trained or weaned before the new baby may forget these skills. After all, with all those adults saying how cute the new baby is when he cried and wet his pants and sucked a bottle, wouldn't you try it? Help parents understand that the best response to these behaviors is no response at all, only increased attention to the child at other times. Often it helps to say out loud, "Oh, would you like to pretend you're a little baby too? Okay, here, I'll give you your bottle; then later you'll decide to be my big girl/boy again."

Suggest that parents help older children see the advantages of being a "big" boy or girl. They might say, "Oh, you want to be a little baby now? Let me rock you; then when you decide to be a big girl/boy again, you can help me make cookies—babies are too little to do that!"

They can also help the big brother or sister recognize and accept both their positive and negative feelings toward the baby. Children usually begin to understand the concept of jealousy about the age of 4 or 5. Younger children will understand the concept of anger. Saying out loud what the child is feeling inside can be very helpful, "I know it makes you feel mad that I'm feeding baby instead of drawing with you. Baby is so little that she doesn't know how to wait yet like big boys do. Thank you for waiting. As soon as I'm done feeding her, I'll draw some pictures with you." Remind parents to never leave a child under 10 alone with the baby—even for just a minute!

A word beforehand to grandparents and others will help them remember to greet the other children first and let the children be the ones to take the visitors into the baby's room. Parents can be prepared to show the visitors not only pictures of the new baby but also some of the big sibling when he or she was a baby.

❋ Honoring the Expectant Mother

Clinicians play an important role in helping pregnant women feel special. In some situations, you may suggest a special ceremony to honor the expectant mother. This ceremony, commonly called a "blessing way," is modeled after a Native American ceremony. Close female friends of the expectant mother usually attend, although male partners and friends can also be invited. In one version, participants offer gifts designed to remind the woman that her friends are thinking of her when she is in labor, sharing with her their strength and wisdom. Each participant may bring an item to put on a necklace that the woman will wear while she labors, or they might bring small objects to put into a wreath that the mother will take to the place of birth. Other gifts might include homemade soup, a casserole, or home-canned vegetables or fruit; an original poem; quilt pieces; plants; a foot massage; or a facial. If the expectant mother likes flowers and gardening, the participants can bring her a plant or a basket of hyacinth or freesia bulbs in a shallow pan of water. Start the bulbs at a time when they will flower a few days after the due date. If the mother has not yet given birth, the flowers may cheer her up when the last days of pregnancy seem endless.

The participants might gather in a circle, united with the expectant mother by a cord (often made of yarn or string) that is passed around a wrist of each person. The participants may tell the mother-to-be what they admire most about her, what they wish for her, and which of their own strengths they will be wishing for her while she is in labor. Each then breaks the cord at her wrist and wears the cord until the baby is born. Often the blessing way ends with the establishment of a telephone tree so that everyone present can be contacted when the honoree's labor begins. Each participant can then focus intently on the mother in the hours ahead.

❋ Health Education Material

Printed Material

Printed material is often given to clients to complement or supplement discussions at prenatal visits. Racks of health education material are often located in an area that is inconvenient, does not allow time for browsing, or does not provide privacy (McVea, Venugopal, Crabtree, & Aita, 2000). Research has shown that clients who have personally received printed material from a physician reported more satisfaction with their care, compared with receiving printed material in the mail or no material at all (Terry & Healey, 2000). Write the client's name on the pamphlet and take the time to review it with her, highlighting or underlining important points.

Clients Who Can't Read

Most health care professionals assume that the majority of their clients are functionally literate (i.e., able to read, write, and perform arithmetic computations at a level that permits them to use them in everyday life). However, in a study conducted in two urban public hospitals, as many as three fifths of the clients were found to have inadequate or marginal literacy in regard to their ability to use the health system to their advantage (Williams et al., 1995). Estimates from the 1992 National Adult Literacy Survey put 40 to 44 million Americans in the functionally illiterate category and another 50 million people in the marginally literate category. This means that many clients cannot read most health education pamphlets, generally written at the 10th-grade level or above. Neither are they able to understand consent forms, which usually have a college or graduate-school readability level (American Medical Association Ad Hoc Committee on Health Literacy, 1999); written discharge instructions; or medication instructions.

Studies have found that clients read three to six grade levels below their last completed grade in school. Generally speaking, adults with less education are less able to understand and use printed information than adults with more education (Kirsch, Jungeblut, Jenkins, & Kolstad, 1993). In the United States, one person in five reads at the fifth-grade level or below. Among inner-city minorities, almost two out of five read below the fifth-grade level, and poor readers obtain much less from health care instructions than do skilled readers. This is true even for materials that have fairly low readability levels. Poor readers may read most or all of the words in an instruction and still obtain little or no meaning from the text (Doak, Doak, & Root, 1996).

"Individuals with limited reading skills take words literally rather than in context. They read slowly and either skip over or become confused by unfamiliar words. They tire quickly and often miss the context in which words are presented. So, written material for such persons must be carefully constructed to assure its comprehensibility. The fifth grade readability level is an appropriate goal for most health care materials intended for the public, but clinicians should keep in mind that even this level will be too difficult for up to one quarter of the population" (National Work Group on Literacy and Health, 1998).

Identifying Literacy Levels

People who find reading difficult frequently are embarrassed because they cannot read. They often go to great lengths to hide this problem, and clinicians, as a result, find it difficult to identify clients with inadequate or marginal literacy skills. While literacy evaluation tests have been used in research studies to identify literacy level, no one test currently available is easily adaptable and sufficiently comprehensive to be useful in clinic and office settings. Consequently, clinicians are left to their own devices as they attempt to make good decisions about how to identify the client's literacy level and how to teach clients whose skills are low. Pamphlets and brochures, perhaps the most common vehicles for client teaching, may be inappropriate. Most health education material is written by good readers for good readers. Health care providers, then, must be aware not only of the client's literacy level, but of the reading level of any written material offered.

Visual Aids

Many people are visual learners. Therefore, visual aids for the clinic or office setting are an important part of midwifery practice.

❋ The Philosophy of the Midwifery Practice

In practices where care is provided by more than one midwife, discussions among the midwives about personal philosophies in regard to labor, birth, and methods of pain relief should occur periodically because feelings often change over time. Questions for discussion might include the following:

When is it appropriate to deny pain medication to women in labor asking for analgesia or anesthesia?
Are a certain group of women giving birth in hospital settings perceived as not needing pain medication in labor?
Should women be offered pain relief medication if they do not ask for it?
Do women whose lives have always been characterized by pain—poor women, for example, or abused women—have any special needs in regard to pain relief in labor?

Hopefully, all birth attendants will remember that the birth belongs to the laboring woman. "Doing" is not always the best thing to "do." Sometimes merely "being" is a very useful—and therapeutic—activity.

❋ Conclusion

When concluding the prenatal revisit, discuss the plan that evolves from the data gathered. Consider the U.S. Public Health Service revisit guidelines when deciding on a date for the next prenatal visit.

As you record your findings, note the health education topics that were discussed as well. Guidelines for charting by novice practitioners can be found in Box 9-2. While expert practitioners dictate their notes or write notes that are

Box 9.2

Charting for Novice Practitioners

SUBJECTIVE

1. Emotional well-being, stress, and fears
2. Common discomforts
3. Use of prescribed and over-the-counter (OTC) drugs and alternative remedies
4. Use of cigarettes, drugs, or alcohol (if applicable)

OBJECTIVE

1. Blood pressure (BP)
2. Urine
3. Weight gain or loss
4. Fetal heart tones
5. Fundal height
6. Presentation (after 34 weeks)

ASSESSMENT

1. IUP at _____ weeks, size ($<$, $=$, or $>$) dates
2. BP: Within normal limits (WNL) or elevated
3. Weight gain (include total gain and gain since last visit)
4. Fetal heart rate: WNL or elevated
5. Urine analysis: WNL or elevated
6. Presentation (after 34 weeks)
7. Psychosocial data
8. Problems (such as anemia, Rh-negative blood)

PLAN

1. Suggestions for relief of common discomforts
2. OTC or prescribed medication
3. Health education (many topics are possible, including the "magic numbers" for fetal movement and preterm labor contractions, risks for vaginal birth after cesarean, danger signs, childbirth education, use of prenatal vitamins, preparation for labor, and discussion of the birth plan)
   a. List all topics discussed. List all danger signs mentioned.
   b. List pamphlets given.
4. Lab work
5. Referrals
6. Return in _____ weeks

significantly briefer, following the suggested format helps new practitioners learn to be thorough in their approach to expectant families.

Good prenatal care requires a combination of knowledge, manual dexterity, respect for both the normal and the abnormal, good judgment, resourcefulness, compassion, and an appreciation of the lives of women. Thoughtful consideration of the uniqueness of each pregnant woman can lead to the provision of meaningful and useful health education.

Appendix 9-1

Topics for Discussion in the Last Month of Pregnancy

1. _____ Review of Birth Plan
2. _____ Student nurse-midwife or medical student in attendance
3. _____ Investigate options for well-baby care
4. _____ Average length of first labor is 16 hours (including latent and active phases) + pushing
5. _____ Early labor
    a. _____ Clues to distinguish latent phase from active phase
    b. _____ Call CNM when/if
        1). _____ contractions are 3–4 minutes apart
        2). _____ you are frightened
        3). _____ your water breaks
        4). _____ there is decreased fetal movement
    c. _____ Management of discomfort in the early phase
        1). _____ Bath/shower
        2). _____ Movement
        3). _____ Massage
        4). _____ Imagery
        5). _____ Breathing techniques
        6). _____ Relaxation techniques
        7). _____ Distraction (movie, shopping)
6. _____ Analgesia/anesthesia available for pain management in the active phase of labor
    a. _____ Narcotic analgesia
        1). _____ Provides relaxation but does not eliminate pain
        2). _____ Potential for respiratory depression in baby
    b. _____ Sterile water papules for severe back pain
    c. _____ Epidural anesthesia
        1). _____ Relieves pain, allows rest
        2). _____ Occasionally prevents Cesarean birth as it allows rest and "buys time" for a baby in a malposition to rotate

      3). _____ Occasionally not 100% effective

      4). _____ Requires IV, continuous fetal monitoring, frequent BP checks, possibly catheterization

      5). _____ Second stage may be longer

      6). _____ Increased incidence of fever requiring antibiotics in labor

      7). _____ May feel intense burning as head emerges

      8). _____ Occasionally not immediately available

      9). _____ If rapid labor, may not have time for administration

      10). _____ Itching is a common side effect

      11). _____ Complications include a drop in BP, respiratory arrest (rare), PP spinal headache, possibly backache for some months following birth

7. _____ If due date passes,

    a. _____ Inductions usually done ONLY for a medical/obstetrical indication

    b. _____ Post-dates testing begins at 41½ weeks, induction offered at 42 weeks

    c. _____ Advantages of sweeping the membranes

    d. _____ Possible use of castor oil but may have only diarrhea and abdominal cramping

8. _____ Hospital practices involving the baby soon after birth

    a. _____ Eye medication

    b. _____ Vitamin K injection

    c. _____ Pediatricians in attendance if meconium-stained fluid

PART 4 The Postpartum Period

Immediately after birth, profound changes take place in the mother's body and, usually, in her heart, soul, and mind, as well. Yet, as wondrous as birth is for many families, the postpartum period is not easy. Bodily changes, hormonal shifts, pain, fatigue, and inevitable alterations in relationships make for a challenging time. As she adjusts to the new baby, the mother must also make decisions about future children and health practices. Part IV looks at these issues. Chapter 10 addresses the transition to parenthood, Chapter 11 discusses common postpartum complications, Chapter 12 contains information about breastfeeding, Chapter 13 speaks to issues in selecting a method of family planning, Chapter 14 deals with routines at the postpartum visits, and Chapter 15 discusses postpartum health education.

Chapter 10

Transition to Parenthood

The initial days of the puerperium can be a time of wonder, relief, joy, astonishment, tenderness, happiness, anxiety, exhaustion, discomfort, sadness, depression, isolation, and bewilderment. A newborn baby in the house can be a shock. Even for families who have had a relatively easy birth and go home to household help and good social support, the adjustment required can be difficult. A prolonged labor or a difficult birth, sore nipples, a fussy baby, an unenthusiastic nurser, or others in the house needing attention will certainly make the situation more difficult. The following suggestions to the new mother may be helpful in the early weeks of parenthood.

✳ Control Pain

Abdominal, breast/nipple, and perineal pain are common after giving birth, whether or not complications are present. Mothers often need to be reminded that pain relief contributes to their ability to sleep and to breastfeed. It also improves one's ability to cope with stressful situations and respond to them with good humor. Perineal pain can be present whether or not lacerations occurred. In fact, women with no visible perineal trauma may report pain for as long as 3 months (Albers, Garcia, Renfrew, McCandlish, & Elbourne, 1999). Reassure mothers that neither ibuprofen nor acetaminophen are known to be harmful to a nursing baby. Soaking in a bathtub for 20 to 30 minutes three to four times a day can be helpful for a sore perineum.

✳ Ask for (and Accept) Help

Sleep deprivation is a constant in many families. Combined with the awesome responsibility of a newborn, parents are easily overwhelmed. Advise new parents to have a ready response to friends and family members who ask, "What can I do to help?" If the parents are reluctant to say what they need, food for the freezer can come in handy on days that seem to get out of hand. "How about a casserole?" is a good response. Other possibilities include grocery shopping, taking or picking up other children, doing the laundry, mowing the lawn, walking the dog, cleaning the house, or chopping veggies. One of the biggest helps can be someone to watch over the baby while Mom naps. When no one volunteers to help, let parents see the legitimacy of asking for assistance.

❋ Lower Your Expectations

How anything as small as a baby can consume the attention of one or even two adults almost every hour of the day is always a mystery. But it happens, and it often seems that nothing else gets done! Help new parents realize that the "good-enough" approach is a philosophy to live by in many areas, particularly housekeeping, body image, and entertaining, in the first few weeks with a new baby.

❋ Don't Plan Anything

The actions of the baby are totally unpredictable. If new parents are scheduled to be somewhere, the baby is bound to spit up, pee, poop, or be inconsolable just as everyone is ready to go out the door. If it is important to be on time, advise parents to get ready 30 minutes earlier than they think will be needed. Better yet, they can help friends and relatives realize that times established for all engagements in the next few weeks are approximate.

❋ Share the Joy

Sometimes new moms forget there are other important people in the baby's life—the other parent, relatives, and special friends. Encourage your client to avoid pushing away these people. Special people in the baby's family need to bond with the new arrival. So encourage the mother to share her joy (and increase the likelihood that these special people will respond graciously when their help is needed).

❋ Get Some Relationship Time

Particularly when a new baby is breastfed, the other parent in the baby's life can feel left out. With the newborn requiring so much attention, important relationships are easily neglected, resulting in hurt feelings. Wise midwives encourage mothers to nurture the bond with their partners by acknowledging their importance, expressing gratitude for their presence, praising the way they care for the baby (even when Mom knows she can do it better), and arranging special adult time together.

❊ New Roles for the Partner

The postpartum period is usually a time when women need assistance and emotional support. Regardless of how independent, self-sufficient, and successful a woman has been before giving birth, the new mother is likely to be in some discomfort, physically exhausted, and emotionally drained. Partners sometimes need help knowing what to do. Suggest that the partner screen phone calls instead of waking the sleeping mother because someone wishes to congratulate her, change the message on the answering machine to announce that calls are eagerly accepted between certain hours, manage the traffic in the house, and entertain those who drop by—outside of the room where the mother is resting. When feasible, the partner can also suggest that out-of-town guests either wait to visit or stay at a nearby motel.

❊ Other Children

How hard it is to have to give up being the youngest child! While some children quickly accept the presence of a younger sibling, many kick and scream through the process. Appendix Q contains suggestions for moving smoothly (maybe somewhat smoothly) through the transition.

❊ Get Some Time Alone

After taking care of the needs of the baby and other family members, it is no wonder the new mother is exhausted. "Mommy time" can mean many things, from getting out of the house and away from the baby for a bit to merely lying down to sleep, knowing that some competent person can respond to the baby's need for a diaper change or holding while Mom restores her body and spirit. Writing thank-you notes, returning phone calls, or relaxing in the shower or tub may help energize the new mother. Going out for a treat, even just coffee or an ice cream, might be enjoyable. Try asking your client, "What would be something that would be fun for you to do for yourself?" Then see if you can help her figure out how to make it happen.

❋ Have a Sense of Humor

As with most things in life, a sense of humor does a lot to reduce stress and make life pleasant. Help parents see the value in laughing and taking the hard parts of new parenthood in stride.

❋ Worries About SIDS

Part of the transition to parenthood involves baby care practices. Clinicians would do well to discuss practices that reduce the risk of sudden infant death syndrome (SIDS). While the cause is unknown, SIDS is associated with the baby lying in the prone position. SIDS is also associated with an overheated baby and maternal smoking during pregnancy. Parents should be told to put their babies on their backs to sleep. The side-lying position is significantly safer than the prone position, but is not as safe as the supine position.

The relationship between sharing a bed with a baby and SIDS is controversial. While the literature contains reports of adults lying on babies, these cases usually involved the use of alcohol or mind-altering drugs. The role of soft sleep surfaces and entrapment and the possibility that the baby rolled by himself or herself into the prone position is not clear. Nor is it clear to what extent other causes of infant death, such as infanticide and cardiac arrhythmias, have been misdiagnosed. There appears to be a significantly greater risk of SIDS when cosleeping occurs among smokers. There is insufficient evidence to conclude that breastfeeding offers some protection against SIDS. A few studies have shown a protective effect from pacifiers (American Academy of Pediatrics, 2000). Clinicians would do well to discuss the recommendations of the American Academy of Pediatrics for reducing the risk of SIDS (Appendix R) with new parents. Remind them that these recommendations should be observed throughout infancy, including the 2- to 4-months-of-age period, during which the incidence of SIDS is the highest.

❋ Conclusion

The image of the shining new mother with flowing tresses in a long, billowy gown and a baby blissfully asleep in her arms conflicts with reality for most new parents. The midwife can be helpful in the days after birth by focusing on the transitions most families undergo at that time.

Chapter 11

Postpartum Complications

Most women who give birth vaginally have few major physical problems in the initial postpartum period. However, complications can occur. Obstetric-related problems include endometritis, mastitis, an infected wound, urinary retention and incontinence, thrombophlebitis, and separated symphysis. Other illnesses can also occur during this time and include urinary tract infection (UTI), pneumonia, and influenza. Accurate diagnosis of these conditions requires a thorough history and physical examination and, sometimes, laboratory tests. This chapter discusses selected common postpartum complications. Postpartum depression is discussed in Chapter 14.

A low-grade fever is common in the first 24 hours postpartum and usually resolves spontaneously. However, any postpartum woman who complains of fever with or without pain after the first 24 hours following childbirth should be evaluated. Evaluation should include the general appearance of the mother, particularly whether she is in any distress. Women with endometritis may be barely able to walk. Evaluate her temperature, pulse, and respirations. Include an examination of the pharynx, auscultation of the lungs, palpation of the costovertebral angle, and palpation and auscultation of the abdomen. Carefully inspect the breasts and nipples, as well as any labial or perineal repair. Examine the lower extremities for signs of thrombophlebitis. Dorsiflex the feet for Homans sign.

Laboratory tests usually include a urine specimen for culture to rule out a UTI. A cervical specimen may be sent to test for chlamydia and gonorrhea. Vaginal cultures are not usually helpful. Although a complete blood count (CBC) may be ordered, results are difficult to interpret if the infection occurs in the early postpartum days, as leukocyte counts are normally high at this time.

❋ Endometritis

Endometritis commonly occurs between the second and the seventh postpartum days. Cesarean birth is the major predisposing factor. A woman with endometritis usually presents with fever and abdominal pain. Foul-smelling lochia may also be present. Examination of the abdomen will reveal a tender uterus.

High fever and rapid pulse speak to the need for hospitalization. The decision to treat a woman with endometritis as an outpatient should be made on the basis of how sick she appears. What is her temperature, and how high is her pulse? Is the leukocyte count unusually high? Is there an adult at home who can look after her while she is ill? A course of antibiotics (Box 11-1) is required.

❋ Mastitis

Mastitis can occur at any time when a woman is breastfeeding but typically not before the tenth postpartum day. The causative organism is usually *Staphylococcus aureus*, and antibiotics are usually required. Symptoms include an area of hardness in the breast, pain, redness, and fever. Your client is likely to tell you she aches all over and feels like she has been "hit by a truck." She typically has a fever of 101°F or more and may confuse symptoms of mastitis with those of flu.

A plugged duct or a yeast infection may be misdiagnosed as mastitis. Although a plugged duct may also present as a painful mass with overlying redness of the skin, the pain is not as intense as that of mastitis. Shooting breast pain without an area of hardness is likely to be caused by a yeast infection. Fever alone does not mean mastitis has developed. Distinguishing between mastitis and a plugged duct can be difficult. If symptoms are not severe and have been present less than 24 hours, the mother can be given a

---

Box 11.1

Recommendations for the Outpatient Treatment of Endometritis

BREASTFEEDING REGIMEN
Clindamycin, 450 mg every 6 hours for 14 days

NONBREASTFEEDING REGIMEN
Doxycycline, 100 mg orally twice a day for 14 days
Metronidazole, 500 mg orally twice a day for 10 to 14 days; it may be given in addition to doxycycline

prescription for antibiotics with the suggestion that she wait before initiating therapy. If her symptoms improve, the antibiotics are not needed. If the symptoms worsen over the next few hours, she should start the antibiotics. If no improvement is noted within 24 hours, antibiotics should also be started.

Treatment of mastitis is summarized in Box 11-2. Women with mastitis should feel significantly better within 24 hours of initiating antibiotics. If they do not, they may need to be hospitalized so they can receive IV antibiotics. Comfort measures include bed rest for at least 24 hours, moist heat to the infected breast for 20 to 30 minutes every 2 to 3 hours while awake, and acetaminophen or NSAIDs for pain and fever. The mother should drink plenty of liquids and discontinue use of a bra for a few days, unless she experiences discomfort without one. A bra, particularly one with an underwire, may increase discomfort.

Mastitis does not contaminate the mother's milk. The baby should continue to nurse from both breasts. In fact, frequent nursing decreases the chances that a breast abscess will form. Feeding from the unaffected breast first is usually helpful. If feeding from the affected breast is too painful, a breast pump or manual expression of the milk may be necessary to prevent engorgement and continue milk production.

✤ Wound Infection

An infected laceration or episiotomy will appear red and swollen. Purulent discharge may be present. The repair may have "broken down." Often sitz baths three to four times a day are all that is needed. In other instances, the wound should be opened by removing the stitches and then cleansed with normal

---

Box 11.2

Recommendations for the Outpatient Treatment of Mastitis

PREFERRED REGIMEN
Dicloxacillin, 500 mg orally four times a day for 7 to 10 days

ALTERNATE REGIMENS
Erythromycin, 250 to 500 mg orally four times a day for 7 to 10 days
or
Clindamycin, 300 mg orally four times a day for 7 to 10 days

saline. Oral antibiotics such as clindamycin should be administered. Note the skin color around the site, as necrosis can occur.

❋ Urinary Retention and Incontinence

Most problems with urinary retention are resolved within 48 hours of giving birth. Occasionally, however, a mother will report frequent voiding and urinary incontinence late in the first postpartum week. Residual urine will be found on postvoid catheterization. The amount of residual urine considered significant is not known. Some clinicians consider more than 100 cc or 150 cc significant, whereas others consider more than one third of the voided amount to be significant. Postpartum women with postvoid residuals considered to be significant should be taught to perform self-catheterization. This should continue until the postvoid residual is no longer significant.

Newly delivered mothers may report urinary incontinence without frequent voiding. They may also note fecal incontinence, as well as difficulty controlling the expulsion of flatus. The extent of these problems is not known but is probably underappreciated. While many women find that symptoms disappear over time, little longitudinal research is available. One recent retrospective study of primiparous women found that at 6 months, postpartum women with midline episiotomies had a 6-times-greater incidence of fecal incontinence compared with women with an intact perineum (Signorello, Harlow, Chekos, & Repke, 2000). In another study, one out of 10 primiparas and one out of five multiparas who delivered vaginally experienced fecal urgency or the involuntary loss of flatus or feces. Symptoms are found even in women without obvious disruption of the rectal sphincter (Toglia & DeLancey, 1994). In one report, only 31% of 180 women studied were asymptomatic at 8 weeks' postpartum (Mason, Glenn, Walton, & Appleton, 1999).

The definitive role of episiotomy or laceration, type of perineal repair, length of second stage, second-stage pushing technique, use of obstetric instrumentation, and birth weight in postdelivery incontinence is unknown.

❋ Thrombophlebitis

The risk of deep vein thrombosis (DVT) is 5.5 times more frequent in pregnant and postpartum women than in nonpregnant women (Laros, 1999). Symptoms of lower extremity DVT include tenderness, swelling, redness, a palpable "cord," and a positive Homan sign (calf pain when the big toe is passively dorsiflexed). Doppler ultrasonography is the preferred diagnostic technique. Physician management for DVT is required, as treatment includes anticoagulation therapy.

❖ Separated Symphysis

Peripartum separation of the pubic symphysis, although rare, is a cause of significant maternal morbidity and, occasionally, long-term disability. It usually presents as pubic tenderness with increased pain on turning in bed or ambulating and becomes apparent almost immediately after delivery. Often the client is not able to walk without assistance. Pubic separation may be palpable.

While a diagnosis can usually be made on the basis of symptoms, an x-ray or ultrasound examination is often requested for confirmation. The size of the interpubic gap necessary for a diagnosis has not been determined. Suggestions of more than 8 mm and more than 10 mm have been made (Cibils, 1971; Hagen, 1974). The size of the gap has not been found to predict sequelae (Scriven, 1995).

Treatment of a separated symphysis involves a pelvic binder, analgesics, and a walker to assist with ambulation. While most women have diminishing symptomatology over a period of weeks or months, symptoms may persist, necessitating use of a wheelchair. Surgery may be required.

❖ Flu

Flu should be part of a differential diagnosis when a postpartum client reports a fever during the winter months. Attack rates may be higher for women exposed to school-age children. "Usually the incubation period is 3 to 4 days, followed by a sudden rise in temperature, often up to 39.2 degrees C (102.5 F), with associated malaise, myalgia, sore throat, nasal congestion, cough, and headache. Malaise may be severe enough to cause the patient to go to bed for several days, and this symptom is often the defining feature that differentiates influenza from other respiratory viruses" (Rhoton-Vlasak, 1999). The development of pneumonia is a potential complication.

Treatment of flu includes bed rest, liquids, and analgesia for myalgia. Although antipyretics may reduce fever, this "is not always desirable since viral replication may be reduced at temperatures above 35 degrees C" (Rhoton-Vlasak, 1999).

❖ Lower Urinary Tract Infection

Infections of the lower urinary tract may also occur in the postpartal period. A urine culture helps distinguish between a UTI and endometritis. Antibiotics, as discussed in Chapter 8, are required.

❊ Critical Findings

Certain rare but potentially fatal conditions may occur postpartally. Some are unique to the postpartum period, and some could occur at any time. In the former category is peripartum cardiomyopathy with symptoms resembling congestive heart failure: dyspnea, orthopnea, chest pain, cough, and palpitations, although initial symptoms can be as vague as severe headache and pedal edema. Peripartum cardiomyopathy has a mortality rate of 75%.

In the second category is cysticercosis, a parasitic disease in which the parasite lodges in the brain. The outcome can also be fatal. Midwives, then, must never be complacent about symptoms reported by clients. Neither should we be paranoid. Rather, vigilance should be our companion, particularly when symptoms do not fit the picture or do not seem to make sense.

❊ Conclusion

Postpartum complications are usually mild. However, pain and/or fever after recent childbirth are wearisome and discouraging. Midwives should attend to them promptly to minimize their impact and to prevent further complications.

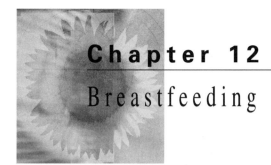

Chapter 12
Breastfeeding

Breastfeeding for women in the United States does not come as naturally as it does for women in many other countries. Most women in this country who have not successfully nursed a baby benefit from early and continuing encouragement from sensitive and well-informed professionals. Practitioners not accustomed to counseling women who breastfeed should purchase a book describing common problems and solutions. A quick reference book with advice about breastfeeding challenges will be useful, such as *The Breastfeeding Triage Tool* (Jolley & Phillips-Angeles, 1998).

❋ Early Breastfeeding Support

Home visits are, of course, ideal for providing support to breastfeeding mothers. Women who give birth in hospitals often lack access to this kind of assistance once they are discharged. When help is not readily available, daily phone calls are appropriate ". . . until the milk is in and the baby is nursing well, with at least 6 wet diapers and 1 to 3 stools in 24 hours" (Jolley & Phillips-Angeles, 1998, p. vii). Telephone consultation combined with early office or clinic visits for women experiencing problems should be instituted to avoid frustration, exhaustion, and disillusionment. A recent study found that approximately 25% of the breastfeeding mothers in the study population (56.3% Black and 34.4% Puerto Rican) stopped nursing in the first postpartum week, and another 10% stopped during the second week (Ertem, Votto, & Leventhal, 2001). These data indicate that a clinic or office visit 1 to 2 weeks after delivery is too late for women with breastfeeding problems.

Midwives often have strong opinions about breastfeeding practices. For example, some decry the use of a pacifier at any time. Some feel a bottle is never appropriate in the first 2 weeks of a baby's life. Some feel that lanolin is the only treatment for sore nipples. As in most things, there is no single guideline or prescription that works for every mother and every baby. Midwives must be sensitive to differences in both the temperament and sucking needs of individual babies and also to the mothers' personal needs or preferences.

❄ The Decision to Stop Breastfeeding

While the majority of women leave the hospital breastfeeding their infants, only 29% are breastfeeding 6 months later. Fewer still continue for the entire year that is recommended by the American Academy of Pediatrics. Many new mothers quit within 2 weeks of giving birth, most doing so only after experiencing frustration, fatigue, pain, fear that the infant isn't getting enough to eat, and repeated attempts to find solutions to the problems (Mozingo, Davis, Droppleman, & Merideth, 2000). The demands of parenthood and consequent physical and emotional fatigue, plus the strange and, for some women, unpleasant feel of a nursing baby, conflicting how-to information, embarrassment at nursing in front of others, unrealistic expectations about how easy it will be to nurse, anticipation of a return to work, and trouble finding time to sit down to nurse, particularly if the baby is a slow nurser, are other obstacles to successful nursing. These factors may be especially problematic for low-income women (Raisler, 2000).

Interestingly, one study has shown that the best predictors of discontinuing breastfeeding are the mother's lack of confidence in her ability to nurse for at least 2 months and her belief that the baby prefers a bottle to the breast (Ertem, Votto, & Leventhal, 2001). Based on these data, midwives should begin efforts to increase the mother's confidence in her ability to nurse her baby during the prenatal period.

Some women who stop nursing soon after giving birth experience feelings of failure, guilt, disappointment, and shame. Others feel mainly relief. Midwives should ask a woman about her feelings once she stops nursing. A counseling referral will be appropriate in some cases.

❄ Problems Involving the Breast

Breastfeeding problems range from those associated with varying degrees of discomfort and morbidity to those affecting the supply of milk. Significant problems require a clinic or office visit to inspect the breasts and nipples and to observe the baby nursing. Be sure to ask permission before touching a woman's breasts and handle them gently. Common problems include engorgement, a plugged duct, nipple pain, flat or inverted nipples, and insufficient milk. Mastitis is discussed in Chapter 11.

Engorgement

Engorgement is a common cause of breast discomfort in the early postpartum days. While it may be difficult to differentiate engorgement from mastitis or a plugged milk duct, engorgement is usually bilateral, comes on gradually, causes a low-grade fever (if any), and is not associated with any systemic symptoms. The breasts are often warm to the touch and have a shiny appearance. Except for the breast discomfort, mothers feel well unless the engorgement is severe. In these cases, the swelling may involve the breast's tail of Spence and extend into the axilla, making it necessary for mothers to hold their arms away from their bodies to avoid pressure on the swollen, painful breast tissue.

Treatment for engorgement in a breastfeeding mother is a mild analgesic, moist heat, and frequent nursing. Unfortunately, the swollen breast can make it difficult for the baby to latch onto the nipple. In these cases, manual expression of milk or a breast pump to remove enough milk to soften the areola can help the baby nurse. Standing under a warm shower while manually expressing or pumping can also be helpful.

Plugged Duct

A plugged duct can cause significant breast pain. The pain is commonly confined to one area of one breast. A lump is palpable, but little or no warmth is present. If fever occurs, it is a low-grade fever, and mothers feel well. Fortunately, the problem usually resolves spontaneously within 24 hours. Applying heat packs before nursing, gently massaging the lump toward the nipple, nursing the affected breast more often, and varying the positions for nursing the baby often help.

❋ Problems Involving the Nipple

Improper positioning of the infant, poor latch-on, and infection are common causes of nipple pain. Breast surgery can interfere with the milk supply.

Nipple Pain

Nipple pain is common in the early days of breastfeeding. In one study, 96 out of 100 mothers reported nipple pain at some time. While it occurred and peaked primarily between the third and seventh days, in some women it lasted for 6 weeks (Ziemer, Paone, Schupay, & Cole, 1990).

Painful nipples may have cracks and blisters, and bleeding can occur. A key component for avoiding trauma to the nipples is correct positioning of the baby. The "belly-to-belly" position emphasizes placing the baby's ears, shoulders, and hips in alignment, facing the mother. To ensure proper latch-on, the baby's mouth should be open wide, sucked-in lips should be pulled out, and as much of the areola as possible should be in the baby's mouth. The baby should be removed from the breast by inserting a finger into the baby's mouth or pulling down on the baby's chin to break the suction.

Research that provides answers about effective treatment for nipple pain is lacking, although some data suggest that warm compresses are helpful when the pain is caused by infants who have not yet learned to latch on or suck properly. Applying black tea bags, which have been steeped and cooled, for 10 minutes after nursing may also be effective (Jolley & Phillips-Angeles, 1998).

Infection

Thrush, a yeast infection, originally in the infant and subsequently transferred to the mother, is another source of nipple pain. It may be readily apparent in the baby, although characteristic white patches in the baby's mouth are not always present. Maternal symptoms include red, itchy, painful nipples throughout the feeding. One milliliter of nystatin suspension every 4 hours for the baby is a common treatment. Treatment for the mother varies. Preferred methods for one group of clinicians and lactation consultants can be adamantly opposed by another group. Recommendations often include nystatin ointment or 1 ml of the baby's nystatin rubbed on to each nipple of the mother immediately after nursing. Warn mothers that nystatin ointment is sticky. Lotrimin cream may also be helpful, applied to the baby's bottom during pediatric therapy and applied to the breast for 24 hours after completion of therapy for the baby.

Burning or shooting pains in the breast often describe intraductal thrush. Mothers with intraductal candidiasis may require oral fluconazole (Diflucan) for 2 to 3 weeks. The initial dose varies from 200 to 400 mg. It is followed by 100 to 200 mg daily. While not approved by the FDA for neonates, fluconazole is increasingly being prescribed for infants because of resistance to other antifungals. Cure rates in pediatric patients have been reported to be 86%, compared to 46% with nystatin (Hale, 2000). Mothers with candidiasis should be instructed to wash all pacifiers and parts of a breast pump with hot water.

Flat Nipples

Flat nipples often occur in women with large breasts. Breast shells applied prenatally are ineffective. Instead, instruct the mother to use them after delivery, applying them to the nipples for about 20 minutes before feeding. This usually causes protrusion of the nipple for a short period of time. The baby should be put to breast as soon as the shells are removed. Applying a cold washcloth or ice to the nipple a few seconds before nursing is also helpful, as the cold causes the areola to contract, firming up the nipple and causing it to protrude. Pumping before nursing will also encourage nipple protrusion (Jolley & Phillips-Angeles, 1998).

Large Nipples

Recent discussion of breastfeeding problems has led some lactation consultants to believe that large nipples (larger than 2.5 cm in diameter, the size of a quarter) may interfere with the baby's ability to compress the milk sinuses and receive milk. In some cases, a supplemental nursing system may be used until the baby's mouth is able to accommodate the nipple (about 3 weeks). Jolley and Phillips-Angeles recommend manual expression of milk or pumping prior to breastfeeding when mothers have large nipples "to make areola and nipple softer and more pliable" (Jolley and Phillips-Angeles, 1998, p. 24).

❊ Insufficient Milk

Causes of an insufficient milk supply include 1) missed hunger cues given by the baby; 2) unrealistic expectations about how often and how long the baby will sleep; 3) difficulty achieving the milk-ejection reflex because of stress, embarrassment, pain, or ineffective sucking; 4) hypothyroidism; 5) selected prescription medications and over-the-counter medications, particularly antihistamines; 6) nicotine; and 7) alcohol (Biancuzzo, 2000). Other causes are mammary agenesis and breast surgery (discussed in Chapter 3). Some mothers expect an abundant supply of milk soon after giving birth. Upon noting the amount of colostrum, they may presume they are deficient. At times, mothers may think that a fussy baby is crying because of inadequate milk. Mothers who feel their supply of breast milk is inadequate are likely to give their babies formula, thereby limiting the frequency and duration of breastfeeding and making the situation worse. Consider each of the common causes of an inadequate milk supply listed previously and address those that seem most likely. Providing information about how milk is produced and the supply-and-demand cycle may be helpful.

Teach mothers to listen for audible swallowing sounds when the baby suckles the breast, an indication that milk is being transferred from the mother to the baby. Until the "milk comes in," breastfed babies may have only one to two wet diapers each day.

Jolley and Phillips-Angeles suggest that mothers who are not confident about their milk supply do "alternate breast massage." "Mom applies pressure where the breast meets the chest and massages the milk toward the nipple. She waits for the infant to take several swallows and then alternates massage of another area of the breast with infant's swallowing" (Jolley and Phillips-Angeles, 1998, p. 19).

❊ Drugs and Breast Milk

Both mothers and clinicians worry that drugs taken by a mother who is breastfeeding will harm the baby. Clinicians can be reassured that the concentration of most medications transferred to the baby through breast milk is "... exceedingly low, and the dose delivered to the breastfed infant is often subclinical" (Hale, 2000, p. 6).

The risks of psychotropic drugs to the baby when mothers breastfeed have not been well studied, so use of these drugs must be weighed against the benefits. Clearly, however, there are times when their use should take precedence over breastfeeding. Fluoxetine (Prozac), although approved for use in pregnancy, may not be appropriate in the postpartum period for breastfeeding women who took the drug prior to giving birth, because plasma levels of fluoxetine rise in the infant each time the baby breastfeeds (Hale, 2000). An alternate selective serotonin reuptake inhibitor (SSRI) medication can be initiated. Lithium prophylaxis for postpartum women with a history of bipolar disorder has been recommended to prevent relapse, estimated to occur in 20% to 50% of these women (Cohen et al., 1995). The American Academy of Pediatrics lists lithium as contraindicated during breastfeeding. However, Hale writes, "Current studies, as well as unpublished experience, suggest that the infant's plasma levels rise to about 30% to 40% of the maternal level, most often without untoward effects in the infant" (Hale, 2000, p. 400). If mothers who take lithium breastfeed, their babies' serum lithium levels should be monitored, and thyroid studies are recommended as lithium can decrease thyroxine production (Hale, 2000).

Guidelines for prescribing drugs for women who are breastfeeding can be found in Box 12-1. A helpful reference book is *Medications and Mothers' Milk* (Hale, 2000). Order from Pharmasoft Publishing, 21 Tascocita Circle, Amarillo, Texas, 79124-7301 (800-378-1317) or order it on-line at www.iBreastfeeding.com ($24.95 + shipping).

❊ Sex and Breastfeeding

If a discussion about sexual activity and breastfeeding has not occurred, the midwife should talk with breastfeeding mothers about the decreased lubrication that some women note during the months that they are breastfeeding. A water-based lubricant can minimize discomfort when lubrication is a problem.

Box 12.1

Guidelines for Prescribing Drugs for Breastfeeding Mothers

1. Although there are wide variations, figure that 1% of the "maternal dose" of a medication will get to the baby.
2. Remember that an infant is unlikely to absorb significant amounts of a drug taken by his or her mother if the drug is absorbed from the mother's gastrointestinal tract (including the aminoglycosides and cephalosporin antibiotics).
3. Choose drugs with shorter half-lives when possible. Suggest that the mother not breastfeed when the medication is at peak level in maternal plasma.
4. Remember that drugs with long pediatric half-lives (including benzodiazepines and fluoxetine) can build up over time in the baby's plasma.
5. Choose a drug with higher protein binding, as the drug does not transfer as readily to the milk.
6. If the drug produces neuroleptic effects in the mother (sedation, depression), it is likely to penetrate the breast milk with similar effects, although these effects will be less intense.
7. Use herbal medicines cautiously. They can contain unknown, dangerous chemicals. Avoid herbal mixtures. If herbal medicines are used, never use more than the recommended dose.

From Hale, T. (2000). *Medications and mothers' milk*. Amarillo, TX: Pharmasoft Publishing.

Mothers should also know that the "let-down" reflex is likely to be activated with orgasm. Accordingly, breastfeeding mothers may wish to wear a bra during sex or place a protective covering over the place of lovemaking. Mothers may wish to offer their partners a bit of breast milk, as many partners are curious about its taste but hesitate to ask if they can do so.

❋ Working Outside the Home and Breastfeeding

Clinicians can help breastfeeding women who will be working outside the home anticipate a variety of reactions to their decision to work and breastfeed. They can also help women realistically prepare for this experience. See Box 12-2 for suggestions for women who anticipate returning to or joining the workforce while breastfeeding.

Box 12.2

Suggestions for Women Who Are Breastfeeding and Employed Outside the Home

1. Stay at home as long as possible.
2. Work part time if possible.
3. Make some "practice runs"—a few hours away from the baby to anticipate problems.
4. Have an extra set of towels, an extra bra, and a change of clothes at the work site.
5. Take a quart of liquid to work and remember to drink it frequently.
6. Practice with a breast pump ahead of time so that you get used to it and the milk will let down quickly.
7. If you are working full time and expressing milk manually or using a manual pump that is objectionable or does not work well, rent a dual hookup electric pump to keep at work.
8. Find a place at work where you can feel comfortable and have some privacy while you pump.
9. Have a backup place at work for pumping in case your first-choice place is not available.
10. If the baby will be in day care, be certain that the day-care provider is supportive of breastfeeding.
11. Arrive early at the day-care provider's site so that you can nurse the baby right before going to work. This will help the baby settle down, and it also allows time for talking with the day-care provider.

❖ Conclusion

Early and repeated conversations with new breastfeeding mothers can be key to whether a woman continues to nurse her child. Making a home visit or asking the new mother to come for a clinic or office visit to watch the baby nurse and evaluate the mother's breasts and the nipples when problems arise is often critical to identifying and solving the problems. Practitioners should also be familiar with resources for helping women breastfeed successfully—breastfeeding support groups (including the La Leche League), helpful web sites, and books on breastfeeding.

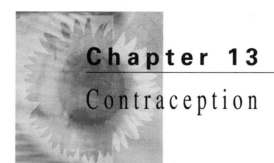

Chapter 13

Contraception

Selection of a contraceptive method is often a complex decision. Parents may need time to consider their options and discuss the many issues involved in selection of a method—effectiveness, complications, benefits, cost, side effects, ease of use, and return of fertility. That is why prenatal discussion of contraception should be encouraged.

This chapter provides practical guidelines for prescribing contraception. Additional information can be found in two books that are particularly useful for clinicians:

Contraceptive Technology, by R. A. Hatcher, J. Trussell, F. Stewart, W. Cates, Jr., G. K. Stewart, F. Guest, and D. Kowal (1998)

A Clinical Guide for Contraception, 3rd edition, by L. Speroff and P. Darney ($29.95) (2001)

 HELPFUL HINT

In some oral contraceptive (OC) users, the low estrogen content of the pill does not allow growth of the endometrium. The result is amenorrhea. Although this is a harmless consequence that some women enjoy, the absence of menses often raises the specter of pregnancy. To avoid expensive, repeated pregnancy testing, advise women to take their basal body temperature (BBT) if they experience amenorrhea. A BBT of less than 98°F at the end of the pill-free week means that conception has not occurred (Speroff & Darney, 2001).

The lowest contraceptive failure rates are found in methods designed for long-term use with little ongoing action required by the user. Failure is more likely to occur in the first 6 months of use, reflecting the difficulty in using a new method correctly and consistently. Figure 13-1 and Table 13-1 illustrate contraceptive failure by method (except for the intrauterine device [IUD]) and duration of use. Additional contributors to method failure are age, marital sta-

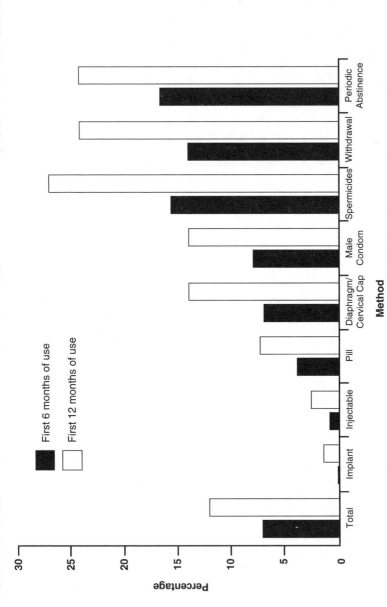

FIGURE 13.1 Contraceptive failure by method. Estimated percentage of U.S. women experiencing contraceptive failure by method and duration of use. (Source: Fu, H., Darroch, J.E. & Ranjit, N. (1999). Contraceptive failure rates: New estimates from the 1995 National Survey of Family Growth. *Family Planning Perspectives*, 31(2).) Model includes correction and standardization for abortion underreporting, duration of use, age, union status, and poverty status.

TABLE 13.1 Percentage of U.S. Women Experiencing Contraceptive Failure, by Duration of Use and Method

Duration and method	Uncorrected*	Corrected* Unstandardized	Corrected* Standardized
First 6 months of use			
Total	5.0	7.1	7.0
Implant	0.0	0.1	0.1
Injectable	1.2	1.1	0.9
Pill	2.6	3.9	3.8
Diaphragm/cervical cap	4.9	6.5	7.8
Male condom	5.1	8.2	8.1
Spermicides	7.0	14.6	15.7
Withdrawal	11.0	13.9	14.1
Periodic abstinence	12.2	13.9	16.7
First 12 months of use			
Total	9.1	12.1	11.8
Implant	1.7	1.8	1.3
Injectable	2.6	3.1	2.5
Pill	6.6	7.6	7.3
Diaphragm/cervical cap	8.4	12.1	14.4
Male condom	9.0	13.9	13.8
Spermicides	15.1	25.7	27.0
Withdrawal	18.2	23.6	24.1
Periodic abstinence	18.9	20.5	24.3

*Correction for abortion underreporting

From Fu, H., Darroch, J. E., & Ranjit, N. (1999). Contraceptive failure rates: New estimates from the 1995 National Survey of Family Growth. *Family Planning Perspectives, 31*(2), p. 60.

tus, and socioeconomic level. The highest failure rates are in adolescents and unmarried women. Lower socioeconomic levels also play a role, probably because of cost, decreased availability of health care, and the "general disadvantage and disruption of poverty" (Fu, Darroch, Haas, 1999). An aggressive follow-up program should be in place for all women using a new method of contraception.

❋ Informed Consent

Informed consent is an important part of prescribing a family planning method. Box 13-1 summarizes the medical and personal information that should be obtained to rule out contraindications to a contraceptive method. This information should be documented and dated in the client record, as should the counseling that was done in relation to the chosen method. Check-off forms listing critical information can be used to ensure that all important information has been included. An outline of topics to be covered in a counseling session can be found in Box 13-2.

❋ Adolescent Contraception

Young adolescents are a particularly vulnerable group for repeat pregnancy. Sexually active teenage girls frequently lack the cognitive, interpersonal, and emotional skills to be successful contraceptive users. A major factor is the fact that adult men are the fathers in 70% of the births that occur to girls through age 18 in this country. "How can young girls enforce abstinence or contraception upon adult men several years their senior . . .?" (Oregon Pregnancy Prevention Task Force, Adolescent Pregnancy Prevention Subcommittee, 1996). A history of abuse, particularly sexual abuse, can also influence a girl's ability to say "no" to sex or to use contraception effectively. The answer to repeat teenage pregnancy is elusive. Until effective programs are in place, longer and

Box 13.1

Information To Be Obtained Prior to Initiating a Method of Birth Control

Medical history
Reproductive history
Previous contraceptive use
Lifestyle, including personal or partner behavior that increases risk for sexually transmitted diseases (STDs)
Relationship status
Future reproductive goals
Smoking history
Fears or concerns about the methods
Ability to adhere to the efficacy and safety requirements

From Kaunitz, A. M., & Zimmer, D. F., Jr. (2000). A medicolegal evaluation of reversible contraceptives. Contemporary OB/GYN, 45(5), 75+. Used with permission.

Box 13.2

Essential Birth Control Counseling Information

How the method works
Effectiveness
Advantages
Risks associated with use, as well as risks associated with pregnancy
Contraindications
Noncontraceptive benefits
Side effects
How to use the method effectively
Medical follow-up required

---

more frequent visits to the provider combined with frequent telephone follow-up should be available to adolescents.

❋ Methods of Family Planning

Oral Contraceptives

Oral contraceptives (OCs) are the most popular reversible method of contraception. They are available in two forms, combination pills that include both estrogen and progestin or pills that contain only progestin (the minipill).

Combination Pills

Combination pills contain estrogen and progestin. Since the 1960 introduction of Enovid, the first "birth control pill," manufacturers have decreased the estrogen content of the combined pill by one fourth and the progestin content by 1/10th. (Enovid contained 150 μg of mestranol and 9.85 mg of norethynodrel.) Almost all combination OCs prescribed today are considered low-dose products, that is, the pills contain less than 50 μg of estrogen. Except for two multiphasic preparations with 40 μg of estrogen in the second phase, most of today's OCs contain between 20 and 35 μg of estrogen. Combination pills are also described in epidemiologic studies as first-, second-, or third-generation pills. These definitions are summarized in Box 13-3.

The combination OC is available as either a monophasic or a multiphasic product. Monophasic pills contain the same amount of estrogen and progestin in each active pill. Multiphasic pills vary the dose of one or both hormones throughout the cycle.

Box 13.3

Definitions of Terms Used to Describe Combined Oral Contraceptives

First-Generation Combination Oral Contraceptives: Products containing 50 μg or more of ethinyl estradiol

Second-Generation Combination Oral Contraceptives: Products containing levonorgestrel, norgestimate, and others in the norethindrone family, as well as 30 or 35 μg of ethinyl estradiol

Third-Generation Combination Oral Contraceptives: Products containing desogestrel or gestodene with 20 or 30 μg of ethinyl estradiol

Low-Dose Oral Contraceptives: Products containing less than 50 μg of estrogen

---

From Speroff, L., & Darney, P. (2001). *A clinical guide to contraception.* Philadelphia: Lippincott Williams and Wilkins, p. 35. Used with permission.

How They Work

The progestin in the combination pill suppresses luteinizing hormone (LH), thereby preventing ovulation. It also prevents buildup of the endometrial lining and thickens the cervical mucus. The estrogen suppresses follicle-stimulating hormone (FSH), preventing the selection of a dominant follicle. Estrogen also enhances the LH suppression action of the progestin (Speroff & Darney, 2001).

Effectiveness

When used correctly, combination OCs practically guarantee protection from pregnancy. Only one woman out of 1,000 becomes pregnant during the first year of combination OC use (Blackburn, Cunkelman, & Zlidar, 2000). However, failure rates of 4% in the first 6 months of typical use and 7% in the first 12 months have been noted (Fu, Darroch, & Haas, 1999).

Advantages

The OC is highly effective at preventing pregnancy. Complications are rare when they are prescribed appropriately. Additionally, OCs have a number of noncontraceptive benefits (summarized in Box 13-4). Because they stop ovulation, they prevent ectopic pregnancy, the leading cause of pregnancy-related death in the first trimester in the United States and a serious cause of maternal mortality in developing countries. Combination OCs also regulate the menstrual cycle and decrease menstrual blood loss (50% to 60% less bleeding, leading to a decrease in iron deficiency anemia) for about two thirds of users. Users experience less dysmenorrhea and fewer premenstrual symptoms. Combination OCs also offer protection against endometrial cancer, even with as lit-

Box 13.4

Noncontraceptive Benefits of Oral Contraceptives

Decrease in dysmenorrhea
Protection against endometrial and epithelial ovarian cancer
Protection against ectopic pregnancy
Fewer premenstrual symptoms
Less anemia
Clearer skin
Regular periods
Shorter, lighter periods
Less cramping with menstrual periods
Ability to periodically avoid menstruation altogether

tle as 1 year of use. Protection against epithelial ovarian cancer, the most common type of ovarian cancer, apparently continues for many years. Combination OCs (except for very-low-dose pills [20 μg]) may increase bone density and/or prevent loss of bone density. Whether current pill formulations protect against ovarian cysts and benign breast disease, as did high-dose OCs (50 μg or more of estrogen), is unknown (Blackburn, Cunkelman, & Zlidar, 2000).

Another major advantage of combination OCs is treatment of acne. Although only Ortho Tri-Cyclen has FDA approval to be advertised for the treatment of acne, in fact, all combined OCs improve acne as they raise sex hormone-binding globulin and decrease free testosterone concentrations (Medical Letter, 2000b).

Disadvantages
The main disadvantage to OCs is the need to take a pill each day. Some women are unable to remember the pill no matter how much they wish to use the OC or how diligently they make a plan to help them remember. In fact, most women may not take the pill on a daily basis despite reporting a pattern of daily use. A 3-month study of 103 women attending two university health services and two publicly funded family planning clinics in Michigan and North Carolina compared women's reports of their pill-taking practices with data obtained from an electronic measuring device that recorded the time and date a pill was removed the package. The reports on the number of days pills were missed agreed only 45% of the time with the data obtained electronically. In each month, the electronic data showed the women missed substantially more pills than they reported (Potter, Oakley, de Leon-Wong, & Canamar, 1996).

The combination OC is not usually prescribed for breastfeeding women because of its association with diminished milk production and concern that the baby may receive harmful amounts of contraceptive steroids.

Risks Associated With Use

Oral contraceptives are associated with morbidity and mortality from heart attacks, strokes, and venous thromboembolism. Other health risks associated with OC use include gallbladder disease in women susceptible to it and rare, nonmalignant liver tumors.

Myocardial Infarction. Cardiovascular risks associated with early pill formulations are significantly decreased—but not eliminated—with newer, low-dose (less than 50 μg of estrogen) pills. A 1996 study reported the maximum estimate of excess risk of myocardial infarction in users of low-dose pills to be one per 100,000 per year. However, the risk rises considerably for women who smoke and for women with hypertension and long-term or uncontrolled diabetes. Still, no risk is noted for women of any age who do not smoke, have their blood pressure checked, and do not have high blood pressure or diabetes (World Health Organization [WHO], 1997).

Ischemic Stroke. A meta-analysis that examined the relationship between ischemic stroke and OC use found that with low-dose estrogen formulations, an OC user's risk for stroke rises from 4.4 to 8.5 per 100,000. This risk, however, is small and, compared to the risk of pregnancy, is probably not significant when the health benefits of OC use are considered.

"If OC use were replaced by the second most popular birth control method, the male condom, an estimated 687,000 additional unintended pregnancies would result per year in the United States, with an associated 26 strokes and 33 deaths based on complication rates of pregnancy and abortion. Although the additional burden of stroke and death due to abortions and full-term pregnancies would not be expected to outnumber the strokes due to OC use, the potential economic and psychological impact of this number of unintended pregnancies is substantial" (Gillum, Mamidipudi, & Johnston, 2000, p. 77).

Women with migraine headaches and focal neurologic symptoms (blurred vision, temporary loss of vision, sights of flashing lights or zigzag lines, or trouble speaking or moving) should not start combination OCs because of a twofold increase in risk of ischemic stroke in this group of women. Women age 35 and older with migraine headaches should not use OCs, even if they do not have focal neurologic symptoms (Blackburn, Cunkelman, & Zlidar, 2000).

Venous Thromboembolism. Idiopathic venous thrombosis occurs 3 to 4 times more often in women who take low-dose OCs. However, most of the increased risk is thought to occur primarily in women with the inherited coagulation problem factor V Leiden mutation. Women with this disorder may have a 30-fold increase in the risk for venous thrombosis. It is best to refer women to a hematologist when they have diagnosed or suspected coagulation disorders, or have a parent or a sibling with this history.

Breast Cancer. A major concern with today's OCs is whether OC use increases the risk of breast cancer. The data currently available generally come from studies of pills containing more estrogen than today's pills and are derived from studies in which the subjects not only initiated OC use later in life, but also used the pill for shorter periods of time than are common today. The cohort of women starting OC use earlier in life, using pills for longer periods of time, and using them to postpone an initial pregnancy (which protects against breast cancer) is just now reaching postmenopausal breast cancer age.

Recent epidemiologic analysis of data collected on more than 53,000 women with breast cancer has led to differing opinions regarding risk. In one study, women using OCs and women who had used them within the past 10 years had a small increased risk of a breast cancer diagnosis. When compared with women who had never used the pill, the tumors found were less likely to have spread beyond the breast. It has been suggested that women who use OCs are screened more often, and their cancer is diagnosed earlier than women who do not use OCs. Additionally, "Ten or more years after stopping the method, an OC user's relative risk of breast cancer is identical to that of a woman who has never used OCs. This argues against a causal association. Oral contraceptives can be used by women with a family history of breast cancer or current benign breast disease" (Contraception Report, 2000, p. 10).

Return of Fertility

After discontinuing OCs, there is a delay in becoming pregnant, with 24 months required before 90% of previous users become pregnant. Of those who have not conceived within 2 years of stopping "the pill," 15% are nulliparas and 7% have given birth previously. This delay is probably due to continuing suppression of the hypothalamic-pituitary system. However, 50% of women who stop the pill to become pregnant conceive within 3 months (Speroff & Darney, 2001).

Contraindications

Nurse-midwives should avoid initiating OC use in women who have any of the conditions listed in Box 13-5. Some clinicians feel that healthy women under age 35 who are hypertensive can take OCs if their blood pressure has responded well to medication. Be cautious and refer such women to a physician.

Side Effects

Breakthrough bleeding is the most common reason women give for stopping the pill, even though this usually disappears after the first months of use. It occurs more often in women who smoke, take the pill inconsistently, or use a product containing 20 μg of estrogen. Other side effects of combined OCs are weight gain, nausea, breast tenderness, amenorrhea, headaches, mood swings, decreased libido, and depression. Many clients are particularly fearful of

Box 13.5

Contraindications to Combination Oral Contraceptives

History of a coagulation abnormality, including thrombophlebitis, conditions predisposing the client to thrombophlebitis, thromboembolism, or a parent or sibling who has had a thromboembolic episode

Cerebral vascular disease, coronary occlusion, or conditions predisposing the client to these conditions

Smoking and age older than 35

Elevated blood pressure

Known or suspected breast cancer

Known or suspected pregnancy

Diabetes-associated vascular disease

Migraine headache with focal neurologic symptoms

Lupus erythematosus with nephritis

Undiagnosed vaginal bleeding

Impaired liver function

Breastfeeding before a good milk supply is established

Time period within 2 to 3 weeks postpartum

Major surgery anticipated within 4 to 6 weeks (except for brief procedures)*

*Considered by some to be periods of high risk

weight gain. While researchers consistently deny an association between OCs and weight gain, many clinicians are convinced that the phenomenon is real and decry the tendency to blame weight gain on lack of exercise, aging, and overeating (when it is the pill that increases appetite).

   HELPFUL HINT

Vomiting and diarrhea appear to be major causes of decreased efficacy in oral contraceptives. As a result, "Even if no pills have been missed, patients should be instructed to use a backup method for at least 7 days after an episode of gastroenteritis" (Speroff & Darney, 2001, p. 40).

Advance discussion of possible OC side effects can help women select a more appropriate method should potential side effects be unacceptable. This discussion can also help some women tolerate a side effect, especially if it is likely to be temporary. An easy introduction to the topic of side effects is,

"What have you heard about the pill?" If none are mentioned, address each side effect anyway. "Some people say the pill made them gain weight (be moody, feel nauseated, or bleed between their periods). Have you ever heard anyone say that? Do you think that might happen to you?"

Drug Interactions

Clinicians must remember that OCs taken with certain drugs may decrease their effectiveness or increase drug metabolism. The drugs in question are primarily drugs affecting liver metabolism. Of particular importance to midwives are antiepileptic drugs. Anecdotal reports of conception occurring when clients on OCs take antibiotics can be found, but "there is no evidence of ovulation" (Speroff and Darney, 2001, p. 97). Box 13-6 summarizes drugs that interact with combination OCs.

Box 13.6

Drugs That Interact With Oral Contraceptives

MEDICATIONS AFFECTING LIVER METABOLISM AND CONTRAINDICATING COMBINATION OC USE

Carbamazepine
Felbamate
Oxcarbazepine
Phenobarbital
Phenytoin
Primidone
Rifabutin
Rifampicin
Topiramate
Vigabatrin
Possibly ethosuximide and griseofulvin

DRUGS THAT MAY BE POTENTIATED BY COMBINATION OCS AND MAY REQUIRE LOWER DOSES

Diazepam (Valium)
Chlordiazepoxide (Librium)
Tricyclic antidepressants
Theophylline

DRUGS THAT MAY NEED TO BE TAKEN IN HIGHER DOSES

Acetaminophen
Aspirin

From Speroff, L., & Darney, P. (2001). *A clinical guide to contraception.* Philadelphia: Lippincott Williams and Wilkins, p. 143. Used with permission.

How to Select a Combination Oral Contraceptive

There are no rules to follow when selecting an OC for a client. In theory, the multiphasic pills mimic the menstrual cycle and should be associated with fewer side effects. In practice, no advantage over monophasic pills has been noted. In fact, no data suggest that any low-dose (sub-50 μg) pill is better than another. The very-low-dose-estrogen products may cause less bloating and breast tenderness, but users risk a higher incidence of breakthrough bleeding. Because there is no way to know in advance how any one woman will respond to the pill prescribed, the only useful guideline is to begin with a low-dose preparation. Demulen 1/35 is a good choice for women who are lactose intolerant, because it contains none of the lactose "fillers" found in other preparations (Nelson, 2001).

Women who are happy with a combined low-dose OC they have previously used should be given the same pill. Women who have experienced a pill-related side effect should be given a different pill. A lower-dose estrogen pill may be appropriate for women who had headaches, nausea, weight gain, or breast tenderness. Progestin is the usual culprit with mood swings and depression. Although there are eight different progestins in today's pill, each comes from one of two families: the norethindrone family or the levonorgestrel family. With a progestin-related side effect, change to the other progestin family.

Instructions for the Client

When to begin. The World Health Organization recommends waiting 6 weeks after delivery before initiating any contraception (WHO, 1996). However, in the United States, recommendations for the initiation of OC often depend on whether the client is breastfeeding or bottle-feeding her baby. Most clinicians do not prescribe combination OCs to breastfeeding women. In the absence of breastfeeding, the combination pill can be started at 3 weeks postpartum (Speroff & Darney, 2001). No backup method is required. Breastfeeding women can wait until they wean their babies to use the combination pill, although combination OCs are sometimes prescribed once a good supply of milk is established.

What to do when a combination OC pill is missed. Missing pills is common. As many as one third of women have missed three or more pills per pack by the third cycle (Speroff & Darney, 2001). Advise clients that if one pill is missed, the missed pill should be taken as soon as it is noted. No backup method is needed. If two pills are missed in the first 2 weeks of the pill pack, take two pills on each of the next 2 days. Use a backup contraceptive method until menstruation occurs. If two pills are missed in the 3rd week of the pill pack or if more than two active pills are missed at any time, use another form of contraception for 7 days. If the missed pill is a Sunday starter, take a pill every day until Sunday and start a new package of pills on Sunday. If it is not a Sunday starter, start a new package of pills as soon as the third missed pill is remembered (Speroff & Darney, 2001). Box 13-7 summarizes these recommendations.

Decreasing the Pill-free/Placebo Interval

For a variety of reasons, women may wish to avoid menses from time to time. This can be accomplished by skipping the placebo pills in a 28-day pill package. Such action causes continuous suppression of FSH and results in amenorrhea. Advantages to this dosage regimen accrue for women with cyclic menstrual symptoms (traditionally referred to as premenstrual syndrome [PMS]), as well as women with a past history of pregnancy while taking pills correctly, women with endometriosis, those with hygiene problems associated with menses (such as women who are mentally retarded), and women wanting to avoid menstruating for a special occasion (Hatcher, 1999). Because there is little long-term experience eliminating or decreasing the pill-free interval, some suggest limiting the regimen to 12 months (Hatcher, 1999).

Medical Follow-Up

A follow-up visit 1 to 2 months after initiation of OC should be scheduled to discuss side effects, identify concerns, examine how the client is taking the pill, go over what to do when a pill is missed, review risks, and emphasize benefits. Box 13-8 summarizes these follow-up activities.

Box 13.7

What To Do When Combination Oral Contraceptive Pills Are Missed

If one pill is missed, take the missed pill as soon as missing it is noted. No backup method is needed.

If two pills are missed in the first 2 weeks of the pill pack, take two pills on each of the next 2 days. Use a backup method until menstruation occurs.

If two pills are missed in the 3rd week of the pill pack

or

If more than two active pills are missed at any time, use another form of contraception for 7 days.

If the missed pill is a Sunday starter, take a pill every day until Sunday. Start a new package of pills on Sunday.

or

If the missed pill is not a Sunday starter, start a new package of pills as soon as the third missed pill is remembered.

From Speroff, L., and Darney, P. (2001). *A clinical guide to contraception*. Philadelphia: Lippincott Williams and Wilkins. Used with permission.

Box 13.8

Follow-up Visit 1 to 2 Months after Initiating Oral Contraception

1. Discuss side effects.
2. Identify concerns.
3. Review pill-taking procedures.
4. Discuss what to do when a pill is missed.
5. Review risks.
6. Emphasize benefits.

Yearly follow-up visits are appropriate thereafter to identify a contraindication to the method that has developed in the interim (such as resumption of smoking in a woman who is now 35 years old). Height should be measured, blood pressure should be determined, and thyroid, breast, and pelvic examinations should be performed.

Progestin-Only Pills

The progestin-only pill (POP) was developed in the 1970s to decrease the thromboembolic effects of estrogen. In the United States, these pills are used primarily for women who are breastfeeding because they do not affect milk production. The POP contains about 25% of the progestin in the combined pill. "There is no evidence for any differences in clinical behavior among the available minipill products" (Speroff & Darney, 2001, p. 139).

How They Work
Progestin-only pills thicken cervical mucus, making it impenetrable to sperm. The endometrium becomes sparse, making the uterine environment unfavorable for implantation. Ovulation is prevented in about half of users (Population Reports, 2000).

Effectiveness
Progestin-only pills are slightly less effective than combination pills for women who do not breastfeed. Among perfect users, five women out of 1,000 will become pregnant during the first year of use, although rates as high as 9.6 out of 100 women per year of use are known (Speroff & Darney, 2001). For breastfeeding women progestin-only pills are as effective as the combined pill (Population Reports, 2000).

Advantages
Progestin-only pills are used postpartally in breastfeeding women because they have no adverse effect on milk volume. They may also be appropriate for women who experience decreased libido, as well as for women who have

unacceptable side effects while taking the combination pill. Progestin-only pills are useful for women in whom estrogen is contraindicated and in women who smoke or have high blood pressure, although it must be noted that ". . . the freedom from estrogen effects, although likely, is presumptive. Substantial data, for example on the associations with vascular disease, blood pressure, and cancer, are not available because relatively small numbers have chosen to use this method of contraception" (Speroff & Darney, 2001, p. 142). Whether the minipill has the same noncontraceptive benefits as the combination pill is unknown at this time.

Disadvantages
The drawback to the POP is the need to take it at the same time every day. About 22 hours after the minipill is taken, the cervical mucus acting as a barrier to sperm decreases, "and by 24 hours sperm penetration is essentially unimpaired" (Speroff & Darney, 2001, p. 140). A difference of more than 3 hours can allow ovulation to occur and requires the use of condoms for each act of intercourse in the next 48 hours (Kaunitz & Zimmer, 2000; Speroff & Darney, 2001).

Strange as it may seem, the minipill is less effective than the IUD at preventing ectopic pregnancy. While it does not increase the incidence of ectopic pregnancy, ". . . when pregnancy occurs, the clinician must suspect that it is more likely to be ectopic" (Speroff & Darney, 2001, p. 140).

Risks Associated With Progestin-Only Pills
Progestin-only pills seem to be safe contraceptive agents in almost all respects. One study, however, found that Latinas who had a history of gestational diabetes mellitus (GDM) and who took the POP had an almost 3-times-greater chance of developing type-2 diabetes than women who used the combination pill (Kjos, Peters, Xiang, Thomas, Schaefer, & Buchanan, 1998). Whether this association is found with additional studies and in additional populations remains to be seen. Until further evidence is available, prudence suggests recommending another contraceptive method for all women who have had GDM.

Contraindications
The FDA requires package labeling for the minipill to include the same list of contraindications required for the combination OC. Others also feel that a history of ectopic pregnancy or functional ovarian cysts constitute a relative contraindication to POPs (Cunningham et al., 2001).

Side Effects
Irregular bleeding is the main problem with the minipill. Menstrual cycles are short and irregular in 40% of users. Ten percent will have irregular bleeding/spotting or amenorrhea (Speroff & Darney, 2001). Some women have a problem with acne.

Drug Interactions

Potential interactions between the minipill and certain medications preclude their use. These drugs are the same ones that should be avoided when using the combination pill (see Box 13-6).

Instructions for the Client

Guidelines vary for initiating POPs for breastfeeding mothers. Speroff and Darney recommend waiting 3 days after delivery "to allow the decline in pregnancy levels of estrogen and progesterone and the establishment of lactation" (Speroff & Darney, 2001, p. 83). Another recommendation is to begin at 3 weeks postpartum for women who are partially breastfeeding and 6 weeks for women who are completely breastfeeding (Kaunitz & Zimmer, 2000). Still others recommend initiating POPs when menstruation returns or at 6 months' postpartum, whichever comes first, noting that only two pregnancies per 100 women will occur in the first 6 months after childbirth (Population Reports, 2000). Inherent in this recommendation is exclusive breastfeeding, a practice not commonly observed in the United States.

The usual time of intercourse must be considered when helping clients determine the optimum time for taking the POP. Because cervical mucus thickening decreases 22 hours after taking the minipill and 2 to 4 hours are required to effect a change in cervical mucus (Speroff & Darney, 2001), the time to take the minipill must be individualized.

Users must understand the importance of taking the pill at the same time every day and should have a supply of condoms on hand to use when intercourse occurs and taking the pill is off by 3 or more hours.

The Intrauterine Device

Today's IUDs are safe and effective. Fears about their use stem from experience with the Dalkon Shield, a device introduced in 1971 that was associated with 200 cases of midtrimester septic abortion and 20 maternal deaths (Boonstra, 2000). Investigation revealed that bacteria accumulated in the spaces between individual filaments within the nylon sheath of the tail of the device. Bacteria traveled up the tail and, as the pregnant uterus grew, the tail was drawn into the uterine cavity. Current IUDs have a monofilament tail so that bacteria do not accumulate.

Uterine perforation was also a problem with the Dalkon Shield and with other first-generation IUDs. The "pull-back" insertion technique used with today's devices diminishes the perforation risk.

Modern IUDs began when developers simultaneously realized that a T-shaped device could accommodate well to the endometrial cavity and that the addition of copper or progesterone to the device increased its effectiveness. Initially, the copper devices were wound with 200 to 250 mm^2 of copper wire.

Some of these devices are still in use. The first hormone-containing IUD worked well for women with heavy menses or dysmenorrhea, but its 1-year life span precluded use by many women. Incorporating a different progesterone, levonorgestrel, into the device, lengthened the life span considerably.

Two IUDs are currently marketed in the United States, the TCu380A (ParaGard) and the LNG-20 (Mirena). Both are T-shaped devices. The TCu380A is made of polyethylene with copper wound on each of the transverse arms and the vertical shaft. A monofilament polyethylene thread is tied through a knob at the tip of the T, resulting in two threads that are 12-cm long. The device can remain in utero for 10 years. The LNG-20 has a collar on the vertical shaft that releases levonorgestrel. This device can remain in utero 5 to 7 years.

Advantages

The TCu380A and the LNG-20 have the advantage of long-term contraceptive efficacy without having to take a pill every day, remembering to take injections at specified intervals, or planning for contraceptive use in association with intercourse. The IUD can be a good choice for women with certain medical complications and for women who smoke. The cost of an IUD is both an advantage and a disadvantage. The high initial cost is prohibitive to many. However, over the life of the device, the cost is low.

Disadvantages

All IUDs are contraindicated in women with or at risk for sexually transmitted infections. Initial cost, as indicated above, is an additional disadvantage. Approximately one out of 20 women will expel the TCu380A during the first year. Expulsion occurs in approximately one out of 20 IUD insertions. Table 13-2 compares expulsion and removal rates for the TCu380A and LNG-20.

TABLE 13.2 Expulsions and Removal Rates for the TCu380A (ParaGard) and LNG-20 (Mirena)

Device	Expulsion rate	Removal rate
TCu380A	5	14
LNG-20	6	17

Adapted from Speroff, L., & Darney, P. D. (2001). *A clinical guide for contraception* (3rd ed.). Philadelphia: Lippincott Williams & Wilkins, p. 231. Used with permission.

Risks Associated With IUD Use

Risks associated with IUD use include uterine perforation and pelvic infection. Perforation risk decreases significantly with attention to insertion technique. Devices using a "withdrawal" technique for insertion are associated with fewer perforations. In randomized trials, the perforation rate with the TCu380A was one in 1,360 (ParaGard T380A Product Monograph, no date). Previous reports that breastfeeding women had a significantly greater chance of a uterine perforation with IUD insertion are probably unfounded, as additional research suggests that perforation in breastfeeding mothers is more likely to be related to the timing of insertion rather than to breastfeeding (Grimes, 1998).

Infection may occur at the time of IUD insertion in spite of aseptic technique. Infection occurring 3 or 4 weeks after insertion or later is usually caused by a sexually transmitted disease (STD). Whether the administration of doxycycline (100 to 200 mg) or azithromycin (500 mg) shortly before insertion provides protection against infection is unknown, as results of studies are controversial. Endometritis (uterine tenderness) without associated symptoms can be treated with 100 mg of doxycycline for 14 days (Box 13-9).

Whether an IUD increases the risk of ectopic pregnancy is debated. While traditional teaching holds that IUDs increase the incidence, Speroff and Darney state that IUDs, except for Progestasert (no longer marketed), protect against ectopic pregnancy because pregnancy is rare in IUD users. Further they state, "The protection against ectopic pregnancy provided by the TCu-380A and the levonorgestrel IUD makes these IUDs acceptable choices for contraception in women with previous ectopic pregnancies" (Speroff & Darney, 2001, p. 233). Remember, however, that a pregnancy that occurs with an IUD in place is more likely to be ectopic than a pregnancy occurring without an IUD.

Contraindications

Contraindications to all IUDs include pregnancy, postpartum endometritis within the previous 3 months, undiagnosed vaginal bleeding, immunosuppres-

---

Box 13.9

Treatment of IUD Insertion-Associated Endometritis

For treatment of endometritis when uterine tenderness occurs without cervical motion, rebound, or adnexal tenderness; adnexal mass; elevated white blood cell count; or elevated sedimentation rate:

Doxycycline, 100 mg twice a day for 14 days

*Note: "No harmful effects have yet been reported in breastfeeding infants" (Hale, 2000, p. 226).

sion, an unresolved abnormal Pap smear, known or suspected uterine malignancy, untreated vaginitis or cervicitis, fibroids, bicornuate uterus, genital actinomycosis, multiple sexual partners, alcohol and drug dependence, a nonmonogamous relationship, and pelvic inflammatory disease (PID) (current, within the previous 3 months, or recurrent). These contraindications are summarized in Box 13-10.

Insertion

Women who exclusively breastfeed have excellent protection against pregnancy for at least 12 weeks postpartum, so clinicians need not worry about pregnancy at the 4- to 6-week postpartum visit in this group of women. A well-involuted uterus at 4 weeks does not contraindicate placement of an IUD. Postpartal IUD insertion is usually easy in women who have had cervical dilatation in labor. A study published 2 decades ago reported that expulsion

---

Box 13.10

Contraindications to IUD Insertion

ALL IUDS

- Pregnancy
- Postpartum endometritis in the preceding 3 months
- Distortions of the uterine cavity
    Fibroids
    Bicornuate uterus
- STD risk factors
    Alcohol or drug abuse
    Multiple sexual partners
    Nonmonogamous relationship
- Current, recurrent, or recent PID
- Immunosuppression
- Uterus that sounds <6 cm or >9 cm
- Unresolved abnormal Pap smear or known or suspected uterine malignancy
- Undiagnosed vaginal bleeding
- Untreated vaginitis or cervicitis (including bacterial vaginosis)
- Genital actinomycosis

THE TCU380A (PARAGARD)

- Heavy menses
- Severe anemia
- Dysmenorrhea
- Bleeding disorder or anticoagulation therapy
- Copper allergy

and removal rates for pain and bleeding decrease when the IUD is inserted in the middle of the menstrual cycle (day 12 through 17) rather than during menses, the time traditionally considered best for insertion (White et al., 1980). Whether this applies to today's IUDs is not known.

When inserting an IUD, remember

1. To perform a bimanual examination to determine the position of the uterus prior to application of a tenaculum to the cervix and measurement of uterine length
2. To insert the IUD only if the uterus measures between 6.0 and 9.0 cm. Inserting the device when the length is less than 6.0 cm increases the incidence of expulsion, pain, bleeding, and perforation. Inserting the device when the length is greater than 9.0 cm may increase the incidence of pregnancy.
3. To advise the client to take ibuprofen (800 mg) 1 hour prior to the time scheduled for insertion

---

 HELPFUL HINT

If you choose not to use a paracervical block with IUD insertion, perform the bimanual examination to determine uterine position with 1% lidocaine gel as the lubricating gel for the examination. This will numb the cervix and decrease the discomfort associated with application of the tenaculum.

Some midwives also place a small amount of the anesthetic gel on a cotton swab and place the swab in the cervix prior to measuring the length of the uterine cavity.

 HELPFUL HINT

Use a pipelle to sound the uterus for size rather than a metal sound.

Informed consent requires a discussion of the effectiveness rate, side effects, and complications associated with IUD use. Charting should include a description of the procedure, medications used prior to insertion (such as a nonsteroidal anti-inflammatory drug [NSAID] and/or antibiotic), indication of the client's ability to feel the IUD strings before leaving the clinic or office, a listing of danger signs that were discussed, and a description of the medical emergency help that was conveyed. Documenting that the client read the consent form prior to insertion is also important. Unfortunately, the consent form that accompanies the TCu380A violates many principles of obtaining informed consent from persons with low literacy skills. It may be more helpful to document specific topics within the consent form that were reviewed with the client. Appendix R contains a form that can be added to a client record to facilitate charting of pre-insertion counseling and the IUD procedure. This type of form also helps the clinician address and document all important points.

 HELPFUL HINT

Pharmaceutical companies usually have patient assistance programs that provide medicines, including intrauterine devices (IUDs), free of charge to clinicians whose clients might not be able to purchase the medicine.

   A yearly list of the companies participating in such programs, along with company addresses and eligibility criteria, is published by the Pharmaceutical Research and Manufacturers of America (1100 Fifteenth St., N.W., Washington, DC, 20005). Web sites containing helpful information include the web site of the Pharmaceutical Research and Manufacturers of America, www.phrma.org and www.rxassist.org.

Instructions for Client Use

A client should be advised to notify the health care provider if she feels pregnant, either she or her partner has an STD, or she is no longer in a mutually monogamous relationship. TCu380A users should also report amenorrhea. All users must know warning signs of infection: uterine tenderness, foul-smelling discharge, fever, or chills. Users should check monthly for the IUD threads. NSAIDs initiated at the onset of menstruation in women with the copper device can minimize cramping and heavy menses. These instructions are summarized in Box 13-11.

   The client should also be able to feel the threads of the IUD in her vagina before she leaves the clinic or office.

Medical Follow-up

Reexamination within 3 months after insertion is recommended for all IUDs to check for full or partial expulsion of the device.

The TCu380A

How It Works

The main mechanism of action of the copper-containing IUD is thought to be an endometrial response that causes the release of white blood cells, prostaglandins,

---

Box 13.11

Client Instructions After IUD Insertion

1. Notify the health care provider if
   a. A period is missed.
   b. The relationship is no longer mutually monogamous.
   c. Signs of infection are present: uterine tenderness, foul-smelling discharge, fever, or chills.
2. Check for strings monthly (after menses when menstruation resumes).
3. Use NSAIDs when menstruation begins for cramping and for heavy menses. Continue use for 3 days.

---

and enzymes. Endometrial fluid is altered, and both sperm motility and integrity are affected. The result is inhibition of fertilization. Copper IUDs damage sperm and "substantially" reduce the number of sperm in the fallopian tubes. Secondarily, IUDs may also inhibit implantation, although this mechanism of action is thought to be infrequent (Grimes, 1998).

Effectiveness
The first-year pregnancy rate of the TCu380A is approximately one per 200 users.

Risks
The TCu380A may cause anemia, particularly with long-term use. Perforation is rare, particularly with attention to uterine position and insertions that do not require that the device be pushed into the uterine cavity, as was the case with the Dalkon Shield, Lippes Loop, and Saf-T-Coil.

Return of Fertility
Studies show that there is no delay in return of fertility following removal of an IUD, regardless of duration of use.

Contraindications
The copper device is contraindicated in severe anemia, heavy menses, dysmenorrhea, anticoagulation therapy, and allergy to copper. Women at risk for bacterial endocarditis should receive prophylactic antibiotics at insertion (and at removal). Intrauterine devices should not be inserted if the uterus measures less than 6 cm. Package insert instructions also say that the uterus should not measure more than 9 cm.

Side Effects
Side effects of the TCu380A include irregular bleeding, heavy menses, prolongation of menses, and dysmenorrhea. Heavy menses and dysmenorrhea, in most cases, respond to ibuprofen, although removal of the device is sometimes

required. Hypermenorrhea and dysmenorrhea are uncommon in women using the LNG-20 IUDs. However, periods may be light or absent (60% amenorrheic when using the LNG-20 for 12 years), and this may be a deterrent to continued use for some women. Most removals of the TCu380A are for pain or bleeding (Speroff & Darney, 2001), but the recent introduction of the LNG-20 allows IUD contraception for women with histories of dysmenorrhea and heavy menses.

The LNG-20 Intrauterine System

The LNG-20 Intrauterine System is another T-shaped IUD with a collar on the vertical arm containing 52 mg of levonorgestrel.

How It Works

The LNG-20 thickens cervical mucus and thins the endometrial lining. In some women it prevents ovulation.

Effectiveness

The LNG-20 is highly effective. The first-year failure rate is 0.1% and the 5-year failure rate is 0.71%.

Advantages

The LNG-20 is associated with an increase in hemoglobin. Oligomenorrhea and amenorrhea, considered advantages by some women, are common— oligomenorrhea within 2 years of insertion in 70% of levonorgestrel IUD users and amenorrhea in 30% (Speroff & Darney, 2001). Dysmenorrhea may be decreased.

Disadvantages

Amenorrhea may be perceived as a disadvantage by some women. Irregular bleeding in the first weeks of use may also be unacceptable.

Side Effects

Erratic bleeding after insertion is common with the LNG-20 and can be heavy as well. Twenty percent of users experience bleeding that lasts longer than 8 days. However, by the third month, prolonged bleeding is experienced by only about 3% of users.

Injectable Contraception

Long-Term Injectable Contraception

Injectable contraception with depot medroxyprogesterone acetate (DMPA, also known as Depo-Provera) has been used worldwide for contraception since the 1960s, although FDA approval in the United States was delayed until 1992. The dosage is 150 mg every 11 to 13 weeks. No backup method is needed if the injection is administered during the first 5 days of the menstrual cycle. When given later in the cycle, a backup method should be used for 5 to 7 days (Nelson, 2001).

How It Works
Depo-Provera acts by blocking the LH surge, thereby preventing ovulation. It also prevents 1) sperm penetration by thickening cervical mucus and 2) implantation of the ovum by altering the endometrium.

Effectiveness
The failure rate of long-term injectable contraception is less than 1% per year (The Contraception Report, 2000). In doses of 150 mg, DMPA provides protection from pregnancy for 14 weeks.

Advantages
In addition to being highly effective, long-term injectable contraception is not associated with intercourse. No pill packages will be found in hidden places, and no implants will be seen or felt. There are no estrogen-related side effects, nor is there a pill to take on a daily basis. Injectable contraception is useful with breastfeeding women and women with seizure disorders. It may be appropriate for women who are smokers over 35 years of age and women with a history of thromboembolism, seizure disorders, or sickle cell disease. A 70% decrease in sickle cell crises has been noted when women with sickle cell anemia use Depo-Provera (Nelson, 2001). DMPA is associated with a decrease in both endometrial and ovarian cancer. In some cultures, the fact that the medicine is administered by way of injection is an advantage.

Disadvantages
The disadvantages of DMPA include the comparatively high up-front cost of the injection every 3 months, the fact that it is an injection (not considered an advantage by some), irregular bleeding patterns, amenorrhea, weight gain, and the need for clients to remember to schedule the injection every 3 months.

While not associated with intercourse, long-term injectable contraception may pose problems to teenagers whose mothers keep track of their daughters' menstrual periods. The mother of an amenorrheic teen using DMPA may suspect pregnancy.

A relatively long period of time is required for the body to clear DMPA (6 to 8 months, longer in heavier women). This means that side effects take time to disappear and the return of menstrual regularity may not be immediate.

Risks Associated With Use
Whether DMPA is associated with an increase in breast cancer is not known. Study results are conflicting. Speroff and Darney recommend that clinicians "... consider informing patients that Depo-Provera might accelerate the growth of an already present occult cancer" (Speroff & Darney, 2001, p. 206.) Whether bone loss occurs that could contribute to osteoporosis later in

life is another unanswered question. Clinicians may want to avoid DMPA for adolescents because of the fact that a rapid increase in bone density occurs during this time. "Almost all of the bone mass in the hip and vertebral bodies will be accumulated in young women by age 18, and the years immediately following menarche are especially important" (Speroff & Darney, 2001, p. 208).

Return of Fertility

Eighteen months after an injection of Depo-Provera, 90% of women wishing to conceive will be pregnant. However, the "delay to conception" is approximately 9 months and likely to be longer in women who are overweight. Women who wish to conceive quickly after discontinuing a method should select a different contraceptive (Speroff & Darney, 2001). Because return of fertility may be delayed, DMPA may not be a good method for older women considering a future pregnancy.

Contraindications

Because of the study that found an increase in type 2 diabetes in Latinas with previous GDM, Depo-Provera should be used cautiously in women with a history of GDM until further studies gather more data.

Side Effects

Side effects of DMPA include intermenstrual bleeding, weight gain, moodiness, depression, breast tenderness, headache, nervousness, fatigue, and decrease or loss of libido. Menstrual irregularities, including irregular bleeding and spotting, cause about one third of clients to stop using the method at the end of 1 year (Grimes, 2000). Amenorrhea after 9 to 12 months of use is common, an advantage to some users but a scary occurrence to others.

For many users, weight gain is a major concern. The package insert accompanying Depo-Provera lists the following as a summary of associated weight gain:

Duration of Use	Average Weight Gain
1 year	5.4 lb
2 years	8.1 lb
4 years	13.8 lb
6 years	16.5 lb

Despite the admission of weight gain in the Depo-Provera package insert, researchers claim that weight gain cannot be documented by research studies. Initially, studies also failed to support an association between DMPA and depression. However, a recent study comparing DMPA users with nonusers over a 3-year period found that continuous DMPA users were 40% more likely than nonusers to report symptoms of depression (Civic, Scholes, Ichikawa, LaCroix, Yoshida, Ott, & Barlow, 2000).

Noncontraceptive Benefits

Like the OC, long-acting injectable contraception has noncontraceptive benefits. These include a decreased risk of endometrial cancer and ectopic pregnancy; less menstrual flow, anemia, and endometriosis; and fewer uterine fibroids.

Instructions for the Client

Clients using long-term injectable contraception must understand that repeat injections should be scheduled every 12 weeks. Make the appointment before the client leaves the clinic or office, as this seems to increase the return rate for subsequent injections.

Medical Follow-up

Precautions to be observed in the administration of DMPA, established by the manufacturer, are summarized in Box 13-12. Yearly breast and pelvic examinations, as well as measurement of height, weight, and blood pressure, are recommended.

Short-Term Injectable Contraception

Short-term (monthly) injectable contraception has been studied since 1968 and used throughout the world, but only recently has it been available in the United States. The injection, administered every 23 to 33 days, contains 25 mg of

---

Box 13.12

Precautions in Relation to the Administration of Depo-Provera to Avoid Accidental Pregnancies

1. If the client is amenorrheic and completely breastfeeding at the postpartum checkup, no pregnancy test is needed prior to the injection. If the client is amenorrheic and partially breastfeeding, perform a pregnancy test before the first injection. If menses has occurred, give the initial injection within 5 days of onset.
2. Administer the medicine
   a. Deep IM (in the arm rather than the hip, particularly in overweight women)
   b. By Z-track technique
   c. Without massage by the health care professional after injection, as well as client activities that could increase absorption (Speroff & Darney, 2001). (I know one woman who bowled a few hours after injection and was soon pregnant. Other anecdotal reports, including pregnancy after weight lifting, suggest the latter precaution is appropriate.)
   d. At 12-week intervals, with 14-week intervals possible

From package insert, "Depo-Provera," Upjohn Corporation.

medroxyprogesterone acetate (MPA) and 5 mg of estradiol cypionate (E_2C). The trade name of the product is Lunelle.

How It Works

Monthly contraceptive injections prevent conception by estrogen suppression of FSH and LH. The progestin suppresses LH, thins the endometrium, and thickens cervical mucus.

Effectiveness

MPA/E_2C is as effective as surgical sterilization. Clinical trials reported 12-month pregnancy rates of 0 to 0.2 per 100 woman-years of use.

Advantages

In addition to being highly effective, MPA/E_2C provides cycle control. It is not associated with the irregular, heavy bleeding and amenorrhea common with Depo-Provera. Regular menses occur for up to 70% of users, although the bleeding may last 1 to 2 days longer than with OCs. Only 1% of users reported amenorrhea after the first month of use, and 4 % reported amenorrhea after 60 weeks of continuous use (Shulman, 2000). Return to fertility is prompt.

Disadvantages

Disadvantages with short-term injectable contraception include breakthrough bleeding in the first 3 months of use, occurring about as frequently as with low-dose OCs (Speroff & Darney, 2001); lack of protection against sexually-transmitted infections; and the necessity of monthly injections, requiring not only the inconvenience of an additional visit to a clinic or office, but also the expenses such a visit generates. Some states permit pharmacists to give the injections.

Because the product contains estrogen, estrogen-related complications may occur. Additionally, women may not understand that the first menses after the initial injection will occur 14 to 21 days after the injection rather than 28 days. They are likely to think they are experiencing breakthrough bleeding rather than menses. Predictable menses will occur after the third cycle.

The combination of estrogen and progestin may inhibit lactation. Until further data are available, avoid monthly injectable contraception for women who are breastfeeding.

Return of Fertility

Return of fertility is similar to that of IUD and diaphragm users. ". . . ovulation returns 2 months after the last injection" (Speroff & Darney, 2001, p. 211). Conception occurs by 5 months in about 60% of women and within 1 year in about 83% of women.

Contraindications

Contraindications to short-term injectable contraception are similar to those for OCs. They are summarized in Box 13-13.

Box 13.13

Contraindications to Short-Term Injectable Contraception (Lunelle)*

Known or suspected pregnancy
Thrombophlebitis or thromboembolic disorders
Current or history of deep vein thrombophlebitis or thromboembolic disorders
Cerebral vascular or coronary artery disease
Undiagnosed abnormal genital bleeding
Women who smoke more than 15 cigarettes per day and are over 35
History of liver dysfunction or disease
Known or suspected estrogen-dependent neoplasia
Severe hypertension
Diabetes with vascular involvement
Headaches with focal neurologic symptoms
Valvular heart disease with complications

---

*Identified by the manufacturers, Pharmacia and Upjohn

Side Effects
Serious side effects are reported by fewer than 2% of women using short-term injectable contraception. Bleeding and breast tenderness are the most common, occurring 3 times as often in users of short-term injection contraception as in OC users. Weight increases occur 4 times as often, acne occurs twice as often, and emotional lability also occurs twice as often. The incidence of nausea and headache is the same in short-term injection users as in OC users.

Client Instructions
Users of short-term injectable contraception need an injection every 23 to 33 days. A thorough discussion about expected bleeding patterns can minimize confusion and dissatisfaction. Clients should understand that bleeding will occur 2 to 3 weeks after the first injection, rather than 4 weeks after as might be anticipated. Regular menses will occur thereafter. Bleeding occurs 22 days after each injection and lasts 5 to 6 days, longer than the bleeding experienced by users of OCs.

Barrier Methods

How They Work
Contraception intended to keep sperm from encountering an ovum by introducing a barrier of some kind between the two has been used for centuries. Some methods were combined with substances thought to kill sperm.

Advantages
Barrier methods of contraception contain no hormones and, therefore, users do not have to cope with hormonal side effects and potential complications. Barrier methods provide some protection against most STDs. However, only the condom also protects against HIV. Barrier methods do not affect fertility after use and may be used with breastfeeding.

Disadvantages
Barrier methods must be used with each act of intercourse and, therefore, require significant motivation on the part of each partner.

Contraindications
Barrier methods should not be used by women who have had toxic shock syndrome.

The Diaphragm With Contraceptive Cream

How It Works
The diaphragm is meant to be used with a spermicidal cream, the diaphragm acting as a barrier to sperm and the cream killing sperm that pass the barrier.

Effectiveness
Pregnancy rates are highly variable and range from a low of 2% to a high of 25%. Efficacy depends on perfect use and appropriate fit.

Advantages
Advantages of the diaphragm-spermicide combination include the fact that it is a method that a woman can choose to use or not use each time she engages in sexual intercourse. The cost of a diaphragm is reasonable for most women, especially considering that it can be used for many years. The major expense is the ongoing need for the spermicide.

Some couples share responsibility for family planning by alternating use of the diaphragm with use of a condom—the "my month, your month" or "my week, your week" approach.

Disadvantages
Among the disadvantages of the diaphragm with spermicide are the need to 1) be fitted by a health care professional, 2) use it with every act of intercourse, 3) anticipate intercourse so that it can be in place at the right time, 4) use more spermicide if a second act of intercourse occurs with the diaphragm in place, 5) leave the diaphragm in place for 6 hours after coitus, and 6) clean and dry the diaphragm after each use.

Risks Associated With Use
Toxic shock syndrome is associated with use of a diaphragm, but because this syndrome occurs so rarely, it should not be an important consideration when it comes to choosing a method of contraception.

Contraindications

The diaphragm will not prevent pregnancy if it does not fit properly. Unfortunately, some women do not have the anatomy required for a proper fit. For a diaphragm to fit properly, the client must have 1) a pubic symphysis whose inner surface will accommodate and hold the diaphragm in front and 2) sufficient muscular integrity that the diaphragm will stay in place. A diaphragm that fits loosely behind the symphysis permits the penis to enter the vagina between the rim of the diaphragm and the symphysis and is likely to result in a deposition of sperm smack in the middle of the diaphragm! Stretching of the muscles surrounding the vagina during childbirth, as well as a cystocele or rectocele, contribute to poorly fitting diaphragms, causing them to be unstable. A program of Kegel exercises (75 times/day) for 3 months may allow for diaphragm use.

Diaphragms are made with one of three types of springs: flat, arcing, or hinged. The flat-spring diaphragm maintains a straight line when squeezed for insertion. This type of spring is useful for women who have an anterior cervix but is not good for women with a posterior cervix, as the diaphragm is easily placed in front of the cervix. The arcing-spring diaphragm is useful for most women. It bends into an arc regardless of where it is squeezed, facilitating placement over the cervix irrespective of cervical position in the vagina.

Diaphragm sizes range from 60 mm to 105 mm in size and are available in 5-mm increments. Most women use sizes between 70 mm and 85 mm. Figure 13-2 illustrates the traditional approach for measuring the size of diaphragm needed. A properly fitting diaphragm hooks "nicely" (not too loose and not too tight) behind the symphysis, fills the vagina, and covers the cervix.

 HELPFUL HINT

When fitting a diaphragm for someone who has never had intercourse, start with one that measures 65 mm. When fitting a diaphragm for someone who has had a vaginal birth, start with a 75-mm ring.

Side Effects

Women who use diaphragms are at increased risk for urinary tract infections. Why this is so is not known. Occasionally, women or their partners are allergic to spermicide or the latex with which the diaphragm is made.

Instructions for the Client

Before leaving the clinic or office, a new diaphragm user should receive instructions on insertion and removal of the diaphragm and should demonstrate her ability to insert and remove it properly before she leaves. Visual aids

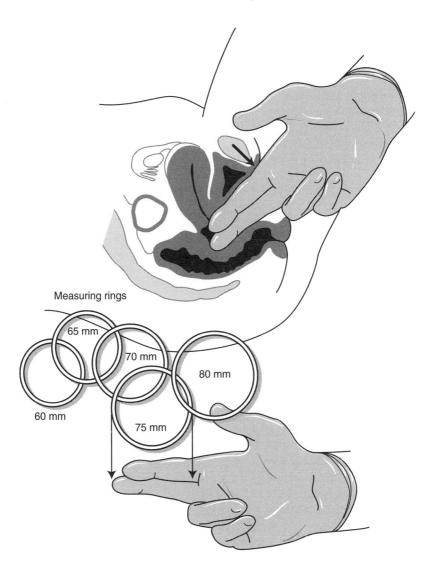

Measuring rings

65 mm

70 mm

80 mm

60 mm

75 mm

FIGURE 13.2 Determining diaphragm size. (Adopted from S. Koperski from Jackson, Berger, Keith, *Vaginal Contraception*, G.K. Hall Publishers.)

in most patient instruction pamphlets are not appropriate for women with low literacy skills.

If a woman is not able to anticipate intercourse and have the diaphragm in place when it occurs, some clinicians, assuming that intercourse will occur at night, advise women to "wash your face, brush your teeth, and put in your diaphragm."

Traditional instructions for client use include 1) inserting the diaphragm between 15 minutes and 1 hour before intercourse, 2) using an extra applicator of diaphragm contraceptive gel if more than an hour elapses between insertion and intercourse, 3) using an extra applicator of diaphragm contraceptive gel for every additional act of intercourse, 4) leaving the diaphragm in place for 6 hours after intercourse, and 5) not leaving the diaphragm in place for more than 24 hours. Unfortunately, the validity and usefulness of these instructions have not been tested.

With each insertion the user must be sure that the diaphragm covers the cervix. The diaphragm should be washed with mild soap and water after each use, rinsed well, dried, checked for holes, kept in the container in which it arrived, and stored in a cool place.

Advise clients to have the fit checked with any significant gain or loss of weight and after childbirth. It also makes sense to have the fit checked after initial sexual experience, but the number of times intercourse should occur before reexamination has not been addressed.

The Cervical Cap

The cervical cap fits over the cervix. It comes in four sizes and is somewhat more difficult to fit than a diaphragm. Effectiveness and side effects are similar to those of a diaphragm. The cap can be left in place for 48 hours.

The Male Condom

Effectiveness

Condoms are estimated to be between 80% and 95% effective in preventing pregnancy. Concurrent use of a spermicide, through use of a spermicide-coated condom or spermicide in addition to a condom, increases protection from both pregnancy and sexually transmitted infections. However, the shelf life of a spermicide-coated condom is only 2 years, while the shelf life of a condom that is not coated with spermicide is 5 years. Additionally, the incidence of bacteriuria with *Escherichia coli* or *Staphylococcus saprophyticus* increases when condoms are used with spermicide (Speroff & Darney, 2001).

Advantages

The male condom protects against sexually transmitted infections, including HIV, as well as pregnancy. Its use provides the male partner with an opportunity to share in the responsibility for preventing pregnancy.

Disadvantages

Condoms are not as effective as some other temporary methods of birth control. Both men and women may report decreased sexual pleasure with condom use. Condoms can slip, and they can break. Slippage rates as high as 5% are reported, while breakage rates range between one and eight for 100 episodes of vaginal intercourse (Speroff & Darney, 2001). Because oil-based lubricants weaken condoms, Vaseline should not be used as a lubricant when condoms are used. In addition, vaginal preparations should not be used to treat vaginal yeast infections when a condom will be worn, as these preparations are oil based (Nelson, 2001).

Some women prefer to assume responsibility for contraception, because only women become pregnant.

Instructions for Client Use

Clients can benefit from knowing kinds and brand names of condoms; how they vary in size, color, texture, taste (now available in vanilla, banana, and strawberry flavors), smell, thickness, and price; and where they are likely to be located in a store. This information can be obtained by purchasing a representative sample of condoms in the pharmacy section of a well-known grocery store. Keep samples in the examining room to use in your discussion with your client.

Counseling should include teaching how to put on the condom. A good way to teach the correct technique is to use a penis model, but any penis-shaped object (a cucumber, banana, zucchini, or yellow squash) will do. After demonstrating the technique to the client, give the client an opportunity to put the condom on the model herself. Interjecting humor by blowing a condom up like a balloon or filling it with water may help. Additional suggestions for helping clients talk about condoms with a partner can be found in Chapter 15.

The Female Condom

How It Works

The female condom is a loose-fitting polyurethane sheath with a flexible ring at each end (Figure 13-3). A small, inner ring lies within the closed end and is used during insertion. When placed behind the pubic bone, it helps keep the condom in place. It does not need to cover the cervix. The outer ring remains on the outside of the vagina covering the vulva and providing some protection to the labia.

Effectiveness

Protection against pregnancy is thought to be similar to that of the diaphragm (Speroff & Darney, 2001; Family Health International, 2000a).

Advantages

The female condom provides protection against sexually transmitted infections as well as pregnancy, although the extent of protection is not fully

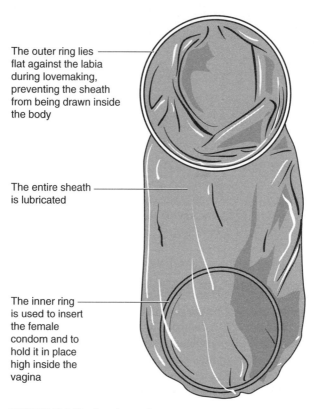

The outer ring lies flat against the labia during lovemaking, preventing the sheath from being drawn inside the body

The entire sheath is lubricated

The inner ring is used to insert the female condom and to hold it in place high inside the vagina

FIGURE 13.3 The female condom.

known. It is prelubricated, causes no allergic reactions, and is stronger than latex. It can be used with both oil-based and water-based lubricants. Use does not depend on an erect penis. The female condom can be inserted up to 8 hours before sexual activity begins, and immediate withdrawal of the penis after ejaculation is not necessary. Unlike male condoms, the female condom does not deteriorate when exposed to heat and humidity. The expiration date (shelf life) is 5 years from the manufacturing date (World Health Organization & Joint United Nations Programme on HIV/AIDS, 2000).

For some women, the female condom is a reasonable alternative to other methods. The World Health Organization and the Joint United Nations Programme on HIV/AIDS are encouraging the introduction of the female condom as part of a public health strategy for reproductive health care. Their guide to designing and implementing programs in a variety of settings describes programs in Africa, Central and South America, and the United States (World Health Organization & Joint United Nations Programme on HIV/AIDS, 2000) and contains useful ideas for discussing the female condom with clients. Whether consistent use can be sustained is unknown.

Disadvantages
The availability of other methods of pregnancy and STD protection in the United States as well as the cost of the female condom make this method significantly less popular than others in this country.

The Sponge

The "Today" sponge was first marketed in 1982, but it was removed from the market in 1995 when the manufacturer decided that correcting manufacturing problems at the old factory where the sponge was made would be too costly. Subsequently, the client and production equipment were sold (1999), the equipment was updated, and FDA approval for the new sponge was granted in 2000.

How It Works
The vaginal contraceptive sponge incorporates the spermicide nonoxynol 9 into its polyurethane disc. The sponge also absorbs semen and acts as a barrier to the cervical canal. Unlike the diaphragm, additional spermicidal gel or cream is unnecessary, and unlike spermicides, no waiting time between insertion and intercourse is required. Release of the spermicide occurs with insertion and continues for 24 hours. Frequency of coitus does not affect effectiveness.

Effectiveness
The method-effectiveness rate is 89% to 91% when used correctly with each act of intercourse. The use-effectiveness rate is 84% to 87%. Data suggest that the more women use the sponge, the more effective it is. Data conflict about whether the number of vaginal births the user has had influences the sponge's effectiveness.

Advantages
Advantages of the contraceptive sponge include the following:

- Over-the-counter availability
- No special fitting
- Disposability (also a disadvantage for environmental reasons)
- A comfortable feel
- A small size ($\frac{1}{2}$-inch thick and $\frac{3}{4}$-inch diameter) for convenient if in a purse
- No hormonal side effects
- Use necessary only when needed

- Immediate spermicidal effect lasting 24 hours regardless of the number of episodes of coitus
- No interference with spontaneity; insertion can occur well in advance of intercourse
- No requirement of additional applications of spermicidal cream or gel for repeated acts of intercourse

Disadvantages
Disadvantages of the contraceptive sponge include a relatively low effectiveness rate and no protection against STDs. Some women (and men) are allergic to the spermicide. Vaginal dryness, soreness, and itching can also occur. Some women find the sponge messy, and some find it difficult to remove.

Risks Associated With Use
There may be a slightly higher incidence of toxic shock syndrome with the sponge, but the risk is low. (Speroff and Darney say there is no risk of toxic shock syndrome.) Some clinicians feel risk, if present, may be lessened by not using the sponge during menses and by removing it before it has been in place 24 hours.

Contraindications
There are no known contraindications to the contraceptive sponge.

Side Effects
Allergic reactions, vaginal dryness, soreness, and itching have been reported with use of the contraceptive sponge. Difficult removal has also been reported.

Instructions for Client Use
The sponge should be moistened and excess moisture squeezed out before insertion. It should be left in place for 6 hours after the last act of intercourse. Intercourse should occur within 24 hours of insertion (Speroff & Darney, 2001).

Lactational Amenorrhea

Amenorrhea associated with lactation is an old method of child spacing. Repeated nursing by the baby causes prolactin levels to rise. As a result, follicles in the ovary fail to develop, and the ovaries do not secrete estrogen (Speroff & Darney, 2001).

Effectiveness

The exact contraceptive effectiveness of this method is variable and probably depends on the intensity of sucking by the baby, the frequency of nursing, and the extent of supplemental feedings. Estimates of effectiveness when an infant is fed exclusively at the breast range from total protection for 10 weeks (Speroff & Darney, 2001) to 2% at 6 months (Tommaselli, Guida, Palomba, Barbato, & Nappi, 2000). Some clinicians feel that women who fully or nearly fully breastfeed (day and night with breastfeeding accounting for at least 85% of the feedings) have little need for contraception for 6 months if menstruation has not resumed (Blackburn, Cunkelman, & Zlidar, 2000). Variables thought to influence the success of lactational amenorrhea (LAM) include 1) breast-feeding at least 6 times daily, 2) not allowing a lapse of more than 10 hours between feedings, and 3) not allowing more than a 6-hour interval between most feedings (Tommaselli, Guida, Palomba, Barbato, & Nappi, 2000). The effectiveness of LAM as a contraceptive method also depends on the presence of amenorrhea and perhaps avoiding a pacifier so that the infant's suck remains strong.

Advantages of Breastfeeding as a Contraceptive Method

Breastfeeding is inexpensive, provides infants with round-the-clock instant access to just-right food at a just-right temperature, protects babies against certain infections, and may facilitate maternal-infant bonding in addition to protecting against pregnancy.

Disadvantages of Breastfeeding as a Contraceptive Method

To be used effectively as a contraceptive method, breastfeeding must be almost exclusively the source of infant nutrition. If frequency and intensity of infant feeding is reduced, as may occur when a baby is ill, the contraceptive effect is lessened. The effect is also lessened when menstruation returns and/or when 6 months have passed since delivery.

Contraindications

There are no known contraindications to LAM.

Side Effects

Breastfeeding is associated with both vaginal dryness and dyspareunia, although it may be difficult to know the extent to which breastfeeding is responsible, because vaginal dryness may be caused by insufficient sexual foreplay dyspareunia may be the result of trauma (seen or unseen) to vaginal or perineal tissue at the time of birth.

Instructions for Client Use

Women who use LAM for contraception need to know that effectiveness depends on frequent and exclusive or almost exclusive breastfeeding. They should also know that effectiveness diminishes as time goes on, particularly past 6 months' postpartum. Effectiveness also diminishes with the return of menses. If an infant becomes sick and is not nursing as frequently or as intensely as normal, ovulation may occur, and a backup method of contraception should be used. Whether protection against pregnancy resumes when infant suckling returns to normal has not been studied.

Periodic Abstinence

How It Works

The most fertile time of the menstrual cycle is from 5 days before ovulation through the day of ovulation. A variety of contraceptive methods take advantage of the infertile phases of the menstrual cycle. Collectively known as natural family planning, these methods attend to length of the menstrual cycle, body temperature, characteristics of cervical mucus, or combinations of these to recommend when coitus should and should not take place. They also consider that sperm live 2 to 7 days in the female reproductive tract, and the ova live from 1 to 3 days (Speroff & Darney, 2001).

The calendar or rhythm method subtracts 18 days from the shortest cycle and 11 days from the longest cycle to identify the days of the cycle on which sexual intercourse is to be avoided. This method is best based on six consecutive and regular menstrual cycles.

The cervical mucus, ovulation, or Billings method uses cyclical changes in cervical mucus to identify abstinence days. Sexual intercourse is to be avoided on consecutive days after menstruation and before ovulation so that seminal fluid does not interfere with assessing the cervical mucus. Intercourse must also be avoided until the 4th day after the last day of sticky, wet mucus.

The symptothermal method combines the cervical mucus method with body temperature to identify the fertile time of the cycle. It requires taking one's temperature before arising. Abstinence begins with wet, sticky mucus. Coitus is resumed the 4th day after the wet, sticky mucus or the night of the 3rd day of a temperature rise of 0.4 to 0.8°F above preovulatory temperatures. The preovulatory temperature is somewhat below normal body temperature.

Effectiveness

The effectiveness of periodic abstinence methods is typically about 80%. Perfect use in a WHO study resulted in a pregnancy rate of 3.1% during the first year, but "imperfect use" resulted in a pregnancy rate of 86.4% (WHO, 1997).

Advantages

Couples who use periodic abstinence methods successfully are often pleased with the positive contributions to their relationship that occur because of increased cooperation and understanding. No cost is another advantage, as is the fact that there are no physical side effects of the method because nothing is inserted into the body in any way.

Disadvantages

The major disadvantages to periodic abstinence for family planning are the high pregnancy rates, the time and intense instruction needed to use the methods well, the relatively long number of days to observe abstinence (17), and the commitment to the method required by both persons in the relationship.

Instructions for Client Use

Couples interested in natural family planning are best referred to a teaching center that specializes in such instruction, unless the midwife has had special preparation in teaching these methods. Multiple meetings between the teacher and the interested couple are required if the couple is to understand how to use a method effectively. Effectiveness increases when periodic abstinence is used in conjunction with a diaphragm and/or spermicide.

❊ Emergency Contraception

"Emergency contraception" is a term referring to methods of preventing unintended pregnancy by acting shortly after unprotected intercourse or contraceptive failure. It can be accomplished with either OCs or insertion of the TCu380A IUD. The use of the LNG-20 for emergency contraception has not been studied.

Advantages

Protocols for the use of emergency contraception have been used for many years and have a record of both safety and efficacy. An added benefit is the potential for substantially reducing the rate of unintended pregnancy and abortion.

The Oral Contraceptive for Emergency Contraception

The OC for emergency contraceptive purposes can be

- High doses of low-dose combination OC pills
- A combination of estrogen and progestin designed and marketed specifically for emergency contraception (four tablets of Preven, each containing 50 µg of ethinyl estradiol and 0.25 mg of levonorgestrel)
- Progestin-only pills, also designed and marketed specifically for emergency contraception (Plan B, containing two 0.75-mg tablets of levonorgestrel)

How It Works

The exact mechanism of action has not been established for high-dose estrogen or progestin pills in preventing pregnancy when taken soon after intercourse. "They can inhibit or delay ovulation. Some studies have shown alterations in the endometrium, suggesting that they could also interfere with implantation of a fertilized egg, but other studies have found no such effects. Other possible mechanisms include interference with fertilization or with tubal transport of the embryo" (Medical Letter, 2000c, p. 10).

Effectiveness

Without emergency contraception, an estimated eight women out of 100 will become pregnant if they have intercourse midcycle. This number is reduced to two out of 100 women if combination emergency contraceptive pills are used (a decrease of 75%). Levonorgestrel alone, as found in Plan B, seems to be more effective than estrogen-progestin combinations, with an 89% reduction in pregnancies as opposed to 75% (Medical Letter, 2000c).

Disadvantages

Disadvantages of emergency contraception include the need to start treatment soon after intercourse, the high incidence of nausea and vomiting that occur when OCs from traditional pill packs are used, the necessity of a short-notice appointment with someone who can write a prescription for the medicine or insert the IUD for women who live in states where pharmacists are not allowed to distribute emergency contraceptive OCs, and the fact that the method is not 100% effective in preventing pregnancy.

Contraindications

Although some feel that pregnancy is the only contraindication to emergency contraceptive pills (Brown, 2001), others feel that the usual contraindications to OCs should be observed. Speroff and Darney emphasize that the high estrogen doses in combination OC emergency contraception preclude prescribing it for women with a personal or close family history of idiopathic thrombotic disease (Speroff & Darney, 2001). The levonorgestrel-only pill (Plan B) can be used for women in whom estrogen is contraindicated.

Side Effects

Adverse effects of emergency contraception tablets include nausea (in as many as 23% clients taking Plan B and 50% of those taking Preven) and vomiting (in as many as 6% of clients taking Plan B and 19% taking Preven). Breast tenderness has been noted with both regimens. No fetal malformations have been reported.

Client Instructions

All OC regimens must be initiated within 72 hours of intercourse, although initiation within 24 hours of intercourse increases efficacy. Because of the high incidence of nausea and vomiting with postcoital contraception, clients should be advised to take an antiemetic 1 hour prior to the first emergency contraception tablet(s). Over-the-counter products are usually effective. Clients who vomit within 1 hour of taking either dose should repeat the dose.

Clients should be asked at the postpartum visit if they would like a prescription that can be used if needed. Providing clients with the product before it is needed facilitates use. Box 13-14 summarizes directions for taking OC products for emergency contraception.

Since 1998, pharmacists in Washington State have been able to have collaborative prescription agreements with physicians, allowing the pharmacist to provide emergency contraception directly to clients (Ellertson, Shochet, Blanchard, & Trussell, 2000). When this program expands to other states, women should be informed of its availability.

Although not desirable, repeated use of the method is not known to have harmful effects. Clinicians should stress that postcoital contraception is not the same as any of the new methods of medical abortion.

The TCu380A (ParaGard) IUD for Emergency Contraception

How It Works

The TCu-380A prevents pregnancy by preventing implantation.

Effectiveness

Insertion of the copper TCu380A within 5 days of unprotected intercourse is more effective than emergency contraceptive pills. While the number of stud-

Box 13.14

Directions for Taking the Emergency Contraceptive Products Used in the United States

REGULAR COMBINATION ORAL CONTRACEPTIVES

1. One hour before taking the pills, take an over-the-counter medicine that prevents nausea and vomiting.
2. Take the following oral contraceptives as indicated:
   a. Ovral: take two tablets as soon as possible after intercourse but before 72 hours have elapsed, followed by two tablets 12 hours later
   b. Alesse: take five tablets as soon as possible after intercourse but before 72 hours have elapsed, followed by five tablets 12 hours later
   c. Lo/Ovral, Nordette, Levlen, Triphasil, Tri-Levlen: take four tablets as soon as possible after intercourse but before 72 hours have elapsed, followed by four tablets 12 hours later
   d. Ovrette, MICRONOR (norgestrel minipill): take 20 tablets as soon as possible after intercourse but before 72 hours have elapsed, followed by 20 tablets 12 hours later

PREVEN

1. One hour before taking the pills, take an over-the-counter medicine that prevents nausea and vomiting.
2. Take two tablets as soon as possible after intercourse but before 72 hours have elapsed.
3. Take two more tablets 12 hours later.
4. If vomiting occurs within 1 hour of taking either dose, take two tablets again.

PLAN B

1. One hour before taking the pills, take an over-the-counter medicine that prevents nausea and vomiting.
2. Take one tablet as soon as possible after intercourse but before 72 hours have elapsed.
3. Take the second tablet 12 hours later.
4. If vomiting occurs within 1 hour of taking either dose, take a tablet again.

ies involving women using the copper Tcu380A for emergency contraception is small, the failure rate is estimated at 0.1%.

Advantages

The device can be left in place up to 10 years to provide ongoing contraception.

Disadvantages

Disadvantages are the same as previously discussed in regard to IUDs plus the need to insert the device within 5 days of unprotected intercourse. Because it works by preventing implantation, this method may not be acceptable to women who believe that life begins with conception and do not believe in abortion.

Risks Associated With Use

Risks are the same as those previously discussed in regard to IUDs.

Contraindications

Contraindications are the same as those previously discussed in regard to IUDs. Consequently, this is not an appropriate method to use for women with multiple sexual partners or women who have been raped.

Side Effects

Side effects are the same as those previously discussed in regard to IUDs.

Instructions for Client Use

Instructions for client use are the same as those previously discussed in regard to IUDs.

✳ Conclusion

Clinicians must recognize the many factors that must be considered before recommending or prescribing a method of contraception. Serious consequences may result from failure to thoroughly address the medical and social issues surrounding a woman's choice of a family planning method. Thorough discussion of contraception during prenatal visits facilitates postpartum selection of a method likely to be used and appreciated by women and their partners. When the entire discussion about contraception is left for the postpartum visit, adequate time is lacking to address concerns and impart essential information.

The importance of early follow-up when a new method of family planning is initiated cannot be overemphasized. Sometimes a brief phone call to provide reassurance and encouragement will make the difference between the client abandoning or continuing the method.

Chapter 14
The Postpartum Visits

The initial postpartum visit has traditionally taken place 6 weeks after the baby's birth, despite the fact that no longitudinal studies identify the advantages of this time. Considering that a significant number of nonbreastfeeding women ovulate before the sixth postpartum week (Speroff & Darney, 2001), and that a new baby requires significant adjustments for most families, an earlier visit is desirable. Some practices are able to offer new mothers two (or more) postpartum visits. Not only are these meetings a time to assess the client's physical and emotional well-being, but also opportunities abound to 1) answer questions; 2) provide emotional support; 3) plan for effective contraceptive use (if desired and not yet initiated); 4) determine if additional follow-up is indicated in the upcoming weeks or months; and 5) provide education about important health topics. This chapter discusses the history, physical examination, and laboratory tests appropriate at these visits. Health education topics are discussed in Chapter 15.

✳ The First Postpartum Visit (1 to 2 Weeks Postpartum)

A growing body of literature notes that postpartum health concerns are commonly unrecognized by health care professionals. Painful perineums and hemorrhoids, urinary incontinence, backache (especially when epidural anesthesia has been used or the baby weighed more than 4000 g), and depression are underreported (Brown & Lumley, 1998). Consequently, an early postpartum visit to identify and discuss these problems should occur sometime in the first 2 weeks when allowed by the practice setting. The early clinic or office visit should include a discussion of physical discomforts and the transition to parenthood (see Chapter 10), a review of symptoms of potential complications (see Chapter 11), discussions about the progress of breastfeeding (see Chapter 12), perception of the birth experience, and screening for postpartum depression. These topics are summarized in Box 14-1.

Box 14.1

Topics for Discussion at the Postpartum Visits
Physical discomforts Transition to parenthood Symptoms of potential complications Progress of breastfeeding Perception of the birth experience Screening for postpartum depression

In lieu of a visit, the midwife should telephone the new mother to offer support and identify problems.

Making Sense of the Birth Experience

Vivid memories of what happened not only to their bodies, but also to their psyches as a result of the childbirth experience stay with women for many years (Simkin, 1991 & 1992). Involuntary body responses (such as shaking and vomiting), the care given by the health care provider attendant at the health care facility, as well as institutional policies can all play a significant role in the mother's perception of the birth (de Vusse, 1999). Women need opportunities to talk about what they have experienced. For some women, this opportunity will only occur if a thoughtful health care provider is willing to address the psychological as well as the physical outcomes of birth.

When the midwife who attended the birth is also the person who conducts the postpartum visit, a unique opportunity exists to fill in the pieces of the experience that are missing for the mother and assure her that she handled her labor well. Simkin suggests an opening statement such as, "Even though I was there, I'm interested in knowing what the experience was like for you." She also suggests that the midwife compliment the mother with a statement such as, "How much I admired you when . . ." or "Do you know what I saw? I saw a woman who was in a very challenging situation and rose to the occasion." When the midwife, the expert on birth, tells the mother she did well, the mother may have a more positive impression of her own actions (Simkin, undated).

Whether or not the midwife at the postpartum visit was the birth attendant, the midwife can help the mother reconstruct the birth experience by reviewing the medical record with her. The intrapartum experience is so intense that mothers cannot remember all that happened.

It is impossible to predict how a given woman will feel about what happened to her. While the midwife may think that a woman who has a short labor will be grateful it was short, it may have been too intense to cope with, and women may respond with anger over being out of control. Self-esteem and self-confidence may have diminished.

Box 14-2 contains suggestions for phrasing questions that can facilitate a discussion about the mother's perceptions of the birth. Recollections of the birth as traumatic, either emotionally or physically, necessitate ongoing discussion, as they can precipitate postpartum depression.

Physical Examination

The early postpartum visit may include parts of a physical examination. If breastfeeding problems are identified, examine the breasts or nipples. Persistent perineal pain requires examination of the perineum. Additional visits, telephone calls, or referrals for counseling are often appropriate.

❖ The 4- to 6-Week Postpartum Checkup

Often the postpartum "checkup" visit consists of a breast and pelvic examination and prescription of a birth control method. Wise midwives use the time to discuss once more the pregnancy and birth, knowing that a woman's ability to make sense of the experience requires both time and reflection. A thoughtful postpartum checkup includes a detailed history and a modified physical exam-

---

Box 14.2

Questions That May Facilitate Discussion of the Birth Experience

1. When you were pregnant, what worried you the most about labor? About the birth itself?
2. How would you describe your labor and the baby's birth?
3. How was it different from what you expected?
4. What was hardest?
5. Was there anything about your behavior that surprised you?
6. How did you feel about the behavior of those who were with you?
7. What helped the most?
8. Did anything happen that scared you?
9. Did anything happen that you did not like?
10. Did you get the help that you needed from family and friends who were with you; from the nurses, midwives, or doctors who cared for you; or from those who are important to you but were not there?
11. What would you like to do differently if you have another baby?

ination. A careful review of the medical record will determine if laboratory tests are indicated and will identify areas for health education.

If the husband or partner comes to the 6-week visit, try to arrange time to determine his or her feelings and perceptions. If you did not have a chance prenatally to ask about the father's or partner's childhood experiences with abuse, do it now. Be sure to ask if any parent or caretaker was an alcoholic or drug user. A referral to a parenting group, a support group, a mental health counselor, or sources of information may be in order.

History

Inquiries about physical and emotional well-being should attempt to identify recent episodes of pain, bleeding, fever, incontinence, dyspareunia, and depression. Breastfeeding mothers often experience spotting off and on during the first 60 postpartum days. This is a normal phenomenon.

Incontinence

Regrettably, few practitioners inquire about urinary or fecal incontinence or inability to control the expulsion of flatus. Many do not know that anal incontinence is a relatively common finding after delivery, particularly when forceps have been used to facilitate birth. It also occurs in noninstrumental deliveries. One out of 10 primiparas and one out of five multiparas who deliver vaginally may experience fecal urgency or the involuntary loss of flatus or feces (Toglia & DeLancey, 1994). Women who experience symptoms may be unable to play with their children, exercise, run for a bus, laugh, cough, sneeze, make love, shovel snow, or dance. They may be deeply troubled by embarrassment, worry, and fear that others will find out. Symptoms often disappear after 6 months. Encourage them to do Kegel exercises, although the exact contribution of Kegel exercises to diminution of symptoms is not known. When symptoms persist, refer the client to a specialist.

Dyspareunia

The incidence of pain during intercourse following either a vaginal or cesarean birth is unknown, but it is probably higher than suspected by clinicians. Accurate evaluation is complicated by three factors: 1) many women have not resumed intercourse prior to the postpartum examination, 2) many clinicians do not routinely ask if intercourse has occurred and whether it was painful, and 3) women are reluctant to initiate a discussion on the topic. When mentioned in textbooks, the discussion of pain with intercourse after having a baby is usually brief. The cause of the pain is commonly attributed to lacerations, episiotomy repair, or vaginal dryness if the woman is breastfeeding. Yet one third of women who report pain or discomfort during intercourse have had no obvious tissue trauma.

A recent study of 53 lactating and nine nonlactating postpartum women revealed the following (Geotsch, 1999):

- The problem was not fully developed at the postpartum visit.
- Of the 23 women who had entry dyspareunia, three had cesarean births, and another three had no episiotomy or repair.
- In women who had some type of perineal repair, the repair site was the source of dyspareunia in only 8% of the women who delivered vaginally, and resolution of the pain required 2 to 7 months.
- The dyspareunia was often described as burning or stretching with penetration and could last for hours or days after intercourse.
- Fifty percent of the women with entry dyspareunia had pain lasting for more than 5 months.

The author concluded, "The typical timing of postpartum visits and instructions to women as to when to resume intercourse have conspired to leave the problem of postpartum dyspareunia unexplored and underdetected. Most patients have no basis for complaints about painful sex at the time of the six-week postpartum visit since usually they are still postponing it" (Goetsch, 1999, p. 967). The fact that postpartum dyspareunia is so common and long lasting begs for additional studies to investigate its frequency, duration, and management. Meanwhile, the least that midwives can do is to identify the problem and to search for specialists able to address it.

Postpartum Depression

Symptoms of postpartum depression, outlined in Box 14-3, may appear at any time during the first year after the baby's birth. For this reason, its occurrence is underestimated. Not only is postpartum depression a source of great distress for a new mother and her partner, but the irritability, fatigue, anger, worry, sadness, and anxiety that are present can also interfere with the mother's ability to respond and relate to her baby and other children and can have long-lasting effects on them. Thoughts of suicide and harming the baby may occur. Prompt identification and treatment of postpartum depression should be a high priority in any practice.

Clinicians must be able to recognize the symptoms, respond to a woman's potential for harming herself or her baby, and make appropriate referrals to mental health professionals, support groups, and/or new mother groups. If the client seems unable to follow through with a referral, the clinician should make the initial contact. Clinicians can also help a new mother mobilize sources of support and should call at intervals to see how she is doing. Considering postpartum depression is likely to continue over a period of months,

---

Box 14.3

Symptoms of Postpartum Depression

- Sleeplessness
- Constant sleeping
- Lack of appetite
- Inability to concentrate
- Tearfulness
- Sadness
- Helplessness
- Hopelessness
- Numbness
- Anxiety

- Despair
- Lack of interest
- Thoughts of hurting the baby
- Lack of energy
- Obsessive thoughts
- Inability to complete activities of daily living
- Suicidal thoughts
- Irrational fears

---

ongoing contact is beneficial. Low-income women should be asked about chronic stressors, such as poor maternal health, a fussy baby, inadequate money for basic needs, and the absence of social support, as these have been found to correlate with postpartum depression in this population 6 months after giving birth (Seguin, Potvin, St. Denis, & Loiselle, 1999).

About 10% of the time, postpartum depression is caused by postpartum thyroiditis, a transient condition that usually resolves spontaneously after 1 to 4 months. However, one in four women with postpartum thyroiditis eventually develop a chronic hypothyroid condition. When postpartum depression occurs, thyroid testing should be requested to rule out a hyperthyroid or hypothyroid state. Medication is often helpful while symptoms are present. Postpartum thyroiditis is likely to recur in subsequent pregnancies.

Psychotropic medication may be indicated in the treatment of postpartum depression. Breastfeeding mothers are likely to be concerned about the excretion of psychotropic drugs in breast milk and the consequent effect on the baby. The few studies reported usually involve small numbers of subjects.

Fluoxetine (Prozac) has a long pediatric half-life and builds up in the baby over time. In three studies involving four, six, and 16 nursing mothers, paroxetine (Paxil) did not have adverse effects in the infants (Hale, 2000). A fourth study of six nursing mothers found "interindividual variation" in paroxetine excretion in breast milk. The authors also reported a time- and dose-dependent rate of excretion and recommended avoiding breastfeeding 4 to 7 hours postdose and possible nighttime administration if the infant does not nurse at night (Ohman, Hagg, Carleborg, & Spigset, 1999).

Research with sertraline (Zoloft) shows "attaining clinically relevant plasma levels in infants is remote at maternal doses less than 150 mg/day" (Hale, 2000, p. 598).

The frequency, causes, and treatment of acute childbirth-related trauma symptoms are rarely studied. However, some data suggest that women who have "operative deliveries" (emergency cesarean births, birth of the baby with forceps, and vacuum-assisted births) and women who express dissatisfaction with care during labor are more likely to develop symptoms.

Postpartum depression should be distinguished from postpartum blues and postpartum psychosis. The former is a short-lived period of emotional lability that usually occurs toward the end of the first postpartum week and lasts a day or two. The latter is a condition involving unipolar depression, bipolar depression, or schizophrenia. Symptoms of postpartum psychosis include severe insomnia, hallucinations, agitation, and bizarre feelings or behavior. This condition requires immediate medical attention.

❊ The Physical Examination

The postpartum physical examination provides an opportunity to identify problems resulting from childbirth, discuss body changes, and detect abnormalities that may have arisen since the prenatal physical examination.

Height

If maternal height was not measured prenatally, a postpartum measurement will provide baseline data to be compared with future measurements that may indicate osteoporosis.

Weight

Few women have regained their prepregnancy weight by the time of the postpartum checkup. Weight at the postpartum visit provides an opportunity to discuss nutrition and exercise at a time when women may be particularly motivated to "get back in shape." Chapter 15 discusses these topics in more depth.

Blood Pressure

Postpartum blood pressure measurements are particularly important for women who were hypertensive while pregnant. Differentiating between chronic hypertension and transient hypertension of pregnancy or gestational hypertension is an important determination. Recommendations for follow-up health care and a future pregnancy depend on an accurate blood pressure diagnosis. Women with an elevated blood pressure at 6 weeks postpartum should have another blood pressure determination at 12 weeks postpartum, because a persistent elevation is likely to indicate chronic hypertension (National High Blood Pressure Education Program Working Group on High Blood Pressure in Pregnancy, 2000).

Recurrence rates for preeclampsia vary according to parity (higher for multiparas) and race (higher in Black women compared with White women when diagnosed after 36 weeks). Women with early-onset preeclampsia, multiparas with either preeclampsia or hypertension, and women with gestational hypertension are at increased risk for cardiovascular disease. A woman who experiences late-onset preeclampsia in an initial pregnancy appears to have no increased cardiovascular risk unless subsequent pregnancies are characterized by hypertension (NIH, 2000). Women with early-onset severe preeclampsia may "harbor metabolic abnormalities or risk factors associated with vascular thrombosis" (National High Blood Pressure Education Program Working Group on High Blood Pressure in Pregnancy, 2000, p. 23). Referral for evaluation of activated protein C resistance (Factor V Leiden), antiphospholipid antibodies, hyperhomocysteinemia, and protein S deficiency may be indicated.

Examination of the Breasts

Breast examination with lactating women can be difficult because of breast size and general lumpiness. Still, a thorough clinical examination (see Chapter 4) is imperative, as breast cancer can occur at any time, even while a woman is breastfeeding. In addition to palpating the breasts for masses, observe the nursing mother's breasts for nipple trauma. Although nipple problems have usually resolved by this time, cracks and bleeding occasionally persist, requiring a discussion with the mother to determine the cause. The breast examination is best accomplished right after a breastfeeding baby has nursed. Any breast abnormality requires further diagnostic workup.

Emphasize the importance of monthly breast self-examination (BSE) to all women, even those who are young and who, in the past, may have been told that their risk for breast cancer is low. New evidence indicating that breast tumors grow more rapidly in younger women (Kerlikowske, 1996) mandates that all women know the importance of this examination.

Considerable time is required to do a good job of examining the breasts. Considerably more time is needed to do a good job of teaching BSE. Women consistently report that instruction in the procedure for performing BSE is inadequate. Some practices designate a nurse in the office or clinic to do this teaching.

The Pelvic Examination

In addition to the regular components of a pelvic examination, the postpartum pelvic should include particular attention to the labia, the perineum, and the anus for signs of healing if lacerations occurred or an episiotomy was done. Occasionally, fusion of the upper portions of the labia will be noted, usually the result of unrepaired bilateral periurethral or labial lacerations. Such fusion is not usually a problem. Practitioners should look for cystoceles and rectoceles and, when noted, should discuss Kegel exercises, although again, the exact contribution of the Kegel to resolution of the cystocele or rectocele is unknown. While no one knows the frequency, duration, or technique that is most effective, it may be useful to give the client a guide, such as 75 times a day for 3 months.

A rectal examination, often "deferred" in childbearing women because of the discomfort and embarrassment associated with it, should always be performed at the postpartum examination to assess the integrity of the rectal sphincter. A rectal examination can also detect masses that are low in the pelvis and may have been missed on vaginal examination.

❖ Laboratory Tests

Laboratory tests that may be appropriate at the postpartum examination include follow-up tests for conditions that were present during the pregnancy and tests that are considered part of good care for women in general or tests indicated because of family medical history. Tests in the first category include a fasting blood sugar for women who were diagnosed with gestational diabetes (to be certain that the women are not true diabetics) and tests of thyroid function for women on thyroid medication. More than half of women diagnosed with gestational diabetes mellitus during pregnancy later develop type 2 diabetes (Gabbe, Hill, Schmidt, & Schulkin, 1998). A diagnosis for type 2 diabetes can be made on the basis of a fasting blood sugar of 126 mg/dL on two separate occasions. Refer these women to a physician. Tests needed because of family history would include measurement of cholesterol and triglyceride levels for women with risk factors for coronary heart disease (see Chapter 15).

❖ Conclusion

Like good prenatal visits, the good postpartum visit requires thoughtful interaction between the clinician and the client. Because of the time it takes to identify the issues that might be important to discuss, it is useful for a client to complete a postpartum history form before seeing the midwife. Appendix T contains a sample form.

Chapter 15

Health Issues for Women

A variety of topics to improve health can be discussed at the postpartum examination. These include health issues unique to a given woman, as well as preventive health recommendations. Smoking cessation, substance abuse, safer sex, weight management, and weapons in the home may be appropriate for some women, while calcium supplementation, symptoms of depression, immunizations, and risks for cancer and heart disease are appropriate for all. *Clinician's Handbook of Preventive Services*, a 1998 publication of the U.S. Public Health Service, summarizes the recommendations of major authorities.

✳ Smoking

Most women who stop smoking while they are pregnant resume smoking in the months following delivery. Despite efforts to help women maintain their quit status after delivery, 25% of spontaneous quitters relapse by 6 weeks postpartum, and 70% to 80% are smoking 12 months later (Severson, Andrews, Lichtenstein, Wall, & Akers, 1997). These statistics should not be surprising when remembering that new mothers have multiple issues to contend with, and smoking is a familiar coping tool.

A study of pediatricians, nurse practitioners, and physician assistants who received training and materials to help new mothers quit smoking or not start again showed that their special efforts had a significant effect on quit status at 6 months but not at 12 months. The best predictors of whether a mother would be smoking at both 6 and 12 months were whether she allowed smoking in the home and whether her partner smoked.

The authors noted, "Many mothers reported that they were more comfortable in getting themselves and others to smoke outside than to quit smoking. This intermediate step of making the house smoke-free is probably an important step toward quitting and could be characterized as a stage of change" (Severson, Andrews, Lichtenstein, Wall, & Akers, 1997, p. 128). Further research to determine whether this truly is an intermediate step would be helpful, as some clinicians are concerned about the message that is sent to children when parents go outside to smoke: "It's okay to smoke, if you do it outside."

Screen for smoking at each postpartum visit, remembering that smoking cessation is a process accomplished over time, and relapses are common. Make a question about smoking a "vital sign," which you ask about as routinely as the last menstrual period. Use the postpartum visit to reinforce the importance of a smoke-free environment for the client and for her children. Remind smokers of the link between parental smoking and lower respiratory illnesses (bronchitis, bronchiolitis, pneumonia); asthma; ear, nose, and throat problems; sudden infant death syndrome (SIDS); and meningococcal disease. Try the "30-second stop-smoking prompt": "Don't smoke while holding your baby or while children are near. Keep your home and auto smoke free. Don't let others smoke around your children" (Oregon Health Division, 1996b, p.1).

Women who are still smoking or who have resumed smoking should be assessed again for stage-of-quitting desire—precontemplation ("I won't"), contemplation ("I might"), preparation ("I will"), or action ("I am"). Some practices use color-coded "quit stickers" to identify the stage. The stickers prompt the clinicians to assess the client at each visit, identifying the current stage and providing appropriate information. Color-coded health education folders allow easy access to teaching materials that can be used in discussions with the client (Spoljoric, 2000).

In the end, remember that it is not possible for every woman to stop smoking, even when intellectually realizing that a child's health is at stake. The lives of many women have been and are filled with pain. While we must be persistent in our efforts to encourage smoking cessation, our clients always deserve gentleness, kindness, and encouragement.

❖ Alcohol Consumption

Discussions about alcohol consumption give the clinician an opportunity to 1) provide clients with guidelines for alcohol use, 2) identify increases in consumption associated with the stresses of new parenthood, 3) interpret findings of research studies on drinking as they become available, and 4) refer clients to community resources when appropriate. Women should be advised that more than seven drinks per week or more than two drinks per occasion can put them at risk for alcohol-related problems.

Research suggesting that "moderate" amounts of alcohol lead to a lower incidence of heart disease may prompt clients to ask for recommendations about daily alcohol intake. Moderate means one daily drink (12 oz of beer, 5 oz of wine, or 1 1/2 oz of 80-proof distilled spirits) for women and refers to daily intake rather than to average intake. The truth is that moderate drinking carries risks as well as benefits. It increases the likelihood that a person will die from liver disease, breast cancer, suicide, and accidents. Increased alcohol consumption is related to hypertension, obesity, stroke, cardiomyopathy, and fetal alcohol syndrome. In persons with a familial predisposition to alcoholism, the possibility of becoming addicted is real. Consequently, some leaders in preventive medicine advise that recommendations to American women to consume one alcoholic beverage each day are premature and may even be misguided.

❊ Safer Sex

Safer sex counseling is appropriate at the postpartum visit. The high divorce rate and high incidence of serial monogamy mean that many women will have a new sexual partner after the baby is born. All women should know that the risk of infection from sexual intercourse can be decreased by avoiding sex with high-risk partners; avoiding anal intercourse; using latex condoms when having sex with anyone other than a single, mutually monogamous partner known to be HIV-negative; and limiting sexual relationships to those with a mutually monogamous partner known to be HIV-negative. However, negotiating safer sex is a complex process. For some women, the cost incurred by asking a partner to use a condom is too high. Loss of the relationship as well as loss of food, shelter, and even one's children or one's life can be at stake.

Midwives can often be helpful to women by helping them think through a discussion of condom use. You might begin a discussion of safer sex by asking, "Would you see any problems with talking to a new partner about using a condom?" or "What do you think would happen if you started talking about them?" or "What do you think other people should do about condoms when they have a new sexual partner?" Other ways to engage the client might include asking, "What do you think about using condoms when you have sex?" You could continue with these questions: "Have you ever used one before?", "How did it go?", and "Have you ever had a bad experience with a condom? Maybe it broke (or interrupted lovemaking, or wouldn't stay on, or didn't taste good, or your partner said it was too tight, or he couldn't feel as much, or he didn't like having to pull out?)".

Acknowledge that the first discussion between a woman and a new sexual partner about using condoms is likely to be awkward and embarrassing. If the client thinks she might have difficulty getting started, suggest she begin by talking about a television show (or newspaper article, movie, radio show comment, billboard, remark by a friend, or pamphlet) she has seen or heard in which condom use was discussed. Help her anticipate common partner responses and possible replies: "They're not romantic" ("AIDS isn't romantic either"), "They decrease the feeling" ("Let me show you how good they can feel"), "They might break" ("Yes, condoms do break, but it's less than one time out of 100"), "You must have been playing around with someone else!"

("You're not my first partner, and I want to be sure you are protected; I'm probably not your first partner, and I know you want to see me protected as well"), and "Don't you trust me?" ("It's not a matter of trust; it's a matter of health").

Sometimes depersonalizing the subject helps. Ask the client, "Why do you think people would have trouble with this?" Then you might move the subject closer to home with something like this statement: "These are the things that put people at risk. Where do you see yourself?" When you know the client, you might begin a discussion of safer sex by returning to information about sexual practices obtained at the first prenatal visit. "I remember that you told me . . ." can be an opener. When the client has not used condoms with a new sexual partner in the past, ask her, "What keeps you from using condoms all of the time?" and "What might you do about that?"

✽ Weight Management

Different situations involving a desire to lose weight may be presented at the postpartum visit. One is the new mother who was an appropriate weight for height at conception and gained the recommended amount of weight during her pregnancy. She wishes to return to her prepregnancy weight. A second situation is the mother whose prepregnancy weight for height was appropriate, but an excessive amount of weight was gained during her pregnancy. She, too, wishes to return to her prepregnancy weight. A third situation is the overweight or obese woman who is still overweight or obese and wants a weight appropriate for her height. (Definitions and classification of obesity and overweight are summarized in Table 15-1.)

TABLE 15.1 Body Mass Index Classification of Overweight

	Obesity class	Body mass index
Underweight		<18.5
Normal		18.5–24.9
Overweight		25.0–29.9
Obesity	I	30.0–34.9
	II	35.0–39.9
	III extreme obesity	at or >40

From World Health Organization and the National Heart, Lung, and Blood Institute.

Losing weight is rarely easy. Research is giving us a clearer picture why: "The simple decisions of what, when and how much to eat may not be completely under people's conscious control" (Kolata, 2000). Genetic factors influencing body weight are just beginning to be understood, and the lifelong struggle of some women with guilt, ridicule, and a sense of failure is just beginning to be appreciated.

Clinicians may focus on the health benefits for women who are overweight, citing the fact that even modest reductions of 5% to 10% can lower blood pressure, serum lipid levels, and glucose levels. However, a more effective approach may be to acknowledge the difficulties involved. Instead of traditional instructions to eat less and exercise more, a kind and thoughtful approach emphasizing one small change at a time may be a useful beginning. Appendix U contains some suggestions for women wishing to embark on a weight-loss program.

 HELPFUL HINT

Clients not accustomed to reading labels often appreciate help in this area. Try removing labels from cans and packages. Place them in plastic casings in a three-ring binder to show to clients, selecting labels that illustrate the points you wish to make. This is a good way to demonstrate that some reduced-fat products have *more* calories than the regular product.

Clinicians might think about the words of a woman who, by height and weight, is categorized as "morbidly obese." "I do eat. I also work, sing, paint, write, volunteer in the community, help my neighbors, garden, walk the dog, love my husband, take care of and love my kids, spend money, call my mother, kiss my granddaughter and have parties once in a while. . . . So why does society want to change a cow into a deer? Why did I try the same things for 35 years myself? I guess I forgot about the important things in life and about people like my Uncle Gene. With the kindest heart in the world, he was adored and admired by everyone who knew him until the day he died. I've never met anyone fatter. . . . We are who we are. I happen to be more than some would want me to be, but that does not make me less" (Madrigal, 1995).

 HELPFUL HINT

Evaluating the diets of women from varying ethnic backgrounds can be difficult. Particular problems may be found in certain groups of low-income women. For example, a study of the diets of 186 Mexican women in Chicago showed inadequate intake of folate, iron, zinc, and calcium. The study also showed poor use of foods thought to decrease cardiovascular disease and cancer (Ballew & Sugerman, 1995). Spending time in ethnic food stores may be helpful as you counsel women about nutrition. Discussions with nutritionists working with ethnic groups can also help.

❊ Guns in the Home

The postpartum visit is a time to reinforce the precautions that should be taken when there are guns in the home. Confirm with women who indicated prenatally that guns and ammunition are kept in a locked place away from the eyes and hands of children that this is, indeed, true. Discuss safety procedures with women who indicated prenatally that appropriate precautions are not being observed. The arrival of a new baby may motivate some parents to adhere to safety guidelines.

❊ Calcium Supplementation

Women between the ages of 19 and 50, including women who are breastfeeding, should consume 1000 mg of elemental calcium daily. Girls of childbearing age 18 and under should consume 1300 mg daily (National Academy of Sciences Food and Nutrition Board, 1997). Calcium supplements are often needed to meet these recommendations. Absorption may be improved by taking any 500-mg (or less) calcium supplement with meals (Medical Letter, 2000a). Clients should be instructed to check product labels for the amount of elemental calcium in a tablet. They should also restrict their buying to products with the United States Pharmacopeia (USP) mark to be certain that the product meets standards for quality and purity. Appendix CC contains patient instructions for taking a calcium supplement.

Calcium supplements are marketed in a variety of forms: calcium carbonate and calcium phosphate (40% elemental calcium), calcium citrate (21% elemental calcium), calcium lactate (13% elemental calcium), and calcium gluconate (9% elemental calcium). Most are well tolerated, but high doses of calcium carbonate can cause constipation, bloating, and flatulence. While calcium gluconate is less constipating, it is considerably more expensive. Calcium citrate can be taken at any time. Because calcium citrate tablets contain less elemental calcium, more tablets must be taken to equal the same amount of elemental calcium in calcium carbonate. Calcium citrate is also significantly more expensive than calcium carbonate. Calcium phosphate, the formulation used in calcium-fortified orange juice, can be taken anytime and does not cause gas or constipation. While more expensive than calcium carbonate, it is less expensive than calcium citrate (Calcium Information Center, no date).

Tums and Rolaids are inexpensive and easy-to-obtain sources of calcium carbonate. In addition to coming in a variety of flavors (spearmint, berry, and tropical fruit), they come in a variety of dosages and are recommended by the National Osteoporosis Foundation. Other brands are less expensive and are available in similar dosages. Bonemeal and dolomite should be avoided as calcium sources, because they may be contaminated with lead.

❖ Exercise/Physical Activity

Data continues to accumulate to support the importance of exercise (planned bodily movement designed to increase physical fitness) and physical activity (any bodily movement) to help prevent coronary artery disease and decrease colon cancer, osteoarthritis, cholesterol, low-density lipoprotein (the bad one), and triglycerides. Exercise/physical activity can be used to prevent and treat hypertension, type 2 diabetes, and obesity; prevent bone loss; and increase bone strength, decreasing the likelihood of falls and the concomitant risk of fractures. Exercise can improve intellectual functioning and increase self-esteem. Mild depression may be alleviated (Shahady, 2000). Stress may be diminished.

Relatively few Americans are engaged in a regular exercise program, and few practitioners go beyond telling clients that they need to be physically active/exercise. Effective counseling probably requires an approach similar to the Five "A" Program to help patients stop smoking: ask, advise, assess, assist, and arrange.

You might begin a discussion of physical activity with women who are relatively sedentary by determining the client's feelings about increasing activity. Have there been previous attempts? What happened? What kind of program might fit into the client's life at present? What would be the obstacles (time, money, embarrassment)? What would it take to get started? Shahady suggests writing a prescription for exercise on a prescription pad. It might read, "Walk for 20 minutes with the baby in a front pack five mornings a week." "The prescription is tailored to what is achievable at the time, given the patient's values, preferences, level of awareness, and abilities. It may not be ideal . . ., but it is a start" (Shahady, 2000, p. 2177).

While limited data are available on women and exercise, current "best practice" recommendations include:

• Individualizing suggestions for type of activity, frequency, duration, and intensity to the client's current level of fitness

- Encouraging a slow start for women at lower levels of fitness. (Women who are sedentary might need to begin with climbing stairs each day or walking for periods as short as 5 to 10 minutes.)
- Encouraging any activity that increases body movement, aiming for 20 to 30 cumulative minutes of physical activity most days of the week

Be creative when discussing physical activity/exercise, particularly with low-income women. Think, for example, about the difficulties in developing an exercise program if you are poor and live in a neighborhood where walking is not an option or you do not have money to join a fitness center or purchase a treadmill for use at home.

❖ Depression

As discussed in Chapter 14, screening for postpartum depression is an essential feature of the postpartum visits. Good midwifery care will include a discussion about depression with all women. As much as 15% of the general U.S. population will experience major depression at some time during their lives (Oregon Health Division, 2000c). Depression is associated with significant maternal morbidity and even mortality. Most women with a history of major depression will experience recurrences throughout their lives. With approximately 15% of people who are depressed committing suicide, depression should be viewed as a potentially fatal illness. "Unfortunately, up to 2/3 of persons with depression either do not seek or do not receive any treatment (often because their illness goes undetected). Of the remaining 1/3 who do receive treatment, many get improper treatment (e.g., benzodiazepines) or insufficient treatment (e.g., sub-therapeutic doses or premature termination of antidepressants or lack of referral to mental health care)" (Oregon Health Division, 2000c). Maternal depression also has a profound effect on babies and children. Without intervention, studies show that by 4 months of exposure to a depressed mother, babies have learned to be depressed. Thus, it is imperative that mothers and families understand that recognition and treatment of depression protect the child.

In addition to screening all women for depression, clinicians should 1) alert all women to the symptoms, 2) make family members mindful of the symptoms (fatigue and feelings of hopelessness may cause the depressed person to avoid seeking help), 3) convey a sense of hope to those who are depressed (90% of individuals with major depression respond to treatment [Oregon Health Division, 2000c]), 4) identify resources for both pharmacologic treatment and psychotherapy, and 5) explore client resistance to pharmacologic measures.

Recent research shows that many cases of depression are the result of a deficiency in amine neurotransmitters. Among other things, these substances lower the level of serotonin, the mood regulator, in the brain. Drugs known as the selective serotonin reuptake inhibitors (SSRIs) increase serotonin. Fluoxetine (Prozac), paroxetine (Paxil), sertraline (Zoloft), and citalopram (Celexa) are SSRIs commonly used to treat depression. Short-term therapy with psychotropic drugs is likely to be helpful in 65% to 80% of people who take the medication. Psychotropic drugs can also benefit women with dysthymia (the chronically unhappy), bulimia, and premenstrual dysphoric disorder. While most midwives are not prepared to prescribe these drugs themselves, they can refer the client to someone who can evaluate the client to determine if use may be appropriate.

Clinicians should be knowledgeable about psychopharmacology so that the women who take psychotropic drugs can receive appropriate support should they have questions or concerns. For example, women taking one of these drugs may ask how long it takes for a response to occur, when is it appropriate to consider changing drugs, and how long pharmacologic therapy should be continued once depressive symptoms are relieved. It is helpful to know that it takes 6 to 12 weeks to discover who will respond to the drugs; that in some ways the SSRIs are like nonsteroidal anti-inflammatory drugs, and a person may respond well to one drug and not to another; that additional pharmaceutical therapy may be necessary for effective treatment; that clients in the initial phase of treatment should be monitored for response; and that drug therapy should probably be continued for 8 to 12 months after depressive symptoms abate.

Additionally, clinicians should recognize that clients who receive treatment may occasionally be given improper medicine, receive subtherapeutic doses, or have the medicine terminated prematurely. Clinicians should also know that the greatest risk of relapse occurs within 4 months of recovery. Midwives without this knowledge may watch women discontinue drug therapy unnecessarily or continue with ineffective therapy. Psychotherapy alone, or in combination with an appropriate drug, may also be useful in the treatment of depression. Advances in short-term psychotherapy (eight to 20 sessions) have been shown to be effective.

Some clinicians suggest St. John's wort (*Hypericum perforatum*), an herb used for centuries to treat mental disorders and nerve pain, for the treatment of mild to moderate depression. St. John's wort is available in capsule, tea, and tincture forms. Early clinical trials found that it compared favorably with the tricyclic antidepressants (the SSRIs were not studied) in the short-term treatment of mild to moderate depression. Unfortunately, the methods used to select, diagnose, and evaluate clients in these clinical trials are open to criticism. A recent study found that St. John's wort was not effective in the treatment of major depression (Shelton et al., 2001).

Until more data are available, some clinicians will choose to use St. John's wort, particularly for clients who choose not to use conventional pharmaceuticals (Kim, Streltzer, & Goebert, 1999; Woelk, 2000)). Potency of products varies dramatically from one product to another, making it difficult to define a recommended dose. Products stating "standardized extract" may be more likely to contain effective dosages (National Institutes of Health, 2000).

Side effects of St. John's wort include mania, dry mouth, dizziness, gastrointestinal symptoms, photophobia, and fatigue (National Center for Complementary and Alternative Medicine, 2000). St. John's wort should not be taken with other antidepressants. New studies suggest that St. John's wort may interfere with the effectiveness of birth control pills (National Center for Complementary & Alternative Medicine, 2000). Be certain to alert clients about this possible drug interaction.

❊ Immunizations

The postpartum period is an opportune time to immunize against rubella and varicella. Rubella vaccine is usually administered prior to hospital discharge for women identified as non-immune by routine prenatal laboratory testing. Side effects of rubella vaccine include a slight fever, rash, enlarged lymph nodes, and arthralgias 3 to 25 days after receiving the vaccine. Those with a history of an anaphylactic reaction to neomycin should not be immunized against rubella, as neomycin is found in this vaccine.

Two subcutaneous doses of varicella vaccine given 4 to 8 weeks apart confer immunity to 94% of those receiving the vaccine. Seroconversion lasts 7 to 13 years in 80% of cases. Side effects include tenderness and erythema at the injection site (25%), as well as a generalized maculopapular rash within 1 month of the injection (Medical Letter, 1995).

The postpartum period is also an excellent time to catch up on other immunizations. Vaccines that should be offered include tetanus-diphtheria (Td) if 10 or more years have elapsed since the last immunization; polio, if the series was incomplete during childhood; hepatitis B for high-risk individuals (see Chapter 1); and mumps, if women have not had the disease or been vaccinated. Every adult needs a tetanus immunization because any wound can become contaminated with tetanus. Tetanus vaccine is given in combination with diphtheria, a disease not well known in developed countries. However, diphtheria struck 80,000 people in Russia in the 1990s, and protection is prudent.

Hepatitis B vaccine should be given in the deltoid muscle rather than in the buttocks because of increased immunogenicity when administered in the arm (CDC, 1991a). Two intramuscular doses are given 4 weeks apart, and the third dose is given at least 2 months after the second (U.S. Public Health Service, Office of Disease Prevention and Health Promotion, 1998). Protection is thought to last 10 years, although "much longer-lasting immunity is likely"

(U.S. Public Health Service, Office of Disease Prevention and Health Promotion, 1998, p. 91).

Postvaccination testing should be conducted for immunocompromised clients and health care workers between 1 and 2 months after completion of the series. Testing is not indicated for persons at low risk of "continued mucosal or percutaneous exposures to blood" (U.S. Public Health Service, Office of Disease Prevention and Health Promotion, 1998, p. 340).

Since 1989, a second dose of the measles, mumps, and rubella vaccine has been recommended for adults who were vaccinated against measles before 1979, as they have a higher risk of getting measles.

Hepatitis A vaccine is now available and should be offered to anyone who wants this immunity, particularly illegal drug users and travelers to Africa, Asia (except Japan), parts of the Caribbean, Central and South America, Eastern Europe, the Mediterranean Basin, and the Middle East.

Appendix DD summarizes the recommendations of the National Coalition for Adult Immunization and provides an example of an adult immunization record, as well as a vaccine-screening questionnaire.

❖ Cancer

Counseling about individual risk for cancer is often appropriate at the postpartum checkup. A significant family history of cancer includes two or more relatives with the same or related cancers, earlier onset than is typical for that cancer, rare cancers, bilateral disease in paired organs (e.g., tumors in both breasts, eyes, kidneys, or ovaries), and multiple, primary cancers (two or more different cancers in one person). "Although any form of cancer has the potential of being familial, the most common familial cancers are those of the breast, ovary, colon, endometrium, lymphoid and hemopoietic tissue, and brain" (Schneider, 1994).

Breast Cancer

Breast cancer is the most commonly diagnosed cancer in women. It is second to lung cancer as a cause of cancer-related deaths.

While annual breast cancer screening is recommended for all women beginning at age 50, guidelines for screening with mammography between the ages of 40 and 49 vary from yearly (American Cancer Society) to every 1 to 2 years (American College of Obstetricians and Gynecologists, National Cancer Institute, American Medical Association). A 1997 National Institutes of Health Consensus Development Conference panel concluded that women should decide for themselves about screening with mammography based on their personal medical history, their perceptions of risks and benefits, and analysis of scientific evidence (National Institutes of Health, 1997). If review groups cannot agree on the interpretation of the data, the latter criterion seems a bit ridiculous.

Risk factors for breast cancer include a personal history of ductal carcinoma in situ or lobular carcinoma in situ; menarche before age 12; first full-term pregnancy after age 30; never having borne a child; breast cancer in a sister, mother, or daughter; and a breast biopsy, particularly one showing atypical hyperplasia. Evidence for other risk factors (age at menopause, dense breast tissue, use of oral contraceptives, a high-fat diet, alcohol, radiation exposure, and environmental pollutants) is either not conclusive or the contribution of such a factor has not yet been determined (National Cancer Institute, 1998). "BRCA [breast cancer] 1 gene is responsible for between 20% and 40% of hereditary breast cancer, and BRCA 2 is responsible for between 10% and 30%" (Olopade & Cummings, 2000, p. 1812). "The BRCA 1 gene is thought to account for 20% to 40% of breast cancer in families with a high incidence of early-onset breast cancer and for almost 90% of breast cancer in families with a high incidence of breast and ovarian cancers. BRCA 1 mutations are also associated with a 40% to 60% risk of a second primary breast cancer" (Olopade & Cummings, 2000, p. 1813).

Table 15-2 shows the lifetime risk of breast and ovarian cancer in the general population and with altered BRCA 1 and BRCA 2 genes.

Women who may wish to consider genetic susceptibility testing because they are at risk for having inherited BRCA 1 or BRCA 2 mutations include the following (Olopade & Cummings, 2000):

- Women with a diagnosis of breast or ovarian cancer before the age of 50
- Women with a history of breast or ovarian cancer in a first-degree relative

TABLE 15.2 Lifetime Risk of Breast and Ovarian Cancer in the General Population and With Altered BRCA 1 and BRCA 2 genes*

	Breast cancer	Ovarian cancer
General population	12%	1.5%
Altered BRCA 1 gene	50–85%	5–40%
Altered BRCA 2 gene	50–85%	10–20%

Source: National Cancer Institute. (1997).

*These figures may be artificially high, as most research has involved large families with many individuals affected.

From National Cancer Institute. (1997). Genetic testing for breast cancer risk: It's your choice. (Fact sheet).

- Women with a relative with a mutation in BRCA 1 or BRCA 2
- Women of Eastern European descent with a personal or family history of breast or ovarian cancer

Because of the profound consequences of a positive result to genetic testing, referral to a genetics counselor should be discussed before a decision is made to test.

All women should be taught and encouraged to perform breast self-examination (BSE). Recent evidence showing that breast tumors in younger women can grow rapidly in less than a year reinforces the need to encourage all women to perform this monthly examination (Kerlikowske, 1996). Women also should know the differences in recommended ages for initial and follow-up mammograms, and they should be encouraged to share this information with female friends and family members. Pamphlets on how to perform BSE can be offered to clients along with a suggestion that they share the pamphlet with female relatives and friends.

Cervical Cancer

The incidence of cervical cancer is highest in Vietnamese women, while the death rate is highest in Black women. Squamous cell cervical cancer is thought to be caused by certain types of human papilloma virus (HPV), although the role of behavioral status (age at first intercourse, multiple male sexual partners, sexually transmitted infections) and socioeconomic status is unclear (Centers for Disease Control and Prevention [CDC], 2000b).

Identification of precancerous lesions through the Pap test allows for timely treatment of cervical cancer. Survival for women with precancerous cervical intraepithelial neoplasia (CIN) is almost 100%. The American College of Obstetricians and Gynecologists and the American Cancer Society recommend that annual screening begin when a woman becomes sexually active or at the age of 18, whichever comes first. Subsequently, women with three consecutive annual Pap tests with normal findings need to be screened only every 3 years. "Scientific data suggest that once a woman has demonstrated no signs of CIN, as evidenced by three consecutive annual Pap tests with normal findings, her chance of developing CIN II or worse within 3 years is extremely low, regardless of other risk factors" (CDC, 2000b, p. 49).

Other Cancers

At the postpartum visit, clinicians should also counsel clients who have hereditary neoplastic syndromes or familial cancers about the need for follow-up by a specialist.

Ovarian Cancer

If a woman has two first-degree relatives who have had ovarian cancer, the National Institutes of Health recommends an annual recto-vaginal-pelvic examination, CA-125 determinations, and a transvaginal ultrasound until age 35 (earlier, if childbearing is completed). Then a prophylactic, bilateral oophorectomy is recommended.

Colon Cancer

Colorectal cancer is the second leading cause of cancer death in the United States. Fortunately, it has a slow-growing precursor lesion, the adenoma (pre-cancerous polyps). Removal of the adenoma prevents progression to cancer. While individuals considered to be at average risk for colon cancer should be screened with colonoscopy at age 50, the American College of Gastroenterology recommends additional screening for high-risk persons: those with positive family histories of familial adenomatous polyposis (FAP) or hereditary nonpolyposis colorectal cancer (HNPCC). Persons with family histories should receive colonoscopy examinations every 2 years, beginning at age 20 to 25 until the age of 40 and annually thereafter. Colonoscopy has not yet been studied in randomized controlled trials or even case control studies. But because this technique has been shown to be more effective than either sigmoidoscopy or barium enema in identifying the precursor lesion, colonoscopy is evolving as the preferred screening strategy.

Women are considered high risk when they have either multiple first-degree relatives with colorectal cancer or a single first-degree relative with colorectal cancer diagnosed before the age of 60. These individuals should be screened every 3 to 5 years, beginning at age 40 or 10 years younger than the age at which the youngest affected relative was diagnosed. Women with only one first-degree relative diagnosed with colorectal cancer at or before the age of 60 should begin screening at age 40 (Rex, Johnson, Lieberman, Burt, & Sonnenberg, 2000).

Skin Cancer

The three kinds of skin cancer—basal cell carcinoma, squamous cell carcinoma, and malignant melanoma—are hazards of exposure to sunlight. Those most at risk have a family history of skin cancer or have sensitive skin (i.e., always burn on exposure to the sun, never tan, or tan only slightly). People who work outdoors are particularly vulnerable to basal cell carcinoma, as risk increases proportionally with the amount and duration of exposure to ultraviolet radiation, although Blereau and Monroe add, "Severe sunburns in childhood and adolescence appear to confer a greater risk of skin cancer in adulthood than cumulative sun exposure" (2000, p. 1694). Unfortunately, few teenagers always use sunscreen, and an alarming number, 33% in one study, never use it (Banks, Silverman, Schwartz, & Tunnessen, 1992). The value of sunscreen in people with very dark skin is debated (Epstein, Kaplan, & Levine, 2000).

In addition to avoiding sun exposure, particularly between 10 AM and 4 PM, a sun protection plan should include using long-sleeved shirts and long pants, wide-brimmed hats, and sunscreen. Research shows that sunscreens prevent actinic keratoses, the precursors of cutaneous squamous cell carcinoma. Data that show sunscreen prevention of basal cell skin cancers are lacking, but many dermatologists believe that use of sunscreens in early childhood can prevent basal cell carcinoma of the skin (Epstein, Kaplan, & Levine, 2000).

Sunscreens should have a sun protection factor (SPF) of at least 15 and protect against both ultraviolet A (UVA) and ultraviolet B (UVB) rays. The SPF numbers refer to protection against UVB rays. (However, UVA rays can also damage skin.) Regular use of a sunscreen with an SPF of 15 for the first 18 years of life (excluding the first 6 months when there should be no exposure to the sun) can significantly decrease a person's lifetime risk of developing nonmelanoma skin cancer. Instruct clients to generously reapply sunscreen about every hour, after swimming or sweating, and every 2 hours otherwise. Because people with light skin sunburn more readily, they should apply thicker layers of sunscreen with higher SPF values (Epstein, Kaplan, & Levine, 2000). Makeup should be applied over sunscreen, and sunblock lip protection should be used. Box 15-1 summarizes sunbathing tips for the prevention of skin cancer.

"Slip, slop, slap" is a theme recommended by the Skin Cancer Foundation to help people remember to slip on long-sleeved clothes, slop on sunscreen, and slap on a hat. In addition to conveying the "slip, slop, slap" message and instructing clients about the correct use of sunscreen, clinicians should be sure clients know that any persistent sore or growth as well as any irritated or scar-like area should be evaluated by a physician. The main message is that chronic exposure to sunlight is dangerous.

Clients may ask about recent studies suggesting that sunscreen may raise the incidence of melanoma. These studies are difficult to interpret, because people who use sunscreens are likely to be those with light skin and, therefore, already at risk. People who use sunscreens may also stay in the sun longer, thinking they have protection from the sun and have not taken into account use of sunscreens as children (Muirhead, 2000). Indoor sunlamps, tanning parlors, and tanning pills should be discouraged.

Self-examination of the skin should occur monthly and can be conducted with the monthly BSE. The American Cancer Society (1993) recommends that the skin examination include:

• Examining the front and back of the body in a mirror
• Raising the arms and examining each side

Box 15.1

Sunbathing Dos and Don'ts: Tips for the Prevention of Skin Cancer

DOS

1. Avoid sunlight between 10 AM and 4 PM.
2. Wear long-sleeved shirts and long pants. When possible, wear special clothing with a high SPF.
3. Wear wide-brimmed hats to protect the face, ears, and neck.
4. Use sunscreen with an SPF of at least 15.
5. Choose sunscreens that protect against both UVA and UVB radiation.
6. Use sunblock lip protection.
7. Apply makeup over sunscreen.
8. Reapply sunscreen often when sweating occurs.
9. Reapply sunscreen after swimming.
10. Stay in the shade or under an umbrella when you're at a beach, river, or lake.
11. Wear sunglasses that protect you from ultraviolet radiation.

DON'TS

1. Don't assume that cloudy days offer protection against the sun's rays.
2. Don't use sunscreen to allow more time in the sun.

- Bending the elbows to look at forearms, upper arms, and palms of the hand
- Sitting to look at the backs of the legs and feet, the soles of the feet, and the spaces between the toes
- Using a hand mirror to examine the back of the neck, the backs of the ears, and the scalp

Clients can also be taught the "ABCD" approach that gives clues to melanoma. "A" refers to asymmetry, "B" refers to borders that are irregular, "C" refers to color variations, and "D" refers to the diameter of the lesion. Those measuring more than 6 mm, the size of a pencil eraser, require referral to a dermatologist or a diagnostic biopsy.

❖ Heart Disease

Heart disease is the number-one killer of women. While one out of eight women will die from breast cancer, one out of two women will die from heart disease. The risk factors for cardiac disease in women are the same as in men, but they do not carry the same weight for both sexes. Risk factors for heart disease include smoking, high blood pressure, diabetes, high levels of low-density lipoproteins (τ130 mg/dL), low levels of high-density lipoproteins (<35 mg/dL), and a family history of premature coronary heart disease (a family history of a heart attack in one first-degree relative or two second-degree relatives before the age of 55 in men and 65 in women). These risk factors are summarized in Box 15-2. If the client is young, her parents may not be old enough to have developed coronary heart disease. In this case, be certain to inquire about a history of coronary heart disease in grandparents.

Women with heart disease present with symptoms that can be different from those found in men. "Men typically experience substernal chest pain that radiates down the left arm. But many women describe a heaviness in the shoulder, jaw, neck, back, throat, or teeth, and not in the chest. They experience nausea, vomiting, and shortness of breath more frequently than the chest pain pattern typical of men. Women are also more likely to have intermittent pain or no pain at all. Silent ischemic events account for up to 25% of MIs [myocardial infarctions] experienced by women" (Halm, 1999, p. S8).

Preventive care guidelines issued by the American College of Physicians state: "Screening for total cholesterol levels is not recommended for . . . women (younger than 45 years of age) unless the history or physical examination suggests a familial lipoprotein disorder or at least two other characteristics increase the risk for coronary heart disease" (American College of Physicians, 1996, p. 516).

Familial dyslipidemia is suggested by early coronary heart disease among close relatives. However, subclinical coronary heart disease is common among women (Robbins, 2001). Table 15-3 illustrates the normal cholesterol-lipoprotein profile.

Box 15.2

Risk Factors for Cardiac Disease in Women

- Smoking
- High blood pressure
- Diabetes
- High levels of low-density lipoprotein (LDL) cholesterol (>160 mg/dL) and low levels of high-density lipoprotein (HDL) cholesterol (<35 mg/dL)
- A family history of premature coronary heart disease (a heart attack in one first-degree relative or two second-degree relatives before age 65 (age 55 in men).

TABLE 15.3 The Normal Cholesterol-Lipoprotein Profile*

Type of cholesterol	Desirable levels (mg/dL)	Borderline-high levels (mg/dL)	High levels (mg/dL)
Total	Less than 200	200 to 239	240 and above
LDL (bad)	Less than 130	130 to 159	160 and above
HDL (good)	More than 60†	60 to 35	Below 35
Triglyceride	Less than 200	200 to 399	400–1000 (high)
			1000 (very high)

*These categories are for people 20 years of age and older
†More than 60 mg/dL tends to lessen risk posed by a high LDL

❖ Referrals

The need for a referral for additional help with problem areas might arise post-partally. Referrals that might be appropriate include:

- A stop-smoking program
- An anger-control program
- Support groups
- Counseling or therapy
- Medical evaluation and treatment for high blood pressure; thyroid enlargement, abnormal laboratory tests; and incontinence still present after 6 months
- Parenting programs

Sometimes it seems that the people most likely to refrain from attending parenting classes are those most likely to need assistance. It is hard to know a good way to tell a mother that you think her ability to parent is lacking. You might try talking about the stress that a new baby brings to a family and then discuss parenting programs in terms of their focus on helping new parents deal with stress.

Support groups can provide valuable emotional care for women in a variety of circumstances. Because the health care provider may have minimal time to discuss emotional responses to a new baby or medical problems with a psychological component, participation in a support group may help a new mother work through her feelings and problems. Increased knowledge about the problem, concern, or feeling may facilitate adaptation to the new situation. Support groups that might be appropriate include:

New mothers groups
Breastfeeding support groups
Sexual abuse support groups
Domestic violence shelters
Alcoholics Anonymous or Al-Anon

Box 15.3

Selected Health Maintenance Screening Recommendations for Women in the Childbearing Years

Glucose testing: Yearly in women who have had gestational diabetes. Frequency of screening for women in other high-risk groups (obese women and over age 40, a strong family history of diabetes, and American Indians, Latinas, and African Americans) has not been determined.

Hepatitis A vaccine: Women at high risk (including international travelers)*

Hepatitis C testing: All women age 13 and older in high-risk groups (including those who have received a blood transfusion anytime since 1992)*

HIV testing: All high-risk women, as well as pregnant women, women seeking preconception counseling, and women with invasive cervical cancer*

Mammograms: Yearly after age 35 if premenopausal cancer has occurred in a first-degree relative, otherwise yearly or every 1 to 2 years between ages 40 and 49

Pap smear: yearly after age 18 or after becoming sexually active; then every 3 years once three consecutive yearly Pap smears are normal

Thyroid testing: Thyroid-stimulating hormone (TSH) test every 5 years, starting at age 35†

Colonoscopy: Every 10 years starting at age 40 if a single first-degree relative was diagnosed with colorectal cancer at age 60 or later. Every 3 to 5 years starting at age 40 *or* 10 years younger than the age at diagnosis of the youngest first-degree relative diagnosed before the age of 60 *or* multiple first-degree relatives diagnosed at any time, whichever is first‡

*American College of Obstetricians and Gynecologists. (1994).

†Ladenson, Singer, Ain, Bagchi, Bigos, Levy, Smith, & Daniels. (2000).

‡Rex, Johnson, Lieberman, Burt, & Sonnenberg. (2000).

❋ Conclusion

The postpartum visit, while often considered to be routine and boring, is an important meeting between the midwife and the new mother. In addition to identifying physical and emotional problems, the midwife can provide an emotional support system and help the client establish health goals for the future. Box 15-3 summarizes selected health recommendations.

The postpartum visit is also a time for closure on one part of a woman's life. In some instances, the visit also closes a chapter on a unique relationship between the midwife and the client. If the midwife is able to invite the client to return for annual health examinations, the postpartum visits may be a continuation of a long-term relationship. If the visit is a time of leave-taking, it may be somewhat sad. The visit is important and worthwhile from a variety of perspectives.

❊ References

Abramowicz, M. (Ed.). 1995. Varicella vaccine. *The Medical Center on Drugs & Therapeutics, 37*(951), 55–57.

Abramowicz, M. (Ed.). (2000a). Calcium supplements. *The Medical Letter, 42,*(1075), 19–31.

Abramowicz, M. (Ed.). (2000b). Oral contraceptives. *The Medical Letter, 42*(1078), 42–44.

Adler, A. I., & Olscamp, A. (1995). Toxic "sock" syndrome: Bezoar formation and pancreatitis associated with iron deficiency anemia. *Western Journal of Medicine, 163,* 480–482.

Albers, L., Garcia, J., Renfrew, M., McCandlish, & Elbourne, D. (1999). Distribution of genital tract trauma in childbirth and related postnatal pain. *Birth, 26*(1), 11–15.

Alexander, J. M., McIntire, D. D., & Leveno, K. J. (2000). Forty weeks and beyond: Pregnancy outcomes by week of gestation. *Obstetrics& Gynecology, 96*(2), 291–294.

Allaire, A. D., Moos, M., & Wells, S. R. (2000). Complementary and alternative medicine in pregnancy: A survey of North Carolina certified nurse-midwives. *Obstetrics & Gynecology, 95*(1), 19–23.

Alpert, E. J. (1995). Violence in intimate relationships and the practicing internist: New "disease" or new agenda? *Annals of Internal Medicine, 123,* 774–781.

American Academy of Pediatrics. (1996). The prenatal visit. *Pediatrics, 97*(1), 141–142.

American Academy of Pediatrics. (1997). Breastfeeding and the use of human milk [Policy statement]. *Pediatrics, 100*(6), 1035–1039.

American Academy of Pediatrics. (1999). Circumcision policy statement. *Pediatrics, 103*(3), 686–693.

American Academy of Pediatrics. (2000). Changing concepts of sudden infant death syndrome: Implications for infant sleeping environment and sleep position [Policy statement]. *Pediatrics, 105*(3), 650–656.

American Association of Clinical Endocrinologists. (1996). *AACE Clinical Guidelines for the Evaluation and Treatment of Hyperthyroidism and Hypothyroidism.* American College of Endocrinology.

American College of Obstetricians and Gynecologists. (1989). *Amenorrhea* (ACOG Technical Bulletin No. 128). Washington, DC: Author.

American College of Obstetricians and Gynecologists. (1991). *Immunization during pregnancy* (ACOG Technical Bulletin No. 160). Washington, DC: Author.

American College of Obstetricians and Gynecologists. (1993). *Thyroid disease in pregnancy* (ACOG Technical Bulletin No. 181). Washington, DC: Author.

American College of Obstetricians and Gynecologists. (1994). *Diabetes and pregnancy* (ACOG Technical Bulletin Number 200.) Washington, DC: Author.

American College of Obstetricians and Gynecologists. (1995a). *Chorionic villus sampling* (ACOG Committee Opinion No. 160). Washington, DC: Author.

American College of Obstetricians and Gynecologists. (1995b). *Preterm labor* (ACOG Technical Bulletin No. 206). Washington, DC: Author.

American College of Obstetricians and Gynecologists. (1996a). *Hypertension in pregnancy* (ACOG Technical Bulletin No. 219). Washington, DC: Author.

American College of Obstetricians and Gynecologists. (1996b). *Management of isoimmunization in pregnancy* (ACOG Educational Bulletin No. 227). Washington, DC: Author.

American College of Obstetricians and Gynecologists. (1996c). *Prevention of early-onset group B streptococcal disease in newborns* (ACOG Committee Opinion No. 143). Washington, DC: Author.

American College of Obstetricians and Gynecologists. (1997a). *Advanced paternal age* (Committee Opinion No.189). Washington, DC: Author.

American College of Obstetricians and Gynecologists. (1997b). *Fetal fibronectin preterm labor risk test* (ACOG Committee Opinion No. 187). Washington, DC: Author.

American College of Obstetricians and Gynecologists. (1997c). *Management of postterm pregnancy* (ACOG Practice Patterns No. 6). Washington, DC: Author.

American College of Obstetricians and Gynecologists. (1997d). *Routine ultrasound in low-risk pregnancy* (ACOG Practice Patterns No. 5). Washington, DC: Author.

American College of Obstetricians and Gynecologists. (1998a). *Antimicrobial therapy for obstetric patients* (ACOG Educational Bulletin No. 245). Washington, DC: Author.

American College of Obstetricians and Gynecologists. (1998b). *Obstetric aspects of trauma management* (ACOG Educational Bulletin No. 251). Washington, DC: Author.

American College of Obstetricians and Gynecologists. (1998c). *Viral hepatitis in pregnancy* (ACOG Education Bulletin No. 248). Washington, DC: Author.

American College of Obstetricians and Gynecologists. (1998d). *Vitamin A supplementation during pregnancy* (ACOG Committee Opinion 196). Washington, DC: Author.

American College of Obstetricians and Gynecologists. (1999a). *Antepartal fetal surveillance* (ACOG Practice Bulletin No. 9). Washington, DC: Author.

American College of Obstetricians and Gynecologists. (1999b). *Domestic violence* (ACOG Educational Bulletin No. 257). Washington, DC: Author.

American College of Obstetricians and Gynecologists. (1999c). *Joint statement of ACOG/AAP on human immunodeficiency virus screening* (ACOG statement of policy). Washington, DC: Author.

American College of Obstetricians and Gynecologists. (1999d). *Management of herpes in pregnancy* (ACOG Practice Bulletin No. 8). Washington, DC: Author.

American College of Obstetricians and Gynecologists. (1999e). *Prevention of RhD alloimmunization* (ACOG Practice Bulletin No. 46). Washington, DC: Author.

American College of Obstetricians and Gynecologists. (1999f). *Thrombocytopenia in pregnancy* (ACOG Practice Bulletin No. 6). Washington, DC: Author.

American College of Obstetricians and Gynecologists. (1999g). *Induction of labor* (ACOG Practice Bulletin No. 10). Washington, DC: Author.

American College of Obstetricians and Gynecologists. (2000a). *Fetal macrosomia* (ACOG Clinical Management Guidelines No. 22). Washington, DC: Author.

American College of Obstetricians and Gynecologists. (2000b). *Genetic screening for hemoglobinopathies* (ACOG Committee Opinion No. 238). Washington, DC: Author.

American College of Obstetricians and Gynecologists. (2000c). *Perinatal viral and parasitic infections* (ACOG Practice Bulletin No. 20). Washington, DC: Author.

American College of Obstetricians and Gynecologists Committee on Obstetric Practice. (1998). *Vitamin A supplementation during pregnancy* (Committee Opinion No. 196). Washington, DC: American College of Obstetricians and Gynecologists.

American College of Physicians. (1996). Guidelines for using serum cholesterol, high-density lipoprotein cholesterol, and triglyceride levels as screening tests for preventing coronary heart disease in adults. *Annals of Internal Medicine, 124,* 515–517.

American Diabetes Association Expert Committee on the Diagnosis and Classification of Diabetes Mellitus. (1997). Report of the expert committee on the diagnosis and classification of diabetes mellitus. *Diabetes Care, 20*(7), 1183–1197.

American Medical Association Ad Hoc Committee on Health Literacy. (1999). Health literacy: Report of the Council on Scientific Affairs. *JAMA, 281*(6), 552–557.

Andrews, W. W., Goldenberg, R. L., Mercer, B., Iams, J., Meis, P., Moawad, A., Das, A., VanDorsten, J. P., Caritis, S. N., Thurnau, G., Miodovnik, M., Roberts, J., McNellis, D., for the National Institute of Child Health and Human Development Maternal-Fetal Medicine Units Network. (2000). The Preterm Prediction Study: Association of second-trimester genitourinary chlamydia infection with subsequent preterm birth. *American Journal of Obstetrics & Gynecology, 183*(3), 662–668.

Anttila, T., Saikku, P., Koskela, P., Blloigu, A., Dillner, J., Ikaheimo, I., Jellum, E., Lehtinen, M., Lenner, P., Hakulinen, T., Narvanen, A., Pukkala, E., Thoresen, S., Youngman, L., & Paavonen, J. (2001). Serotypes of *Chlamydia trachomatis* and risk for development of cervical squamous cell carcinoma. *JAMA, 285*(1), 47–51.

Arndt, J. (2000, June 5). Sick building syndrome. *Business Week.*

Ballew, C., & Sugerman, S. B. (1995). High-risk nutrient intakes among low-income Mexican women in Chicago, Illinois. *Journal of the American Dietetic Association,* 95(12), 1409–1413.

Banks, B. A., Silverman, Schwartz, R. H., & Tunnessen, W. W. (1992). Attitudes of teenagers toward sun exposure. *Pediatrics, 89,* 40–42.

Baratte-Beebe, K. R., & Lee, K. (1999). Sources of midsleep awakenings in childbearing women. *Clinical Nursing Research,* 8(4), 386–397.

Baron, F., & Hill, W.C. (1998). Placenta previa, placenta abruptio. *Clinical Obstetrics & Gynecology, 41*(3), 527–532.

Barton, M. B., Harris, R., & Fletcher, S. W. (1999). Does this patient have breast cancer? The screening clinical breast examination: Should it be done? How? *JAMA, 282*(13), 1270–1280.

Benowitz, N. L. (1997). Treating tobacco addiction—Nicotine or no nicotine? *New England Journal of Medicine, 337*(17), 1230–1231.

Biancuzzo, M. (2000). Not enough milk: Reasons, rationale, and remedies. *Advance for Nurse Practitioners, 8*(2), 67–68.

Blackburn, R. D., Cunkelman, J., & Zlidar, V. M. (2000, Spring). Oral contraceptives—An update. *Population Reports,* Series A, No. 9. Baltimore: Johns Hopkins University School of Public Health, Population Information Program.

Blackwell, S., & Hendrix, P. C. (2001). Common anemias: What lies beneath. *Clinician Reviews, 11* (3), 53–62.

Blatt, S. D., Meguid, V., & Church, C. C. (2000). Prenatal cocaine: What's known about outcomes? *Contemporary OB/GYN, 45*(9), 67+.

Blereau, R. P., & Monroe, J. (2000). Basal cell carcinoma. *Consultant, 40*(9), 1693–1694.

Boehlen, F., Hohlfeld, P., Extermann, P., Perneger, T. V., & de Moerloose, P. (2000). Platelet count at term pregnancy: A reappraisal of the threshold. *Obstetrics & Gynecology, 95*(1), 29–33.

Boggess, K. A., Myers, E. R., & Hamilton, C. D. (2000). Antepartum or postpartum isoniazid treatment of latent tuberculosis infection. *Obstetrics & Gynecology, 96*(5), 757–762.

Boonstra. (2000). The "Boom and Bust phenomenon:" The hopes, dreams, and broken promises of the contraceptive revolution. *Contraception, 61,* 9–25.

Bowen, L.A. (1994). Trauma and pregnancy, *Clinician Reviews, 4*(3), 49+.

Bowman, J. M. (1978). The management of Rh-isoimmunization. *Obstetrics & Gynecology, 52,* 1–4.

Bracken, M. B., Hellenbrand, K. G., & Holford, T. R. (1990). Conception delay after oral contraceptive use: The effect of estrogen dose. *Fertility and Sterility, 53*(1), pp. 21–27.

Brett, R. L. (1999). Utilization of developmental basic science principles in the evaluation of reproductive risks from pre and post conception environmental radiation exposures. *Teratology, 59,* 182.

Briggs, G. G. (1997a). A guideline for treating hyperemesis gravidarum. *Contemporary OB/GYN, 42*(4), 70+.

Brown, J. E., & Kahn, E. S. B. (1997). Maternal nutrition and the outcome of pregnancy: A renaissance of research. *Clinics in Perinatology, 24*(2), 433–449.

Brown, M. S., Wheeler, L., & Malby, P. (1999). Is there a right way? *Midwifery Today, 49*(Spring), 40–41.

Brown, S., & Lumley, J. (1998). Maternal health after childbirth: Results of an Australian population based survey. *British Journal of Obstetrics and Gynaecology, 105,* 156–161.

Busch, W., & Himes, P. (1995). Maternal serum screening for chromosome disorders and open neural tube defects. *Genetics Northwest, 10*(2 and 3), 4–6.

Butler, E. L., Cox, S. M., Eberts, E. G., & Cunningham, F. G. (2000). Symptomatic nephrolithiasis complicating pregnancy. *Obstetrics & Gynecology, 96*(5), 753–756.

Calcium Information Center. (No date*). How to choose an over-the-counter calcium supplement.*

California Department of Health Services. (No date). *Examination of the lymph nodes.*

Carey, J. C., Klebanoff, M. A., Hauth, J. C., Hillier, S. L., Thom, E. A., Ernest, J. M., Heine, R. P., Nugent, R. P., Fischer, M. L., Leveno, K. J., Wapner, R., & Varner, M. (2000). Metronidazole to prevent preterm delivery in pregnant women with asymptomatic bacterial vaginosis. *New England Journal of Medicine, 342,* 534–540.

Carlat, D. J. (1998). The psychiatric review of symptoms: A screening tool for family physicians. *American Family Physician, 58*(7), 1617–1624.

Carson, C. C., Boggess, K. A., Colgan, R., Hooton, T. M., & Kerr, L. A. (2000). Current management of UTI in women. *Patient Care for the Nurse Practitioner,* Fall, 22.

Centers for Disease Control and Prevention (1991a). Weapon-carrying among high school students: United States, 1990. *MMWR 1991, 40,* 681–684.

Centers for Disease Control and Prevention. (1991b). Hepatitis B virus: A comprehensive strategy for eliminating transmission in the United States through universal childhood vaccination: Recommendations of the Immunization Practices Advisory Committee (ACIP). *MMWR 1991; 40* (RR-13), 1–19.

Centers for Disease Control and Prevention. (1993). Reported vaccine-preventable diseases: United States, 1993, and the childhood immunization initiative. *MMWR 1993a, 43,* 57–60.

Centers for Disease Control and Prevention. (1996). Outbreak of primary and secondary syphilis: Baltimore City, Maryland, 1995 [Editorial note]. *MMWR 1996, 45*(8), 166–169.

Centers for Disease Control and Prevention. (1997). Alcohol consumption among pregnant and childbearing-aged women—United States, 1991 and 1995. *MMWR 1997; 46*(6), 346–350.

Centers for Disease Control and Prevention. (1998). 1998 Guidelines for treatment of sexually transmitted disease. *MMWR 1998; 47*(RR-1), 3–8.

Centers for Disease Control and Prevention. (2000a). Gonorrhea—United States, 1998. *MMWR 2000; 49*(24), 538–542.

Centers for Disease Control and Prevention. (2000b). Implementing recommendations for the early detection of breast and cervical cancer among low-income women. *MMWR 2000, 49*(RR-2), 37–55.

Centers for Disease Control and Prevention. (2000c). National syphilis elimination effort moves full steam ahead. *STD Prevention Letter,* 2, January, 1–3.

Centers for Disease Control and Prevention. (2000d). Preventing congenital toxoplasmosis. In *CDC recommendations regarding selected conditions affecting women's health. MMWR 2000, 49* (RR-2), 57–73.

Centers for Disease Control and Prevention Advisory Committee on Immunization Practices. (1998).

Chalmers, B., & Hashi, K. O. (2000). 432 Somali women's birth experiences in Canada after earlier female genital mutilation. *Birth, 27*(4), 227–234.

Chan, C. C. W., & To, W. W. K. (1999). Antepartum hemorrhage of unknown origin—What is its clinical significance? *Acta Obstetricia et Gynecologica Scandinavica, 78,* 186–190.

Chang, E., & Ramsey-Goldman, R. (2001). Managing systemic lupus erythematosus during pregnancy. *Women's Health [Gynecology edition], 1*(1), 53+.

Chapman, L. L. (1992). Expectant fathers' roles during labor and birth. *JOGNN, 21,* 114–120.

Chapman, S. J. (1998). Varicella in pregnancy. *Seminars in Perinatology, 22*(4), 339–346.

Chien, P. F. W., Owen, P., & Khan, K. S. (2000). Validity of ultrasound estimation of fetal weight. *Obstetrics & Gynecology, 95*(6, Part 1), 856–860.

Cibils, L. A. (1971). Rupture of the symphysis pubis. *Obstetrics & Gynecology, 38,* 407.

Civic, D., Scholes, D., Ichikawa, L., LaCroix, A. Z., Yoshida, C. K., Ott, S. M., & Barlow, W. E. (2000). Depressive symptoms in users and non-users of depot medroxyprogesterone acetate. *Contraception, 61*:385–390.

Clapp, J.F., III. (2001). Recommending exercise during pregnancy. *Contemporary OB/GYN, 46*(1), 30+.

Cnattingius, S., Bergstrom, R., Lipworth, L., & Kramer, M. S. (1998). Prepregnancy weight and the risk of adverse pregnancy outcomes. *New England Journal of Medicine, 338*(3), 147–152.

Colie, C. (1997). Protocols—High-risk pregnancy: Occupational hazards. *Contemporary OB/GYN, 42*, 15+.

Corey, L., & Handsfield, H. H. (2000). Genital herpes and public health: Addressing a global problem. *JAMA, 283*(6), 791–794.

Coronado, G. D., Marshall, L. M., & Schwartz. (2000). Complications in pregnancy, labor, and delivery with uterine leiomyomas: A population-based study. *Obstetrics & Gynecology, 95*(5), 764–769.

Cotch, M. F., Pastorek, J. G., II, Nugent, R. P., Hillier, S. L., Gibbs, R. S., Martin, D. H., Eschenbach, D. A., Edelman, R., Carey, J. C., Regan, J. A., Krohn, M. A., Klebanoff, M. A., Rao, A. V., Rhoads, G. G., & The Vaginal Infections & Prematurity Study Group. (1997). *Sexually Transmitted Diseases, 24*(6), 353–360.

Coustan, D. R. (2000). Making the diagnosis of gestational diabetes mellitus. *Clinical Obstetrics and Gynecology, 43*(1), 99–105.

Creasy, R. K., & Resnik, R. (1999). Intrauterine growth restriction. In R. K. Creasy & R. Resnik (Eds.), *Maternal-Fetal Medicine: Principles and Practice* (4th ed.). Philadelphia: W. B. Saunders.

Crowe, S. M., Mastrobattista, J. M., & Monga, M. (2000). Oral glucose tolerance test and the preparatory diet. *American Journal of Obstetrics and Gynecology, 182*(5), 1052–1054.

Cunningham, F. G., & Leveno, K. J. (1995). Childbearing among older women: The message is cautiously optimistic. *New England Journal of Medicine, 333*, 1002–1004.

Cunningham, F. G., Gant, N. F., Leveno, K. J., Gilstrap, L. G., III, Hauth, J. C., & Wenstrom, K. D. (2001). *Williams obstetrics* (21st ed.). New York: McGraw-Hill.

Dacus, J. V., Meyer, N. L., & Sibai, B. M. (1995). How preconception counseling improves pregnancy outcome. *Contemporary OB/GYN, 40*(6), 111+.

Doak, C. C., Doak, L. G., & Root, J. H. (1996). *Teaching patients with low literacy skills* (2nd ed.). Philadelphia: J.B. Lippincott.

Doerr, L. (2000). Butts out: Incorporating smoking cessation into your practice. *Advance for Nurse Practitioners, 8*(6), 44+.

Dunn, D., Wallon, M., Peyron, F., Peterson, E., Peckham, C., & Gilbert, R. (1999). Mother-to-child transmission of toxoplasmosis: Risk estimates for clinical counselling. *Lancet, 353*, 1829–1833.

Eisenberg, D. M., Davis, R. B., Ettner, S. L., Appel, S., Wilkey, S., VanRompay, M., & Kessler, R. C. (1998). Trends in alternative medicine use in the United States, 1990–1997. *JAMA, 280*(18), 1569–1575.

El-Torkey, M., & Grant, J. M. (1992). Sweeping of the membranes is an effective method of induction of labour in prolonged pregnancy: A report of a randomized trial. *British Journal of Obstetrics and Gynecology, 99*, 455–458.

Ellertson, C., Shochet, T., Blanchard, K., & Trussell, J. (2000). Emergency contraception: A review of the programmatic and social science literature. *Contraception, 61*(3), 145–186.

Enkin, M., Keirse, M. J. N. C., Neilson, J., Crowther, C., Duley, L., Hodnett, E., & Hofmeyr. (2000). *A guide to effective care in pregnancy and childbirth* (3rd ed.). New York: Oxford University Press.

Epstein, J., Kaplan, L., & Levine, N. (2000). The value of sunscreens. *Patient Care for the Nurse Practitioner, 3*(6), 17+.

Ertem, I. E., Votto, N., & Leventhal, J. M. (2001).The timing and predictors of the early termination of breastfeeding. *Pediatrics, 107*(3), 543–548.

Etchells, E. (2000). The significance of systolic murmurs. *The Clinical Advisor, 3*(7/8), 43+.

Etherington, I. J., & James, D. K. (1993). Reagent strip testing of antenatal urine specimens for infection. *British Journal of Obstetrics and Gynecology, 100*, 806–808.

Ezmerli, N. M. (2000). Exercise in pregnancy. *Primary Care Update for OB/GYNs, 7*, 260–265.

Fagan, E. A. (1999). Diseases of the liver, biliary system, and pancreas. In R. Creasy and R. K. Resnik (Eds.), *Maternal-Fetal Medicine: Principles and Practice* (pp. 1054–1081). Philadelphia: W.B. Saunders.

Family Health International. (2000). Female condom reuse examined. *Network, 20*(2), 18–22.

Family Violence Prevention Fund. (1999). Screening for domestic violence changed my practice: An interview with Leigh Kimberg. *Health Alert, 6*(2), 1–3.

Ferenczy, A. (1995). Epidemiology and clinical pathophysiology of condylomata acuminata. *American Journal of Obstetrics and Gynecology, 172*, 1331–1339.

Filly, R. A. (1994). Ultrasound evaluation during the first trimester. In Callen, P. W. (Ed.), *Ultrasonography in obstetrics and gynecology* (pp. 63–78). Philadelphia: W.B. Saunders.

Fishwick, N. J. (1998). Assessment of women for partner abuse. *JOGNN 27*(6), 661–670.

Fleming, D. T., McQuillan, G. M., Johnson, R. E., Mahmias, A. J., Aral, S. O., & Lee, F. K. (1997). Herpes simplex virus type 2 in the United States: 1976 to 1994. *New England Journal of Medicine, 337*(16), 1105–1111.

Foong, L. C., Vanaja, K., Tan, G., & Chua, S. (2000). Membrane sweeping in conjunction with labor induction. *Obstetrics & Gynecology, 96*(4), 539–542.

Foster, H. W. (1997). The enigma of low birth weight and race. *New England Journal of Medicine, 337*(17), 1232–1233.

Franko, D. L., & Spurrell, E. B. (2000). Detection and management of eating disorders during pregnancy. *Obstetrics & Gynecology, 95*(6, Part 1), 942–946.

Fu, H., Darroch, J. E., & Ranjit, N. (1999). Contraceptive failure rates: New estimates from the 1995 National Survey of Family Growth. *Family Planning Perspectives, 31*(2), 56–63.

Gabbe, S., Hill, L., Schmidt, L., & Schulkin, J. (1998). Management of diabetes by obstetrician-gynecologists. *Obstetrics & Gynecology, 91*(5, Part 1), 643–647.

Gall, S. A. (1995). Immunizations for patients and personnel. *Contemporary OB-GYN, 40*, 29+.

Gardiner, S., & Holahan, K. (1999). *Northwest Division Kaiser Permanente guide to clinical laboratory services: 1999.* Hudson, OH: Lexi-Comp.

Garry, D., Figueroa, R., Guillame, J., & Cucco, V. (2000). Use of castor oil in pregnancies at term. *Alternative Therapies, 6*(1), 77–79.

Gazmarian, J. A., Lazorick, J., Spitz, A. M., Ballard, T. J., Saltzman, L. E., & Marks, J. S. (1996). Prevalence of violence against pregnant women. *Journal of the American Medical Association, 275*, 1915–1920.

Gibbs, R. S., & Sweet, R. L. (1999). Maternal and fetal infectious disorders. In R. K. Creasy & R. Resnik (Eds.), *Maternal-fetal medicine* (pp. 659–724). Philadelphia: W.B. Saunders.

Gifford, D. S., Morton, S. C., Fiske, M., Keesey, J., Keeler, E., & Kahn, K. L. (2000). Lack of progress in labor as a reason for Cesarean. *Obstetrics & Gynecology, 95* (4), 589–595.

Gilliland, F. D., Berhane, K., McConnell, R., Gauderman, W. J., Vora, H., Rappaport, E. B., Avol, E., & Peters, J. M. (2000). Maternal smoking during pregnancy, environmental tobacco smoke exposure and childhood lung function. *Tobacco, 55*, 271–276.

Gillum, L. A., Mamidipudi, S. K., & Johnston, S. C. (2000). Ischemic stroke risk with oral contraceptives. *JAMA, 284*(1), 72–78.

Given, P. M. (2000). Spontaneous mandible displacement. *Patient Care for the Nurse Practitioner, 3*(6), 76.

Goetsch: M. F. (1999). Postpartum dyspareunia: An unexplored problem. *Journal of Reproductive Medicine, 44*(11), 963–968.

Gold, M. (1999). *Marijuana's effect on relationships* [On-line]. Lifescape web site. Available:

Goldenberg, R. L., & Dolan-Mullen, P. (2000). Convincing pregnant patients to stop smoking. *Contemporary OB/GYN 45*(11), pp. 35+.

Goldenberg, R. L., Iams, J. D., Mercer, B. M., Meis, P. J., Moawad, A. H., Copper, R. L., Das, A., Thom, E., Johnson, F., McNellis, D., Miodovnik, M., Van Dorsten, J. P., Caritis, S. N., Thurnau, G. R., Bottoms, S. E., & The NICHD MFMU Network. (1998). The preterm prediction study: The value of new vs standard risk factors in preventing early and all spontaneous preterm births. *American Journal of Public Health, 88,* 233–238.

Gordon, M., Rich, H., Deutschberger, J., & Green, M. (1973). The immediate and long-term outcome of obstetric birth trauma. I. Brachial plexus paralysis. *American Journal of Obstetrics & Gynecology, 117,* 51–56.

Graham, H. (1988). Health education. In A. McPherson (Ed.), *Women's problems in general practice.* New York: Oxford University Press.

Grant, S. S. (2000). Prenatal genetic screening. *Online Journal of Issues in Nursing,[On-line serial], 5*(3), Manuscript 3. Available: http://www.nursingworld.org/ojin/topic13/ tpc13_3.html

Green, J. (1999). Commentary: What is this thing called "control"? *Birth, 26*(1), 51–52.

Greene, M. F. (1997). Screening for gestational diabetes mellitus. *New England Journal of Medicine, 337*(22), 1625–1626.

Greenland, V. C., Delke, I., & Minkoff, H. L. (1989). Vaginally administered cocaine overdose in a pregnant woman. *American Journal of Obstetrics and Gynecology, 74,* 476–477.

Gribble, R. K., Meier, Paul, R., & Berg, R. L. (1995). The value of urine screening for glucose at each prenatal visit. *Obstetrics & Gynecology, 86,* 405–410.

Grimes, D. A. (Ed.). (2000). Contraceptive implants and injectables: Recent developments. *Contraception Report, 10*(6), 26–30.

Grimes, D. A., Hanson, V., & Sondheimer, S. (2001). Emergency contraception. *Contemporary OB/GYN, 46*(6), 89+.

Gunn, T. R., & Wright, I. M. R. (1996). The use of black and blue cohosh in labour [Letter to the editor]. *New Zealand Medical Journal, 109*(1032), 410–411.

Gupta, R., Vasishta, K., Sawhney, & Ray, P. (1998). Safety and efficacy of stripping of membranes at term. *International Journal of Obstetrics and Gynecology, 60,* 115–121.

Gurley, B. J., Gardner, S. F., & Hubbard, M. A. (2000). Content versus label claims in ephedra-containing dietary supplements. *American Journal of Health-System Pharmacists, 57,* 963–969.

Gyetvai, K., Hannah, M. E., Hodnett, E. D., & Ohlsson, A. (1999). Tocolytics for preterm labor: A systematic review. *Obstetrics & Gynecology, 94*(5, Part 2), 869–877.

Hadlock, F. P. (1994). Ultrasound determination of menstrual age. In P. W. Callen (Ed.), *Ultrasonography in obstetrics and gynecology* (pp. 86–96). Philadelphia: W.B. Saunders.

Hager, W. D., Schuchat, A., Gibbs, R., Sweet, R., Mead, P., & Larsen, J. W. (2000). Prevention of perinatal group B streptococcal infection: Current controversies. *Obstetrics & Gynecology, 96*(1), 141–145.

Hagerman, R. (1994). *Fragile X Syndrome. The ARC's Q and A on fragile X* [On-line]. Available: http://The Arc.org/faqs/fragqa.html

Hale, T. (2000). *Medications and mothers' milk.* Amarillo, TX: Pharmasoft Publishing.

Halm, M. (1999). Exploding myths about women and heart disease. *The Nurse Practitioner, 24*(9), S8.

Hanford Health Information Network. (1994). *Genetic effects and birth defects from radiation exposure* [A collaboration of three states and nine Indian nations]. HHIN Resource Center.

Harlap, S., & Shiono, P. H. (1980). Alcohol, smoking, and incidence of spontaneous abortions in the first and second trimester. *Lancet, 2,* 173–176.

Hatcher, R. A. (1999). Talk given at Oregon Health Sciences University.

Hatcher, R. A., Trussell, J., Stewart, F., Cates, W., Jr., Stewart, G. K., Guest, F., & Koval, D. (1998). *Contraceptive technology* (17th ed.). New York: Ardent Media.

Henderson-Martin, B. (2000). No more surprises: Screening patients for alcohol abuse. *American Journal of Nursing, 100*(9), 26–33.

Heritage, C. (1998). Working with childhood sexual abuse survivors during pregnancy, labor, and birth. *JOGNN, 27*(6), 671–677.

Hibbard, J. U., Tart, M., & Moawad, A. H. (2000). Cervical length at 16–22 weeks' gestation and risk for preterm delivery. *Obstetrics & Gynecology, 96*(6), 972–978.

Hillis, S. D., Marchbanks, P. A., Tylor, L. R., & Peterson, H .B. (1999). Poststerilization regret: Findings from the United States Collaborative Review of Sterilization. *Obstetrics & Gynecology, 93*, 889–895.

Himes, P. (1998). Screening for hemoglobinopathies in pregnancy. *Genetics Northwest, 12*(1), 4.

Himes, P. (1999). Early prenatal diagnostic testing: Risks associated with chorionic villus sampling and early amniocentesis and screening options. *Journal of Perinatal and Neonatal Nursing, 13*(2), 1–13.

Hoffman, I. F., & Schmitz, J. L. (1995). Genital ulcer disease. *Postgraduate Medicine, 98*(3), 67+.

Holst, B., & Ritter, D. (2001). Managing viral hepatitis. *Clinician Reviews, 11*(1), 51–62.

Iams, J. (1998). Prevention of preterm birth. *New England Journal of Medicine, 338*(1), 54–56.

Joffe, G. M., Jacques, D., Bemis-Heys, R., Burton, R., Skram, B., & Shelburne. (1999). Impact of the fetal fibronectin assay on admissions for preterm labor. *American Journal of Obstetrics and Gynecology, 180*(3), 581–586.

Jolley, S., & Phillips-Angeles, E. (1998). *The breastfeeding triage tool*. Seattle: Seattle King County Department of Public Health.

Jolly, M. C., Sebire, N., Harris, J., Robinson, & Regan, L. (2000). Obstetric risks of pregnancy in women less than 18 years old. *Obstetrics & Gynecology, 96*(6), 962–966.

Jones, T. K., & Lawson, B. M. (1998). Profound neonatal congestive failure caused by maternal consumption of blue cohosh herbal medication. *The Journal of Pediatrics, 132* (3), 550–552.

Jordan, P. (2000). The art of fathering. *FirstTime* Dad, 1(1), 7.

Kane, B., & Sands, D. Z. (1998). Guidelines for the clinical use of electronic mail with patients. *Journal of the American Medical Informatics Association, 5*(1), 104–111.

Katz, V. L., Farmer, R., & Kuller. (2000). Preeclampsia into eclampsia: Toward a new paradigm. *American Journal of Obstetrics and Gynecology, 182*(6), 1389–1396.

Katz, V. L., Kuller, J. A., McMahon, M. J., Warren, M. A., & Wells, S. R. (1995). Varicella during pregnancy: Maternal and fetal effects. *Western Journal of Medicine, 163*, 446–450.

Kaunitz, A. M., & Zimmer, D. F., Jr. (2000). A medicolegal evaluation of reversible contraceptives. *Contemporary OB/GYN, 45*(5), 75+.

Kendrick, J. S., Atrash, H. K., Strauss, L. T., Gargiullo, P. M., & Ahn, Y. W. (1997). Vaginal douching and the risk of ectopic pregnancy among black women. *American Journal of Obstetrics & Gynecology, 176*(5), 991–997.

Kerlikowske, L. (1996). *JAMA, 275*.

Khine, M. L., Winklestein, A., & Copel, J. A. (1999). Selective screening for gestational diabetes mellitus in adolescent pregnancies. *Obstetrics & Gynecology, 93*, 738–742.

Kilpatrick, S. J., & Laros, R. K., Jr.(1999). Maternal hemorrhagic disorders. In R. K. Creasy & R. Resnik (Eds.), *Maternal-fetal medicine* (pp. 935–963). Philadelphia: W.B. Saunders.

Kim, H. L., Streltzer, J., Goebert, D. (1999). St. John's wort for depression: A meta-analysis of well-defined clinical trials. *Journal of Nervous and Mental Disease, 187*(9), 532–539.

Kirsch, I. S., Jungeblut, A., Jenkins, L., & Kolstad, A. (1993). *Adult literacy in America: A first look at the results of the National Adult Literacy Survey*. Washington, DC: U.S. Government Printing Office.

Kjos, S. L., Peters, R. K., Xiang, A., Thomas, D., Schaefer, U., & Buchanan, T. A. (1998). Contraception and the risk of Type 2 diabetes mellitus in Latina women with prior gestational diabetes mellitus. *JAMA, 280*(6), 533–538.

Kolata, G. (2000, December 21). Testing obesity: New research—Molecular keys to the appetite offer new hope. *The Oregonian*, p. A14.

Kosterman, R., Hawkins, J. D., Guo, J., Catalano, R. F., & Abbott, R. D. (2000). The dynamics of alcohol and marijuana initiation: Patterns and predictors of first use in adolescence. *American Journal of Public Health, 90*(3), 360–366.

Krishnana, S. P., Hilbert, J. C., VanLeeuwen, D., & Kolia, R. (1997). Documenting domestic violence among ethnically diverse populations: Results from a preliminary study. *Family and Community Health, 20*(3), 32–48.

Lacroix, R., Eason, E., & Melzack, R. (2000). Nausea and vomiting during pregnancy: A prospective study of its frequency, intensity, and patterns of change. *American Journal of Obstetrics and Gynecology, 182*(4), 931–937.

Ladenson, P. W., Singer, P. A., Ain, K. B., Bagchi, N., Bigos, S. T., Levy, E. G., Smith, S. A., & Daniels, G. H. (2000). American thyroid association guidelines for detection of thyroid dysfunction. *Archives of Internal Medicine, 160*, 1573–1575.

Lamar, M. E., Kuehl, T. J., Cooney, A. T., Gayle, J., Holleman, S., & Allen, S. R. (1999). Jelly beans as an alternative to a fifty-gram glucose beverage for gestational diabetes screening. *American Journal of Obstetrics & Gynecology, 181*(5, Part 1), 1154–1157.

Landers, D.V. (2000). Uncomplicated anogenital gonorrhea. *Contemporary OB/GYN, 45*(7), 127+.

Laros, R. K., Jr. (1999). Thromboembolic disease. In R. Creasy and R. K. Resnik (Eds.), *Maternal-fetal medicine: Principles and practice* (pp. 821–831). Philadelphia: W.B. Saunders.

Lawrence, R. A., & Lawrence, R. M. (1999). *Breastfeeding: A guide for the medical profession.* St. Louis: Mosby.

Lawson, H. W., Henson, R., Bobo, J. K., & Kaeser, M. K. (2000). Implementing recommendations for the early detection of breast and cervical cancer among low-income women. *MMWR 49*(RR-2), 37–55.

Lee, K. (2000). The toll of HIV/AIDS on minority women. *HIV Impact,* Spring.

Lee, W., Lee, V. L., Kirk, J. S., Sloan, C. T., Smith, R. S., & Comstock, C. H. (2000). Vasa previa: Prenatal diagnosis, natural evolution, and clinical outcomes. *Obstetrics & Gynecology, 95*(4), 572–576.

Leguizamon, G., & Reece, A. (1997). Is serologic screening of all pregnant women for cytomegalovirus warranted? *Contemporary OB/GYN, 42*(8), 49+.

Leiblum, S. R. (2000). Redefining female sexual response. *Contemporary OB/GYN, 45*(11), 120+.

Lemen, P. M., Wigton, T. R., Miller-McCarthey, A. J., & Cruikshank, D. P. (1998). Screening for gestational diabetes mellitus in adolescent pregnancies. *American Journal of Obstetrics & Gynecology, 178*(6), 1251–1256.

Liesnard, C., Donner, C., Brancart, F., Gosselin, F., Delforge, M. L., & Rodesch, F. (2000). Prenatal diagnosis of congenital cytomegalovirus infection: Prospective study of 237 pregnancies at risk. *Obstetrics & Gynecology, 95*(6, Part 1), 881–888.

Little, R. E. (1977). Moderate alcohol use during pregnancy and decreased infant birth weight. *American Journal of Public Health, 67*, 1154–1156.

Lydon-Rochelle, M., Holt, V. L., Easterling, T. R., & Martin, D. P. (2001). Risk of uterine rupture during labor among women with a prior cesarean delivery. *New England Journal of Medicine, 345*(1), 3–8.

Madrigal, E. (1995, January 30). Get off my back. I have enough to carry already. *The Oregonian.*

Mancuso, K. M., Yancey, M. K., Murphy, J. A., & Markenson, G. R. (2000). Epidural anesthesia for cephalic version: A randomized trial. *Obstetrics & Gynecology, 95*(5), 648–651.

Manning, F. A. (1999). Fetal biophysical profile. *Obstetrics & Gynecology Clinics of North America, 26*(4), 557–577.

Markovic, N., Ness, R. B., Cefilli, D., Grisso, J. A., Stahmer, S., & Shaw, L. M. (2000). Substance use measures among women in early pregnancy. *American Journal of Obstetrics & Gynecology, 183*(3), 627–632.

Marijuana Anonymous. (2001, April 7). *Twelve questions: Am I an addict?* Available: http://www.marijuana-anonymous.org/Pages/12quest.html

Mason, L., Glenn, S., Walton, I., & Appleton, C. (1999). The experience of stress incontinence after childbirth. *Birth, 26*(3), 164–171.

Mattar, F., & Sibai, B. M. (2000). Eclampsia: VIII. Risk factors for maternal morbidity. *American Journal of Obstetrics and Gynecology, 182*(2), 307–312.

McFarlin, B. L., Gibson, M. H., O'Rear, J. O., & Harman, P. (1999). A national survey of herbal preparation use by nurse-midwives for labor stimulation: Review of the literature and recommendations for practice. *Journal of Nurse-Midwifery, 44*(3), 205–216.

McVea, K., Venugopal, M., Crabtree, B. F., & Aita, V. (2000). The organization and distribution of patient education materials in family medicine practices. *Journal of Family Practice, 49*(4), 319–326.

Mead, P. B.(1997). Parvovirus B19 infection. *Contemporary OB/GYN, 42*(8), 15+.

Medical Letter. (2000c). Plan B: Progestin-only emergency contraceptive. *The Medical Letter, 42*(1070), 10.

Medical Letter. (2001). Drugs for vulvovaginal candidiasis. *Medical Letter, 43*(1095), 3–4.

Meniru, G. I., Hecht, B. R., & Hopkins, M. P. (2000). Female circumcision: At our doorsteps and beyond. *Primary Care Update for Ob/Gyns, 7*, 231–237.

Meyer, N. L., Mercer, B. M., Friedman, S. A., & Sibai, B. M. (1994). Urinary dipstick protein: A poor predictor of absent or severe proteinuria. *American Journal of Obstetrics and Gynecology, 170*, 137–141.

Mikhail, M. S., & Anyaegbunam, A. (1995). Lower urinary tract dysfunction in pregnancy: A review. (1995). *Obstetrical and Gynecological Survey, 50*, 675–683.

Millar, P., Wing, D. A., Paul, R. H., & Grimes, D. A. (1995). Outpatient treatment of pyelonephritis in pregnancy: A randomized controlled trial. *Obstetrics & Gynecology, 86*, 560.

Miller, E., Craddock-Watson, J. E., & Pollock, T. M. (1982). Consequences of confirmed maternal rubella at successive stages of pregnancy. *Lancet 2*, 781–783.

Mills, J. L. (2000). Fortification of foods with folic acid—How much is enough? *New England Journal of Medicine, 342*(19), 1442–1445.

Modern IUDs: Part 2. (1998). *Contraception Report, 9*(5), 4–14.

Mold, J. W., & Dalbir, D. K. (2000). Management of laboratory test results in family practice. *Journal of Family Practice, 49*(8), 709–715.

Moore, T. R. (1997). Clinical assessment of amniotic fluid. *Clinical Obstetrics and Gynecology, 40*(2), 303–313.

Mourad, J., Elliott, J. P., Erickson, L., & Lisboa, L. (2000). Appendicitis in pregnancy: New information that contradicts long-held clinical beliefs. *American Journal of Obstetrics and Gynecology, 182*(5), 1027–1029.

Mozingo, J. N., Davis, M. W., Droppelman, P. G., & Merideth, A. (2000). "It wasn't working:" Women's experiences with short-term breastfeeding. *MCN 25*(3), 120–126.

Mozurkewich, E. I., Luke, B., Avni, M., & Wolf, F. M. (2000). Working conditions and adverse pregnancy outcome: A meta-analysis. *Obstetrics & Gynecology, 95*(4), 623–635.

Nahum, G. G. (2000). Detecting and managing fetal macrosomia. *Contemporary OB/GYN, 45*(6), 89+.

National Academy of Sciences, Institute of Medicine. (1992). *Nutrition during pregnancy and lactation: An implementation guide.* Washington, DC: National Academy Press.

National Academy of Sciences Food and Nutrition Board. (1997). Dietary Reference Intakes for Calcium, Phosphorous, Magnesium, Vitamin D, & Fluoride. Washington, D.C.: National Academy Press.

National Cancer Institute. (1997). Genetic testing for breast cancer: It's your choice. (Fact sheet).

National Cancer Institute. (1998*). Estimating breast cancer risk [On-line].* National Cancer Institute web site. Available: http://rex.nci.nih.gov/massmedia/pressreleases/riskassess. html

National Center for Complementary and Alternative Medicine (NCCAM). (1999). *St. John's wort* (Publication No. Z02). Silver Spring, MD: NCCAM Clearinghouse.

National Institute on Alcohol Abuse and Alcoholism. (1995). *The physician's guide to helping patients with alcohol problems* (NIH Publication No.95-3769). Bethesda, MD: U.S. Department of Health and Human Services.

National Institute on Drug Abuse, National Institutes of Health. (2000). *Marijuana*. National Institute on Drug Abuse web site. Available:

National Institutes of Health. (1997). *NIH consensus statement: Breast cancer screening for women ages 40–49* (Vol. 15, No.1, pp. 1–35). Bethesda, MD: U.S. Department of Health and Human Services, National Institutes of Health.

National Institutes of Health. (1999). DES: Future directions. Research update, 1999. NIH Publication No. 00-4722. Bethesda, MD: U.S. Department of Health & Human Services. National Institutes of Health.

National Institutes of Health, National High Blood Pressure Education Program Working Group on High Blood Pressure in Pregnancy. (2000). *Report of the National High Blood Pressure Education Program Working Group Report on High Blood Pressure in Pregnancy*. Washington, DC: U.S. Department of Health and Human Services. (Also in the *American Journal of Obstetrics & Gynecology, 183*, S1-S22.)

National Tay-Sachs & Allied Diseases Association. [On line].

National Work Group on Literacy and Health. (1998). Communicating with patients who have limited literacy skills: Report of the National Work Group on Literacy and Health. *The Journal of Family Practice, 46*(2), 168–176.

Nelson, A. (2001, June 6). *New developments in contraception*. Talk given in Portland, OR.

New England Regional Genetics Group. (1999). *Position statement: Carrier testing for Canavan disease* [On-line]. Available: http://www.acadia.net/nergg/canavan.html

Nour, N. N. (2000). Female circumcision and genital mutilation: A practical and sensitive approach. *Contemporary OB/GYN, 45*(3), 50–55.

Nichol, K. L., Lind, A., Margolis, K. A., Murdoch, M., McFadden, R., Hauge, M., Magnan, S., & Drake, M. (1995). The effectiveness of vaccination against influenza in healthy, working adults. *New England Journal of Medicine, 333*, 889–893.

Odegard, R. A., Vatter, L. J., Nilson, S. T., Salveson, K. A., & Austgulen, R. (2000). Preeclampsia and fetal growth. *Obstetrics & Gynecology, 96*(6), 950–955.

Ohman, R., Hagg, S., Carleborg, L., & Spigset, O. (1999). Excretion of paroxetine into breast milk. *Journal of Clinical Psychiatry, 60*(8), 519–523.

Olavarrieta, C. D., & Sotelo, J. (1996). Domestic violence in Mexico. *JAMA, 275*, 1937–1941.

Olopade, O. I., & Cummings, S. (2000). Breast and ovarian cancer, Part 2: Counseling patients about risk. *Consultant,*1930+.

Oregon Health Division. (1994). Hepatitis B. *Investigative Guidelines*, 1–10.

Oregon Health Division. (1995). Pelvic inflammatory disease. *CD Summary, 44*(14), 1.

Oregon Health Division. (1996a). Medical aftermath of the Hanford Project. *CD Summary, 45*(1), 1–2.

Oregon Health Division. (1996b). Secondhand smoke: Another reason for parents to quit. *CD Summary, 45*(8), 1–2.

Oregon Health Division. (2000a). Fertile women need to take multivitamins with folic acid (MVF), *CD Summary, 49*(26), 1–2.

Oregon Health Division. (2000b). Lead poisoning has not gone away. *CD Summary, 49*(24).

Oregon Health Division. (2000c). Treating depressed patients. *CD Summary, 49*(18).

Oregon Health Division, Oregon Breast and Cervical Cancer Program. (1999). *Breast cancer diagnosis and follow-up protocols*.

Oregon Pregnancy Prevention Task Force, Adolescent Pregnancy Prevention Subcommittee. (1996). Tough questions about adult men who have babies with babies. *Rational Enquirer*, 6.

Oriel, K. A., & Fleming, M. F. (1998). Screening men for partner violence in a primary care setting. *Journal of Family Practice, 46*(6), 493–498.

Oxorn, H. (1986). *Oxorn-Foote:* Human labor and birth (5th ed.). Norwalk, CT: Appleton-Century-Crofts.

Padilla, L. A., Radosevich, D. M., & Milad, M. P. (2000). Accuracy of the pelvic examination in detecting adnexal masses. *Obstetrics & Gynecology, 96*(4), 593–598.

ParaGard T380A Product Monograph. (No date).

Pearlman, M. D., & Cunningham, F. G. (1996). Trauma in pregnancy. *Williams Obstetrics Supplement, 21*, 1–14.

Pharmacia and Upjohn. (1999). Depo-Provera Contraceptive Injection. (Package insert).

Pollack, H., Lantz, P. M., & Frohna, J. G. (2000). Maternal smoking and adverse birth outcomes among singletons and twins. *American Journal of Public Health, 90*(3), 395–400.

Poma, P. A. (1999). Cervical ripening: A review and recommendations for clinical practice. *Journal of Reproductive Medicine, 44*(8), 657–668.

Poss, J. E., & Rangel, R. (1995). Working effectively with interpreters in the primary care setting. *Nurse Practitioner, 20*(12), 43–47.

Potter, I., Oakley, D., de Leon-Wong, E., & Canamar, R. (1996). Measuring compliance among oral contraceptive users. *Family Planning Perspectives, 28*(4), 154–158.

Power, M. L., Holzman, G. B., & Schulkin, J. (2000). Knowledge and clinical practice regarding folic acid among obstetricians-gynecologists. *Obstetrics & Gynecology, 95*(6, Part 1), 895–898.

Pritchard, J. A. (1965). Changes in the blood volume during pregnancy and delivery. *Anesthesiology, 26*, 393–399.

Raisler, J. (2000). Against the odds: Breastfeeding experiences of low income mothers. *Journal of Nurse-Midwifery & Women's Health, 45*(3), 253–263.

Ramsey, L. A., Ross, B. R., & Fischer, R. G. (2000). Efficacy, safety, and reliability: Common concerns about herbal products. (2000). *Advance for Nurse Practitioners, 8*(2), 31+.

Redman, C., & Walker, I. (1992). *Pre-eclampsia: The facts.* New York: Oxford University Press.

Rex, D. K., Johnson, D. A., Lieberman, D. A., Burt, R. W., & Sonnenberg, A. (2000). Colorectal cancer prevention 2000: Screening recommendations of the American College of Gastroenterology. *American Journal of Gastroenterology, 95*(4), 868–877.

Rhoton-Vlasak, A. (1999). Viral influenza in women. *Primary Care Update Ob/Gyn, 6*(1), 1–7.

Robbins, D. C. (2001). Management of dyslipidemia: Reaching NCEP goals. *Clinician Reviews Supplement, 115*, 4–9.

Roberts, J. M. (1999). Pregnancy-related hypertension. In R. K. Creasy and R. Resnik (Eds.), *Maternal-fetal medicine: Principles and practice* (4th ed., pp. 833–872). Philadelphia: W.B. Saunders.

Roe, V. A. (1999). Antimicrobial agents: Pharmacologic and clinical application in obstetrics, gynecology, and perinatal infections. *JOGNN, 28*(6), 639–648.

Rothman, K. J., Moore, L. L., Singer, M. R., Nguyen, N. D. T., Mannino, S., & Milulsky, A. (1995). Teratogenicity of high vitamin A intake. *New England Journal of Medicine, 333*, 1369–1373.

Rouse, D. J., Andrews, W. W., Goldenberg, R. L., & Owen, J. (1995). Screening and treatment of asymptomatic bacteriuria of pregnancy to prevent pyelonephritis: A cost-effectiveness and cost-benefit analysis. *Obstetrics & Gynecology, 86*, 119–123.

Schieve, L. A., Cogswell, M. E., Scanlon, K. S., Perry, G., Ferre, C., Blackmore-Prince, C., Yu, S. M., Rosenberg, D., for the NMIHS Collaborative Working Group. (2000). Prepregnancy body mass index and pregnancy weight gain: Associations with preterm delivery. *Obstetrics & Gynecology, 96*(2), 194–200.

Schneider, K. A. (1994). Counseling about cancer. *Genetics Northwest, 9*(1), 1–3.

Schoenfeld, A., Ziv, E., Stein, L., Zaidel, D., & Ovadia, J. (1987). Seat belts in pregnancy and the obstetrician. *Obstetrical and Gynecological Survey, 42*, 275–282.

Scioscia, A. L. (1999). Prenatal genetic diagnosis. In R. K. Creasy & R. Resnik (Eds.), *Maternal-fetal medicine* (4th ed., pp. 40–62), Philadelphia: W.B. Saunders.

Seguin, L., Potvin, L., St. Denis, M., & Loiselle, J. (1999). Depressive symptoms in the late postpartum among low socioeconomic status women. *Birth, 26*(3), 157–163.

Severson, H. H., Andrews, J. A., Lichtenstein, E., Wall, M., & Akers, L. (1997). Reducing maternal smoking and relapse: Long-term evaluation of a pediatric intervention. *Preventive Medicine, 26*, 120–130.

Shahady, E. J. (2000). Exercise as medication: How to motivate your patients. *Consultant, 40*(13), 2174–2177.

Shelton, R. C., Keller, M. B., Gelenberg, A., Dunner, D. L., Hirschfeld, R., Thase, M. E., Russell, J., Lydiard, R. B., Crits-Cristoph, P., Gallop, R., Todd, L., Hellerstein, D., Goodnick, P., Keitner, G., Stahl, S. M., & Halbreich, U. (2001). Effectiveness of St. John's wort in major depression: A randomized controlled trial. *JAMA, 285*(15), 1978–1986.

Shulman, L. P. (2000). Monthly contraceptive injection. *The Female Patient, 26*, 14–18.

Sibai, B. M. (1998). Prevention of preeclampsia: A big disappointment. *American Journal of Obstetrics and Gynecology, 179*(5),1275–1278.

Sibai, B. M., McCubbin, J. H., Anderson, G. D., Lipshitz, J., & Dilts, P. V., Jr. (1981). Eclampsia I. Observations from 67 recent cases. *Obstetrics & Gynecology, 58*, 609–613.

Signorello, L. B., Harlow, B. L., Chekos, A. K., & Repke, J. T. (2000). Midline episiotomy and anal incontinence: Retrospective cohort study. *British Medical Journal, 320*, 86–90.

Silver, R. M., & Branch, D. W. (1997). Autoimmune disease in pregnancy. Systemic lupus erythematosus and antiphospholipid syndrome. *Clinics in Perinatology, 24*(2), 291–320.

Simkin, P. (1991). Just another day in a woman's life? Women's long-term perceptions of their first birth experience. Part I. *Birth, 18*(4), 203–210.

Simkin, P. (1992). Just another day in a woman's life? Part II: Nature and consistency of women's long-term memories of their first birth experiences. *Birth, 19*(2), 64–82.

Simkin, P. (1994). Memories that really matter. *Childbirth Educator Magazine,* 220+.

Simkin, P. (2000). Commentary: The meaning of labor pain. *Birth, 27*(4), 254–255.

Simkin, P. (Undated). Processing the birth experience with women.

Simon, E. P., & Schwartz. (1999). Medical hypnosis for hyperemesis gravidarum. *Birth, 26*(4), 248–254.

Slaughter, R., & Kanter, L. (1993). Women being alive. In *Domestic violence: Is it happening to you?*

Smith, J. R., & Herrera, J. L. (2001). Chronic hepatitis B: Diagnosis and current treatment options. *Consultant, 41,* (5), 782-786.

Spaeth, K. R. (2000). Don't hold your breath: Personal exposures to volatile organic compounds and other toxins in indoor air and what's (not) being done about it. *Preventive Medicine, 31*, 631–637.

Speroff, L., & Darney, P. (2001). *A clinical guide to contraception.* Philadelphia: Lippincott Williams & Wilkins.

Spoljoric, D. (2000). How to implement an effective smoking cessation plan. *Patient Care for the Nurse Practitioner, 3*(7), 59+.

Steinberg, P. (2000). Anaphylaxis: 33 commonsense ways to reduce the risk. *Consultant, 40*(5), 873+.

Stewart, J. (2000). Becoming advocates for battered women. *Clinician Reviews, 10*(6). 25–28.

Streissguth, A. P., Sampson, P. D., & Barr, H. B. (1989). Neurobehavioral dose-response effects of prenatal alcohol exposure in humans from infancy to adulthood. *Annals of the New York Academy of Sciences, 562*, 145–158.

Tedeschi, C. (1999). Ties that bind: Mothers, daughters and sons continue to feel effects of DES. *Advance for Nurse Practitioners, 7*(11), 28+.

Terry, P. E., & Healey, M. E. (2000). The physician's role in educating patients. *Journal of Family Practice, 49*(4), 314–318.

Thorp, J. M., Jr., Norton, P. A., Wall, L. L., Kuller, J. A., Eucker, B., & Wells, E. (1999). Urinary incontinence in pregnancy and the puerperium: A prospective study. *American Journal of Obstetrics & Gynecology, 181*(2), 266–273.

Thorstensen, K. A. (2000). Midwifery management of first trimester bleeding and early pregnancy loss. *Journal of Midwifery and Women's Health, 45*(60), 481–497.

Titus, K. (1996). When physicians ask, women tell about domestic abuse and violence. *JAMA* (Medical News and Perspectives), *275*, 1863–1865.

Toglia, M. R., & DeLancey, J. O. L. (1994). Anal incontinence and the obstetrician-gynecologist. *Obstetrics & Gynecology, 84*(4, Part 2), 731–740.

Tommaselli, G. A., Guida, M., Palomba, S., Barbato, M., & Nappi, C. (2000). Using complete breastfeeding and lactational amenorrhea as birth spacing methods. *Contraception, 61*, 253–257.

Toubia, N. (1999). *Caring for women with circumcision*. New York: Rainbo.

Turnquest, M. A., & Brown, H. L. (1999). Human parvovirus B19 infection during pregnancy. *The Female Patient, 24*, 75–81.

Turrentine, M. A., & Newton, E. R. (1995). Amoxicillin or erythromycin for the treatment of antenatal chlamydial infection: A meta-analysis. *Obstetrics & Gynecology, 86*, 1021–1025.

U.S. Public Health Service, Office of Disease Prevention and Health Promotion. (1998). *Clinician's handbook of preventive services* (2nd ed.). Washington, DC: Superintendent of Documents.

U.S. Public Health Service. (2000). *Treating tobacco use and dependence*. Washington, DC: U.S. Department of Health and Human Services.

Van de Vusse, L. (1999). The essential forces of labor revisited: 13 Ps reported in women's stories. *MCN, 24*(4), 176–184.

Vo, Q. T., Stettler, W., & Crowley, K. (2000). Pulmonary tuberculosis in pregnancy. *Primary Care Update in Obstetrics and Gynecology, 7*(6), 244–249.

Wald, A., Zef. J., Sleke, S., Warren, T., Ryncarz, A. J., Ashley, R., Krieger, J. N., & Corey, L. (2000). Reactivation of genital herpes simplex virus type 2 infection in asymptomatic seropositive persons. *New England Journal of Medicine, 342*(12), 844–850.

Wang, J. (2000). Trichomoniasis. *Primary Care Update for Obstetricians and Gynecologists, 7*(4), 148–153.

White, M. K., Ory, H. W., & Rooks, J. B. (1980). Intrauterine device termination rates and the menstrual cycle day of insertion. *Obstetrics & Gynecology, 55*, 220–224.

Wilcox, A. J., Dunson, D., & Baird, D. D. (2000). The timing of the "fertile window" in the menstrual cycle: day specific estimates from a prospective study. *British Medical Journal, 321*, 1259–1262.

Wilhelm, J., Morris, D., & Hotham, N. (1990). Epilepsy and pregnancy: A review of 98 pregnancies. *Australia and New Zealand Journal of Obstetrics and Gynecology, 4*, 290.

Williams, M. V., Parker, R. M., Baker, D. W., Parikh, N. S., Pitkin, K., Coates, W. C., & Nurss, J. (1995). Inadequate functional literacy among patients at two public hospitals. *JAMA, 274*(21), 1677–1682.

Wing, D. (1998). Pyelonephritis. *Clinical Obstetrics & Gynecology, 41*(3), 515–526.

Wisner, K. L., Gelenberg, A. J., Leonard, H., Zarin, D., & Frank, E. (1999). Pharmacologic treatment of depression during pregnancy. *JAMA, 282*(13), 1264–1269.

Witlin, A. G., Saade, G. R., Mattar, F., & Sibai, B. M. (1999). Risk factors for abruptio placentae and preeclampsia: Analysis of 445 consecutively managed women with severe preeclampsia and eclampsia. *American Journal of Obstetrics and Gynecology, 180*(6, Part 1), 1322–1329.

Woelk, H., for the Remotiv/Imipramine Study Group, Universitat Giessen, Giessen, Germany. (2000). Comparison of St. John's wort and imipramine for treating depression: Randomised controlled trial. *British Medical Journal, 321*, 536–539.

Wolfe, H. (1998). High prepregnancy body-mass index—A maternal-fetal risk factor. *New England Journal of Medicine, 338*(3), 191–192.

World Health Organization. (1996). *Improving access to quality care in family planning: Medical eligibility criteria for contraceptive use*. Geneva, Switzerland: Author.

World Health Organization. (1997). *Cardiovascular disease and steroid hormone contraception: Report of a WHO scientific group* (WHO Technical Report Series, No. 877). Geneva, Switzerland: Author.

World Health Organization & Joint United Nations Programme on HIV/AIDS. (2000). *The female condom: A guide for planning and programming*. Geneva, Switzerland: World Health Organization.

Ziemer, M. M., Paone, J. P., Schupay, J., & Cole, E. (1990). Methods to prevent and manage nipple pain in breastfeeding women. *Western Journal of Nursing Research, 12,* 732–744.

Zuckerman, A. J. (1995). Occupational exposure to hepatitis B virus and human immunodeficiency virus: A comparative risk analysis. *American Journal of Infection Control, 23*(5), 286–289.

Appendix A

Environmental Exposure History Form

1. Have you ever worked at a job or hobby in which you came in contact with any of the following by breathing, touching, or ingesting (swallowing)? If yes, please place a check beside the name.

☐ Acids
☐ Alcohols (industrial)
☐ Alkalies
☐ Ammonia
☐ Arsenic
☐ Asbestos
☐ Benzene
☐ Beryllium
☐ Cadmium
☐ Carbon tetrachloride
☐ Chlorinated naphthalenes
☐ Chloroform
☐ Chloroprene
☐ Chromates
☐ Coal dust
☐ Dichlorobenzene
☐ Ethylene dibromide
☐ Ethylene dichloride
☐ Fiberglass
☐ Halothane
☐ Isocyanates
☐ Ketones
☐ Lead
☐ Manganese
☐ Mercury
☐ Methylene chloride

☐ Methylene diphenylene diisocyanate (MDI)
☐ Nickel
☐ Perchloroethylene
☐ Pesticides
☐ Phenol
☐ Phosgene
☐ Polybrominated biphenyls (PBBs)
☐ Polychlorinated biphenyls (PCBs)
☐ Radiation
☐ Rock dust
☐ Silica powder
☐ Solvents
☐ Styrene
☐ Talc
☐ Toluene
☐ Toluenediisocyanate (TDI)
☐ Trichloroethylene
☐ Trinitrotoluene
☐ Vinyl chloride
☐ Welding fumes
☐ X-rays
☐ Other (specify)

2. Do you live next to or near an industrial plant, commercial business, dump site, or nonresidential property?

3. Which of the following do you have in your home? Please circle those that apply.

Air conditioner	Air purifier	Central heating
Gas stove	Electric stove (gas or oil?)	Fireplace
Woodstove	Humidifier	

4. Have you recently acquired new furniture or carpet, refinished furniture, or remodeled your home?
5. Have you weatherized your home recently?
6. Are pesticides or herbicides (bug or weed killers; flea and tick sprays, collars, powders, or shampoos) used in your home or garden or on pets?
7. Do you (or any household member) have a hobby or craft?
8. Do you work on your car?
9. Have you ever changed your residence because of a health problem?
10. Does your drinking water come from a private well, city water supply, or grocery store?
11. During approximately what year was your home built?

If you answered *yes* to any of the previous questions, please explain.

From Agency for Toxic Substances and Disease Registry. (1992). *Case studies in environmental medicine: Taking an exposure history.* Atlanta: U.S. Department of Health & Human Services, Public Health Service.)

Appendix B

Guidelines to Responding to a Disclosure of Childhood Sexual Abuse

1. Invite disclosure. Ask appropriate questions and let the survivor know that you are willing to discuss whatever she feels comfortable telling you about her past. Let her set the limits regarding details; if you push details, do so gently.
2. Comment on her courage. It is often very difficult to talk about past abuse and long-held secrets. She was courageous to have survived her past and she is courageous to discuss it now with you. Let her know that you are sorry that she had to go through such things.
3. Try to be calm and matter-of-fact. She does not need a highly emotional response, but she does need accepting, encouraging support.
4. A child is *never* to blame for the abuse, no matter what the circumstances. Emphasize that for her, and be careful of questions that sound blaming. ("Did you tell anyone?")
5. Believe her. Don't try to deny what happened. Survivors can be experts of minimizing or denial. Gently let her know that you think what happened is important, and that you will not participate in her denial. She is a valuable person, and whatever happened to her was not "OK," or "Not so bad."
6. Take time to listen. Don't try to rush her. It may take a long time for her to disclose the details of her abuse. This may happen slowly over many appointments. Respect her ability to set the pace, no matter how long it takes.
7. Have faith in her ability to heal. She really does not know what is her best path to healing, but she may need your help and support in identifying her needs. Ask "Do you know what would help you?" Ask for permission before you offer a hug or a touch.
8. Become an expert in referral. Know the resources in your area and encourage her to seek therapy if she has not already done so. Groups can be especially helpful for survivors. Remember you are not a therapist, but you can be a sensitive support person. Offer her hope.
9. Respect her confidentiality. Never discuss her disclosure with anyone without her permission. Let her know what you are writing in her chart

and why. If she leads you to believe there are other children still at risk for abuse, you are obligated to report this. Discuss with her the necessity of reporting, but do so gently with lots of support.

10. Check in with her periodically to find out how she is doing, what support she might need, and what else is coming up. If she does not want to talk about it, respect that, but don't let the dialogue stop because you are not open to it.

11. Do your own healing work. Your support will come from a stronger place if you have dealt with your own feelings.

(By Christine Heritage, CNM, Cottage Grove, Oregon. Reprinted with permission.)

Appendix C

Guidelines for Pregnancy Management in DES-Exposed Women

Patient Education and Counseling
- Inform (remind) patient of risk associated with DES exposure, regardless of whether cervical, vaginal or uterine changes are present
- Discuss patient concerns
- Provide National Cancer Institute literature about DES

NO PREGNANCY

Contraception
- Issue caution about choosing IUDs due to possible uterine abnormalities
- Possible problems fitting barrier devices if anatomic anomalies exist
- No evidence precludes other contraception options

Preconception Counseling
- Advise to call clinician as soon as pregnancy is suspected
- Inform about increased risk for ectopic pregnancy

POSSIBLE PREGNANCY

Fertility Evaluation Only When Indicated
- Caution with hysterosalpingogram, endometrial biopsy and hysterectomy due to possible anatomic differences (shorter distance between fundus and cervix)
- Laparoscopy interpretation should consider DES abnormalities (internal configuration of uterus may not manifest on external view)
- Caution regarding uterine surgeries (no established treatment to correct typical T-shaped uterus)
- Consider referral to DES expert
- Refer to psychological counseling and support groups as appropriate

Rule out Ectopic Pregnancy
- Pregnancy test as soon as pregnancy is suspected
- Transvaginal ultrasound 6 weeks after LMP (when gestational sac can be detected)
- If ultrasound does not confirm intra-uterine pregnancy, serial beta-HCG every 48 hours until intrauterine pregnancy confirmed by sonography
- If ultrasound confirms intrauterine pregnancy, start prenatal care listed below

UTERINE PREGNANCY

Ectopic Pregnancy
- Consider surgical vs. medical treatment
- Refer for psychological counseling and support groups as appropriate

High-Risk Prenatal Care for All Pregnancies
- Begin digital palpation of cervix at 12 weeks' gestation
- Office visit every 2 weeks during second trimester to evaluate cervix for effacement and dilation
- Office visit every week during third trimester
- Teach signs of premature labor
- Routine cerclage not indicated; perform only for standard indications

Source: the National DES Education Program

387

Appendix D

Sample Prenatal Genetic Screen*

1. Will you be 35 years or older when the baby is due?
2. Have you, the baby's father, or anyone in either of your families ever had any of the following disorders?

   - Down syndrome (mongolism)
   - Other chromosomal abnormality
   - Neural tube defect, i.e., spina bifida (meningomyelocele or open spine), anencephaly
   - Hemophilia
   - Muscular dystrophy
   - Cystic fibrosis

   If yes, indicate the relationship of the affected person to you or to the baby's father:
3. Do you or the baby's father have a birth defect?
   If yes, who has the defect and what is it?
4. In any previous marriages, have you or the baby's father had a child, born dead or alive, with a birth defect not listed in question 2 above?
   If yes, what was the defect and who had it?
5. Do you or the baby's father have any close relatives with mental retardation?
   If yes, indicate the relationship of the affected person to you or to the baby's father:
   Indicate the cause, if known:
6. Do you, the baby's father, or a close relative in either of your families have a birth defect, any familial disorder, or a chromosomal abnormality not listed above?
   If yes, indicate the condition and the relationship of the affected person to you or to the baby's father:
7. In any previous relationships, have you or the baby's father had a stillborn child or three or more first-trimester spontaneous pregnancy losses?
   Have either of you had a chromosomal study?
   If yes, indicate who and the results.

8. If you or the baby's father are of Jewish ancestry, have either of you been screened for Tay-Sachs disease?

   If yes, indicate who and the results.

9. If you or the baby's father are black, have either of you been screened for sickle cell trait?

   If yes, indicate who and the results.

10. If you or the baby's father are of Italian, Greek, or Mediterranean background, have either of you been tested for beta-thalassemia?

    If yes, indicate who and the results.

11. If you or the baby's father are of Philippine or Southeast Asian ancestry, have either of you been tested for alpha-thalassemia?

    If yes, indicate who and the results.

12. Excluding iron and vitamins, have you taken any medications or recreational drugs since being pregnant or since your last menstrual period? (Include nonprescription drugs.)

    If yes, give name of medication and time taken during pregnancy.

*Any patient replying "YES" to questions should be offered appropriate counseling. If the patient declines further counseling or testing, this should be noted in the chart. Given that genetics is a field in a state of flux, alterations or updates to this form will be required periodically.

(Reprinted with permission from American College of Obstetricians and Gynecologists. (1991). *Antenatal diagnosis of genetic disorders* (Technical Bulletin No. 108). Washington, DC: Author.)

Appendix E

Food Guide Pyramids: Guides to Daily Food Choices

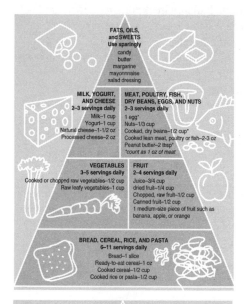

FIGURE 1 Food guide pyramid. (Adapted from National Center for Nutrition and Dietetics; The American Dietetic Association.)

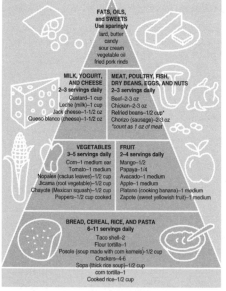

FIGURE 2 Food guide pyramid with popular Mexican fare. (Adapted from National Center for Nutrition and Dietetics; The American Dietetic Association.)

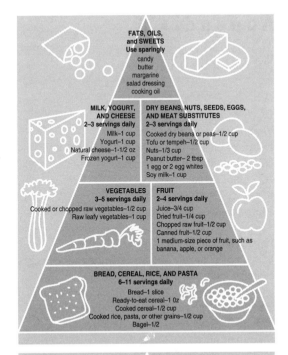

FIGURE 3 Food guide pyramid for vegetarian meal planning. (Adapted from National Center for Nutrition and Dietetics; The American Dietetic Association.)

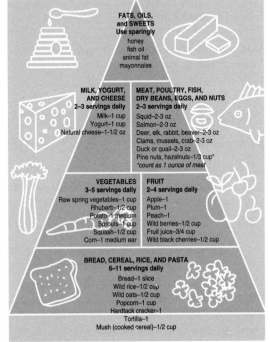

FIGURE 4 Food guide pyramid with popular Native American Fare. (Adapted from National Center for Nutrition and Dietetics; The American Dietetic Association.)

Appendix F

Serving Sizes*

Breads, Cereals, Rice, and Pasta
1 slice of bread
1/2 cup of cooked rice or pasta
1/2 cup of cooked cereal
1 ounce of ready-to-eat cereal
1 large bagel = two to three servings

Vegetables
1/2 cup of nonleafy chopped raw or cooked vegetables
1 cup of leafy raw vegetables

Fruits
1 medium piece of fruit or 1 melon wedge
3/4 cup of juice
1/2 cup of canned fruit
1/4 cup of dried fruit

Milk, Yogurt, and Cheese
1 cup of milk or yogurt
1-1/2 to 2 ounces of cheese

Meat, Poultry, Fish, Dry Beans, Eggs, and Nuts
2 to 3 ounces of cooked lean meat, poultry, or fish
1/2 cup of cooked beans, lentils, pinto beans, kidney beans, or peas
1 egg
2 tablespoons of peanut butter

Fats, Oils, and Sweets
Limit calories from these, especially if you need to lose weight

*The amount you can eat may be more than one serving. For example, a dinner portion of spaghetti would count as two or three servings of pasta.

392

Appendix G

Guidelines for Working
With an Interpreter

1. Meet regularly with the interpreter to keep communications open and facilitate an understanding of the goals and purpose of the interview or counseling session. Certainly you should meet with the interpreter before meeting with the client.

2. Encourage the interpreter to meet with the client before the interview to find out about the client's educational level and attitudes toward health and health care. This information can aid the interpreter in the depth and type of information and explanation that will be needed.

3. Speak in short units of speech—not long, involved sentences or paragraphs. Avoid long, complex discussions of several topics in a single interview.

4. Avoid technical terminology, abbreviations, and professional jargon.

5. Avoid colloquialisms, abstractions, idiomatic expressions, slang, similes, and metaphors.

6. Encourage the interpreter to translate the client's own words as much as possible rather than paraphrasing or "polishing" it into professional jargon. This gives a better sense of the client's concept of what is going on, his or her emotional state, and other important information.

7. Encourage the interpreter to refrain from inserting his or her own ideas or interpretations, or omitting information.

8. To check on the client's understanding and the accuracy of the translation, ask the client to repeat instructions or whatever has been communicated in his or her own words, with the translator facilitating.

9. During the interaction, look at and speak directly to the client, not the interpreter.

10. Listen to the client and watch his or her nonverbal communication. Often you can learn a lot regarding the affective aspects of the client's response by observing facial expressions, voice intonations, and body movements.

11. Be patient. An interpreted interview takes longer. Careful interpretation often requires that the interpreter use long explanatory phrases.

Even if you are using an interpreter, there are ways you can become more actively involved in the communication process.

1. Learn proper forms of address in the client's language. Use of these titles conveys respect for the client and demonstrates your willingness to learn about his or her culture.
2. Learn basic words and sentences of the client's language. Become familiar with special terminology used by clients. Even though you can't speak well enough to communicate directly, the more you understand, the greater the chance you will pick up on misinterpretations and misunderstandings in the interpreter—client interchange.
3. Use a positive tone of voice that conveys your interest in the client. Never be condescending, judgmental, or patronizing.
4. Repeat important information more than once. Always give the reason or purpose for a treatment or prescription.
5. Reinforce verbal interaction with materials written in the client's language and with visual aids.

Nonverbal Communication

Much of what is communicated is not verbalized but conveyed through facial expressions and body movements that are specific to each culture. It is important to understand the cross-cultural variations in order to avoid misunderstandings and unintentional offenses.

Silence. Some cultures are quite comfortable with long periods of silence while others consider it appropriate to speak before the other person has finished talking. Learn about the appropriate use of pauses or interruptions in your client's culture.

Distance. Some cultures are comfortable with close body space, while others are more comfortable at greater distance. In general, Anglo Americans prefer to be about an arm's length away from another person while Hispanics prefer closer proximity and Asians prefer greater distance. Give your client the choice by inviting him or her to "have a seat wherever you like."

Eye contact. Some cultures advise their members to look people straight in the eye while others consider it disrespectful, a sign of hostility or impoliteness. Observe the client when talking and listening to get cues regarding appropriate eye contact.

(From Randall-David, E. (1989). *Strategies for working with culturally diverse communities and clients,* pp. 32–33. Reproduced with permission of The Association for the Care of Children's Health, 7910 Woodmont Ave., Suite 300, Bethesda, MD, 20814)

Appendix H

Body Mass Index Table

TABLE 1 Body Mass Index Table

BMI	19	20	21	22	23	24	25	26	27	28	29	30	31	32	33	34	35	36
Height (inches)	Body weight (pounds)																	
58	91	96	100	105	110	115	119	124	129	134	138	143	148	153	158	162	167	172
59	94	99	104	109	114	119	124	128	133	138	143	148	153	158	163	168	173	178
60	97	102	107	112	118	123	128	133	138	143	148	153	158	163	168	174	179	184
61	100	106	111	116	122	127	132	137	143	148	153	158	164	169	174	180	185	190
62	104	109	115	120	126	131	136	142	147	153	158	164	169	175	180	186	191	196
63	107	113	118	124	130	135	141	146	152	158	163	169	175	180	186	191	197	203
64	110	116	122	128	134	140	145	151	157	163	169	174	180	186	192	197	204	209
65	114	120	126	132	138	144	150	156	162	168	174	180	186	192	198	204	210	216
66	118	124	130	136	142	148	155	161	167	173	179	186	192	198	204	210	216	223
67	121	127	134	140	146	153	159	166	172	178	185	191	198	204	211	217	223	230
68	125	131	138	144	151	158	164	171	177	184	190	197	203	210	216	223	230	236
69	128	135	142	149	155	162	169	176	182	189	196	203	209	216	223	230	236	243
70	132	139	146	153	160	167	174	181	188	195	202	209	216	222	229	236	243	250
71	136	143	150	157	165	172	179	186	193	200	208	215	222	229	236	243	250	257
72	140	147	154	162	169	177	184	191	199	206	213	221	228	235	242	250	258	265
73	144	151	159	166	174	182	189	197	204	212	219	227	235	242	250	257	265	272
74	148	155	163	171	179	186	194	202	210	218	225	233	241	249	256	264	272	280
75	152	160	168	176	184	192	200	208	216	224	232	240	248	256	264	272	279	287
76	156	164	172	180	189	197	205	213	221	230	238	246	254	263	271	279	287	295

Continues

TABLE 1 Body Mass Index Table *(Continued)*

BMI	37	38	39	40	41	42	43	44	45	46	47	48	49	50	51	52	53	54
Height (inches)	Body weight (pounds)																	
58	177	181	186	191	196	201	205	210	215	220	224	229	234	239	244	248	253	258
59	183	188	193	198	203	208	212	217	222	227	232	237	242	247	252	257	262	267
60	189	194	199	204	209	215	220	225	230	235	240	245	250	255	261	266	271	276
61	195	201	206	211	217	222	227	232	238	243	248	254	259	264	269	275	280	285
62	202	207	213	218	224	229	235	240	246	251	256	262	267	273	278	284	289	295
63	208	214	220	225	231	237	242	248	254	259	265	270	278	282	287	293	299	304
64	215	221	227	232	238	244	250	256	262	267	273	279	285	291	296	302	308	314
65	222	228	234	240	246	252	258	264	270	276	282	288	294	300	306	312	318	324
66	229	235	241	247	253	260	266	272	278	284	291	297	303	309	315	322	328	334
67	236	242	249	255	261	268	274	280	287	293	299	306	312	319	325	331	338	344
68	243	249	256	262	269	276	282	289	295	302	308	315	322	328	335	341	348	354
69	250	257	263	270	277	284	291	297	304	311	318	324	331	338	345	351	358	365
70	257	264	271	278	285	292	299	306	313	320	327	334	341	348	355	362	369	376
71	265	272	279	286	293	301	308	315	322	329	338	343	351	358	365	372	379	386
72	272	279	287	294	302	309	316	324	331	338	346	353	361	368	375	383	390	397
73	280	288	295	302	310	318	325	333	340	348	355	363	371	378	386	393	401	408
74	287	295	303	311	319	326	334	342	350	358	365	373	381	389	396	404	412	420
75	295	303	311	319	327	335	343	351	359	367	375	383	391	399	407	415	423	431
76	304	312	320	328	336	344	353	361	369	377	385	394	402	410	418	426	435	443

Calculation of body mass index (BMI) is recommended by the National Heart, Lung, and Blood Institute as a practical means of assessing body fat. Persons with a BMI of 18.5 to 24.9 are considered to be of normal weight. Those with a BMI of 25.0 to 29.9 are overweight. Patients with a BMI of 30.0 to 34.9 or 35.0 to 39.9 are in obesity class I or II, respectively; and those with a BMI of 40 and over are considered extremely obese (obesity class III).

From National Heart, Lung, and Blood Institute (1998). *Clinical guidelines on the identification, evaluation, and treatment of overweight and obesity in adults: The Evidence Report.* Bethesda, MD: National Institutes of Health.

Appendix I

Areas of the World Where Female Circumcision is Found

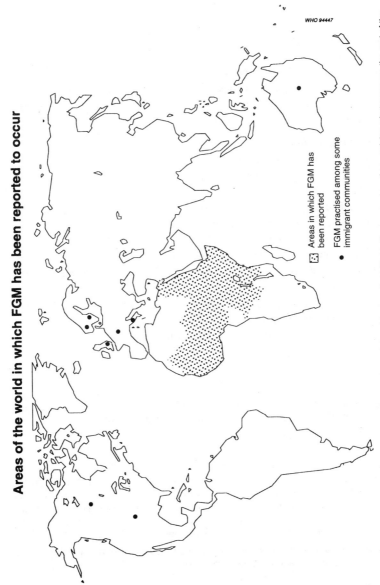

Areas of the world in which FGM has been reported to occur

WHO 94447

⬚ Areas in which FGM has been reported

• FGM practised among some immigrant communities

The designations employed and the presentation of material on this map do not imply the expression of any opinion whatsoever on the part of the World Health Organization concerning the legal status of any country, territory, city or area or of its authorities, or concerning the delimitation of its frontiers or boundaries. Information on the map is based mainly on partial and incomplete data.

Appendix J

Criteria for Tuberculin Positivity by Risk Group*

≥5 mm of induration*
HIV-seropositive persons
Recent contacts of clients with active TB[†]
Clients with fibrotic changes on chest radiograph consistent with healed TB
Organ transplant recipients and other immunosuppressed persons (receiving the equivalent of ≥15 mg/d of prednisone for 1 month or more)

≥10 mm of induration
Injection drug users (HIV-seronegative)
Recent immigrants (within the last 5 years) from countries with high TB prevalence
Residents and employees[‡] in high-risk settings, such as prisons, long-term care facilities, hospitals, homeless shelters
Mycobacteriology laboratory personnel
Persons with diabetes mellitus; chronic renal failure; leukemias; lymphomas; weight loss ≥10% of ideal body weight; carcinoma of the head, neck, or lung; or silicosis
Persons with a history of gastrectomy or jejunoileal bypass
Children younger than 4 years
Children and adolescents exposed to adults at high risk

≥15 mm of induration[§]
Persons with no risk factors for TB

*Adapted from The American Thoracic Society & the Centers for Disease Control and Prevention. (2000). Targeted tuberculin testing and treatment of latent tuberculosis infection *MMWR, 49,* 1–54.

[†]TB, tuberculosis.

[‡]Measure induration transverse to the long axis of the forearm. Place the tip of a ballpoint pen about 2 cm from the edge to the wheal caused by the PPD. Draw a line toward the wheal. Use enough pressure to slightly indent the skin. This causes the pen to stop at the edge of induration. Repeat the procedure with the ballpoint pen on the opposite side of the wheal. Measure the distance in millimeters across the wheal from the inside ends of the two lines (where the pen stopped on each side of the wheal).

[§]For persons who are otherwise at low risk and are tested at the start of employment, a reaction =15 mm of induration is considered positive.

Appendix K

Normal Laboratory Values in Pregnancy

Test	Norms	Comments
Antibody screen	Negative	Tests for "irregular" antibodies as well as Rh antibodies. Remember, "Kell kills, Lewis lives."
Blood type	Any type is within normal	Blood type is not necessary if typing has been done previously at the institution. Typing errors are common. Consequently, institutions prefer two tests, each giving the same results.
Chlamydia	Negative	
Ferritin	10 to 300 ng/mL	<20 indicates iron deficiency anemia, >100 ng/mL is not usually caused by iron deficiency
Glucose tolerance test: a. (1-hr, 50-g load)	<140 mg/dL	This is the screening test. Results determine whether to order the 3-hr, 100-g test for a definitive diagnosis. Some institutions use lower limits (usually 130 or 135 mg/dL) as the threshold for ordering the 3-hr test.
		Some institutions defer the 3-hr test if the 1-hr glucose test is >182 mg/dL because of a 95% chance the 3-hr test will be positive. Others prefer not to label women with GDM unless a true diagnosis is present.
b. (3-hr, 100-g load)	Fasting: <105 mg/dL 1 hour: <190 mg/dL 2 hours: <165 mg/dL 3 hours: <145 mg/dL	Two abnormal values on the 3-hr, 100-g GTT diagnose gestational diabetes. Some institutions use lower limits for the fasting blood sugar.

(Continued)

Test	Norms	Comments
Gonorrhea	Negative	
Group B beta-hemolytic strepto-cocci (S. agalactiae)	Negative	Positive vaginal cultures as well as positive urine cultures require IV antibiotics in labor.
Hematocrit	First trimester: >33% Second trimester: >32% Third trimester: >33%	Guidelines from the Institute of Medicine, 1992.
Hemoglobin electrophoresis	Hemoglobin A: 95% to 98% Hemoglobin A_2: 1.5% to 3.5% Hemoglobin F: <2%	Used to diagnose sickle cell anemias (Hb S) and other hemoglobinopathies
Hepatitis B surface antigen	Negative	+ HB_sAg is the earliest marker of acute infection. When present after 6 months, it indicates chronic persistent or active hepatitis.
	If positive, order hepatitis B e antigen (HB_eAg)	+ HB_eAg = high levels of virus; more likely to transmit virus than women who are HB_sAg-positive but negative for HB_eAg. Infants of these mothers are more likely to become chronic carriers than infants with mothers who are HB_eAg-negative.
HIV	Negative	
Indices (red blood cell)	MCV: 80 fL to 100 fL	MCV <80 = microcytic anemia MCV >80 = macrocytic anemia (consider B_{12} or folate deficiency, liver disease, or hypothyroidism) MCV in the 60s may indicate a hemoglobinopathy.
	MCH: >27% MCHC: 31 to 36 g/dL	
Platelets	150,000 to 400,000 cells/mL	Gestational thrombo-cytopenic purpura is usually the most common cause of low platelets in pregnancy and is usually benign—counts do not usually fall below 70,000/μL; counts <70,000/μL are probably caused by idiopathic thrombocytopenic purpura (ITP). No treatment is usually initiated until the count is <50,000/μL. Watch for preeclampsia or the HELLP syndrome if platelets are <100,000/μL.

Test	Norms	Comments
PPD (Mantoux)	Read in 48 to 72 hours, but positive reactions may still be measurable up to 1 week after testing. Only induration is significant, not redness.	**Criteria for Determining a Positive TB Skin Test*** 1. Positive if induration of 5 mm or more and one of these: a. Close, recent contact b. X-ray suggesting old, healed lesion c. Known or suspected HIV infection d. Intravenous drug user (if HIV status unknown) 2. Positive if induration of 10 mm or more and one of these: a. Risk factors that increase TB risk (excluding HIV) b. Birth in high-prevalence area (Asia, Africa, Latin America) c. Poor medical care, low income, and especially African American, Hispanic, and Native American ancestry d. Intravenous drug user (if HIV-negative) e. Member of locally identified high-prevalence groups
Preeclampsia	Creatinine: <0.9 mg/dL Uric acid: <5.4 mg/dL at term AST: <40 U/L Hematocrit: <38% Platelets: >150,000 cells/μL 24-hour urine: <300 mg	Old guidelines defined severe preeclampsia as between 300 mg and 5 g of protein in a 24-hour urine specimen. New NIH guidelines suggest that greater than 2 g should be considered severe. These guidelines also delete blood urea nitrogen (BUN) level as one of the lab tests for preeclampsia.
Quad screen	The quad screen tests for inhibin A in addition to triple screen markers. It improves the pickup rate for Down syndrome from about 66% to about 75%; a 5% false-positive rate exists.	The quad screen will probably replace the triple screen in the next 5 years.

(Continued)

Test	Norms	Comments
Rh factor	A positive result is preferred so there will be no concern about harm to the baby	
Rubella titer	>1:10 = immunity	If the client is nonimmune, counsel her about avoiding infectious individuals and the need for postpartum immunization.
Sickle cell screen		This test only identifies Hb S and will not identify Hb C or beta-thalassemia trait.
Syphilis (RPR or VDRL)	Negative	Both the RPR and VDRL are nontreponemal tests, meaning a more specific test is required for diagnosis. The next test is the FTA-ABS fluorescent treponema antibody screen.
Thyroid screening: TSH	0.23 to 4.00 μIU/mL	TSH is a good screening test for both hypothyroidism and hyperthyroidism (increased in hypothyroidism and decreased in hyperthyroidism). Follow an abnormal value with a free T4 test.
Triple screen (uses three analytes to screen for neural tube defects, Down syndrome, and trisomy 18); it was called the AFP test or MSAFP test when only AFP was analyzed.	Within normal limits	Screening test only Open NTDs: Elevated MSAFP Down syndrome: low MSAFP, high hCG, and low uE3 Trisomy 18: low MSAFP, low hCG, low uE3
Ultrasound	Nuchal translucency: varies depending on gestational age; nomograms still being constructed; <3 mm considered normal until nomograms are available	Identifying nuchal translucency at 11 to 14 weeks picks up 65% of Downs, although the detection rate varies depending on the expertise of the sonographer and whether the radiology department uses an absolute cutoff or multiples of the median (MoMs)
	Nuchal fold: 6 mm or more	

Test	Norms	Comments
		Gestational age guidelines for accuracy:
		6 to 12 weeks: ± 3 days
		12 to 20 weeks: ± 7 days
		20 to 32 weeks: ± 1.5 weeks
		32+ weeks: ± 2.5 weeks
		Anomaly screen done at 18 to 22 weeks
		"Serial" ultrasounds are performed at 2- to 3-week intervals to follow growth when IUGR is suspected
Urine culture	Negative	Needs colony count of >100,000, unless the organism is *Proteus* or *Klebsiella*, in which case treat with colony count <100,000
		Common contaminants: diphtheroids, lactobacilli, alpha-hemolytic streptococci; mixed flora—even 100,000 colonies usually mean contamination
Urine drug screen	Negative	The length of time that an illicit drug can be found in urine depends on the dose, the size of the person, activity level of the person, concentration of the urine specimen, and whether the drug is fat soluble. Generally, figure the drug was consumed in the last 28 hours, except for fat-soluble marijuana, which can be found in the urine for 7 days and longer than 7 days in a chronic user.
Urine protein (24-hour measurement)	<300 mg in 24 hours	300 mg to 5 g = mild preeclampsia >5 g = severe preeclampsia

Appendix L

Medicolegal and Administrative Guidelines for Using E-mail in a Clinical Setting

Consider obtaining patient's informed consent for use of e-mail. Written forms should:
Itemize terms in Communication Guidelines.
Provide instructions for when and how to escalate to phone calls and office visits.
Describe security mechanisms in place.
Indemnify the health care institution for information loss due to technical failures.
Waive encryption requirement, if any, at patient's insistence.
Use password-protected screen savers for all desktop workstations in the office, hospital, and at home.
Never forward patient-identifiable information to a third party without the patient's express permission.
Never use patient's e-mail address in a marketing scheme.
Do not share professional e-mail accounts with family members.
Use encryption for all messages when encryption technology becomes widely available, user-friendly, and practical.
Do not use unencrypted wireless communications with patient-identifiable information.
Double-check all "To:" fields prior to sending messages.
Perform at least weekly backups of mail onto long-term storage. Define "long-term" as the term applicable to paper records.
Commit policy decisions to writing and electronic form.

(From Kane, B., & Sands, D.Z. (1998). Guidelines for the clinical use of electronic mail with patients. *Journal of the American Medical Informatics Association, 5*(1), p. 106. Used with permission.)

Appendix M

Long Chart Review Guide

Long Chart Review Guide

Perform the following steps before the client arrives:

1. Have a blank piece of paper at your side. As you review the client's record, write down the information you wish to obtain at this visit. There will be topics you wish to pursue, clarify, or expand. If you find your questions are answered with further record review, it is easy to cross off list items. If you write your questions, you will be organized, efficient, and thorough during the prenatal visit.

2. Review demographic data and social history.
   a. Note the client's age. Does it put her in a high-risk group? Should special testing be discussed?
   b. Does she seem to have social support?
   c. What are the stressors in her life?
   d. Is intimate partner violence occurring? Is there any history of emotional or sexual abuse?
   e. How many hours per week is she working for pay? What are the working conditions?

3. Review obstetric dating data and conclusions. (Consider everything.)
   a. Last menstrual period (LMP) (certain/uncertain) with estimated date of birth (EDB) by Nägele's rule (not with the "wheel")
   b. Length, frequency, and regularity of menstrual cycles
   c. Dates, results, and kinds of pregnancy tests
   d. Hormonal contraception prior to conception: kind and date of last use
   e. Date of quickening (usually 16 to 20 weeks in a primipara or multipara and 18 to 20 weeks in a primigravida)
   f. Uterus at the umbilicus (usually at 20 weeks, despite the fact that the length of the abdomen can vary by several inches from one woman to another)
   g. Fetal heart tones (FHTs)
      1). Doppler FHTs commonly heard at 10 to 12 weeks and sometimes as early as 8 weeks

405

        2). Fetoscope FHTs commonly heard at 18 to 20 weeks and sometimes at 17 weeks

    h. Sonographic information

        1). 6 to 12 weeks: +/− 3 days

        2). 12 to 20 weeks: +/− 7 days

        3). 20 to 24 weeks: +/− 12 days

        4). 24 to 30 weeks: +/− 15 days

        5). 32+ weeks: +/− 2.5 days

4. Review the obstetric history.

    a. Is any information missing?

    b. Is any complication likely to recur? If yes, has this information been placed on a problem list?

    c. Have possible emotional sequelae of selected outcomes been addressed (such as early pregnancy loss—miscarriage or elective abortion, cesarean birth, difficult labor, stillbirth)?

5. Review the family history.

    a. Are there any inheritable disorders (including those that might result from ethnicity)? If yes, has counseling been offered, scheduled, or completed?

    b. Is there any drug or alcohol use by family members?

    c. Is there any mental illness in the family? If yes, has a clinician inquired on the effect this might have had on the client? (This is not commonly done.)

    d. Is the client the daughter of a mother who took diethylstilbestrol (DES) when pregnant?

    e. Has her mother or a sister had severe preeclampsia?

    f. Is any information missing?

    g. Is any necessary follow-up completed or in progress?

6. Review the client's medical history.

    a. Is there any chronic illness?

    b. Are there any illnesses that might affect the baby or be exacerbated by pregnancy?

    c. Have any pertinent laboratory tests been ordered?

    d. Is any information missing?

    e. Has any necessary follow-up been completed, or is it in progress, such as copies of records from previous health care providers?

7. Note drug, alcohol, and cigarette history.

    If yes, inquire about current use.

    If the client smokes,

    a. Has a note been made about interest in cutting down or quitting?

    b. Has stage of readiness to quit been established?

    c. Has use of the five "A's" been documented?

d. Have any referrals been made?

e. Is the client involved in a smoking-cessation program?

f. Is the client's chart marked with a smoking sticker?

If the client has quit smoking recently,

a. Is her chart marked with a former smoker sticker?

b. Does her record indicate she has been having strong or prolonged withdrawal symptoms?

c. Does her record indicate she has good support for quitting?

d. What kind of social support has been identified?

e. If previous drug use has been identified, is a urine drug screen indicated today?

8. Review initial physical examination findings.

a. In addition to noting possible problems, you will occasionally find that the physical examination has not been done or has been only partially done.

b. Note abnormal findings:

1). Heart murmur of 3/6 or more

2). Pulse greater than 110 bpm

3). Cervical length <1 cm on pelvic exam

4). Any cervical dilatation before 28 weeks

c. Note normal findings:

1). A slightly enlarged thyroid gland

2). A grade 1/6 or 2/6 systolic murmur

3). 4+ reflexes

d. Have appropriate follow-up tests or referrals been done for abnormal findings?

9. Note body mass index (BMI).

a. Has BMI been determined?

b. Have weight gain recommendations been documented?

10. Review all test results.

a. Have all routine labs tests been done?

b. Are all findings within normal limits? Be sure to attend to all findings from the test (such as mean corpuscular volume [MCV], mean corpuscular hemoglobin [MCH], and mean corpuscular hemoglobin concentration [MCHC] on a complete blood count; placental localization; amniotic fluid volume; structural findings; and recommendations for follow-up as well as gestational age on a sonogram).

c. Has appropriate follow-up been done for any abnormal results?

d. If the client is obese, was a 1-hr glucose screen done at the initial visit?

e. Does gestational age today mean additional tests might be indicated (such as a triple screen between 15 and 20 weeks or a 1-hour glucose screen at 28 weeks)?

f. Has refusal of any recommended test been documented?

g. Are results available for any tests requested at the last visit?

11. Review the problem list.

a. Is it accurate?

b. Is it complete?

12. Review progress notes for previously noted concerns, complaints, or discomforts and any treatment recommended.

a. Have symptoms been relieved with suggested remedies?

b. If time for review of the record is limited, review the notes from the initial visit and the last visit. Note the plan identified at the most recent visit.

13. Review *Important Data and Key Moments in Prenatal Care* in Table 7-1. This guide summarizes data that should be obtained at a variety of gestational ages. It also suggests times for introducing health education topics. Note the suggested actions for today's gestational age.

Appendix N

Short Chart Review Guide and Conduct of an Antepartum Visit

Before today's data are obtained:

1. Have paper to make notes.
2. Review social history.
3. Review dating data.
    Nägele's rule
    Menstrual cycle frequency and duration
    Recent use of hormonal contraception
    Pregnancy test: when and results
    Fetal heart tones (FHTs):
    Doppler: (10 to 12 weeks)
    Fetoscope: (18 to 20 weeks)
    Quickening: (16 to 20 weeks)
    Uterus at umbilicus: (20 weeks)
    Ultrasound: 6 to 12 weeks: +/− 3 days
              12 to 20 weeks: +/− 7 days
              20 to 32 weeks: +/− 1.5 weeks
              > 32 weeks: +/− 2.5 weeks
4. Review the obstetric history.
5. Review the family history.
6. Review the client's medical history.
7. Review the client's drug, alcohol, and cigarette history.
8. Note any history of abuse.
9. Review the initial physical examination findings.
10. Note the client's body mass index and recommended weight gain.
11. Review all lab results.
12. Review the problem list.
13. Note any medicines being taken.
14. Review previous progress notes.

After today's data are obtained:

1. Note blood pressure (BP), urine tests, and weight.
2. Review the revisit questionnaire in Appendix O.
3. Review the information in Table 7-1, *Important Data and Key Moments in Prenatal Care.*
4. Enter the examining room with your paper from the chart review.
   a. Greet everyone, try social talk, and answer any questions from anyone.
   b. Ask questions from the chart review.
   c. Share new test results, as appropriate, with others in the room.
   d. Comment on today's BP, urine, and weight.
   e. Ask questions generated from the revisit questionnaire or ask Healthy Pregnancy Questions.
   f. Ask if the client is taking daily prenatal vitamins or iron tablets.
5. Conduct your examination.
   a. Fundal height and estimated fetal weight
   b. FHTs
   c. Presentation when >34 weeks
6. Offer tummy drawing.
7. Present health education (less is more)
   a. "Magic numbers" for preterm labor and fetal movement.
   b. Pertinent danger signs
8. Discuss plan.
9. Discuss next visit.

(U.S. Public Health Service traditional guidelines)

Antepartum Revisit Form for Patients to Complete

1. Since your last visit have you had:

___ Headaches

___ Problems with your eyes (blurred vision, blind spots, flashing lights or lines)

___ Swelling of your   ___ face   ___ hands   ___ legs   ___ feet

___ Pain in your   ___ chest   ___ back   ___ legs   ___ abdomen

___ Problems with urination (peeing) such as
    ___ burning   ___ leaking urine
    ___ not being able to wait   ___ pain
    to use the toilet

___ Bleeding or spotting from your vagina (birth canal)

___ Leaking fluid from your vagina (water from the bag of waters)

___ Vaginal discharge:
    ___ burning   ___ itching
    ___ change in the discharge   ___ bad smell to discharge
    ___ increase in amount

___ Sores or growths in the genital area (private parts)

___ Illnesses or fever

___ Exposure to children or adults who were sick with an infection

___ Skin rashes or itching

___ Signs of labor such as
    ___ contractions   ___ cramping
    ___ pelvic pressure   ___ low backache

___ Accidents or falls *or* being hit, pushed, shoved, beaten by someone (even if it was just one time)

___ Changes in the way the baby moves

___ Cravings for anything to eat or to smell

___ Visits to another doctor, nurse, clinic, emergency room, or hospital

2. Please write the names of any medicines you have used. Include prescription medicines, over-the-counter medicines, prenatal vitamins, and iron tablets. _____

3. Write the names of any plants, herbs, or herbal teas you have used to help you feel better or treat an illness. _____

4. Write the names of any street or recreational drugs you have used.

_____

_____

5. What alcoholic drinks have you had since your last visit?

_____

_____

6. How many packs of cigarettes have you smoked each day? _____

7. Do you need any   ___ prenatal vitamins   ___ iron tablets
                ___ any other medicines?

8. There are many common discomforts of pregnancy. If there is a particular
one that is bothering you or you want information, help, or suggestions for
how to work with or relieve the discomfort, please place a mark below. If
none of these worry or bother you, skip this section.

___ Nausea (feeling sick to your stomach)
___ Vomiting (throwing up)
___ Diarrhea
___ Constipation
___ Hemorrhoids
___ Not feeling hungry
___ Heartburn
___ Breast tenderness
___ Varicose veins
___ Trouble sleeping
___ Shortness of breath
___ Numbness or tingling of hands or legs or feet
___ Tired all the time (fatigue)
___ Leg cramps
___ Sciatica (sharp pains down your leg)
___ Backache
___ Heart jumping, skipping, or beating very fast
___ Sadness or crying for "no reason"
___ Unusual or intense dreams
___ Changes in desire for sex or way sex feels
___ Anger or irritability
___ Heart skipping or pounding
___ Any other concern not in this list

9. On a scale of 1 (awful) to 10 (wonderful), how are you doing right now?
___ If things are not so good, what would help?

10. Please tell us about anything else that is worrying you or about any
information you want to convey.

(From a tool devised by Linda Glenn, CNM, Portland, Oregon, based on the Healthy
Pregnancy Questions)

Appendix O

Models for Drawing on the Maternal Abdomen

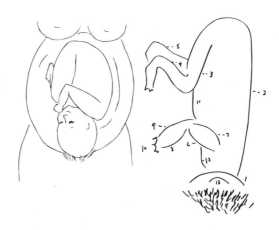

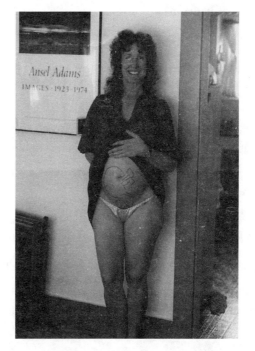

Appendix P

Guidelines for Selecting Printed Material

Organization

1. Is the cover attractive?
2. Are desired behavior changes stressed?
3. Are there no more than three or four main points?
4. Are headers and summaries used to show organization and provide message repetition?
5. Is a summary that stresses what to do included?

Writing Style

6. Is the text conversational in style? Is active voice used? Is the tone friendly?
7. Is technical jargon limited?

Appearance

8. Do the pages appear uncluttered? Are there ample white spaces?
9. Are lowercase letters used (capitals only where grammatically needed)?
10. Is there a high degree of contrast between the print and the paper?
11. Is the print size at least 12 point, serif type, without stylized letters?
12. Are the illustrations simple (preferably line drawings)? When body parts are illustrated, are they placed within the context of the entire body?
13. Do the illustrations amplify the text?

Appeal

14. Is the material culturally, gender, and age appropriate?
15. Does the material closely match the logic, language, and experience of the intended audience?
16. Is interaction invited via questions, responses, suggested action, etc.?

(Reprinted with permission from Doak, C. C., Doak, L. G., & Root, J. H. (1996). *Teaching patients with low literacy skills.* Philadelphia: J.B. Lippincott, p. 43.)

Appendix Q

Recommendations for Reducing the Risk of SIDS

1. Place infants in a nonprone position for sleep.
2. Use cribs that conform to the standards of the Consumer Product Safety Division.
3. Do not put infants to sleep on water beds or other soft surfaces.
4. Do not place pillows, quilts, comforters, or sheepskins under a sleeping baby.
5. Keep soft gas-trapping objects such as pillows, quilts, comforters, sheepskins, and stuffed toys away from the infant's place of sleep.
6. Avoid loose blankets and sheets. Instead, use sleep clothing without other coverings or tuck blankets around the crib mattress with the blankets reaching only to the baby's chest and the baby's feet at the foot of the crib.
7. Avoid entrapment possibilities by moving the bed away from walls and other furniture. Remember the potential dangers of headboards and footboards.
8. Avoid sharing the adult bed with other siblings when the baby is in the bed.
9. Do not smoke or use alcohol or drugs that might contribute to overlying the baby or interfere with responding to the baby.
10. Keep the baby lightly clothed during sleep.

(From the American Academy of Pediatrics, 2000.)

Appendix R

IUD Charting Form

Insertion of Paragard IUD

Pamphlet reviewed with client

_____ Failure = 1 in 200

_____ Complications: uterine perforation, severe pelvic infection

_____ Side effects: heavy menses, dysmenorrhea, irregular spotting initially

_____ Danger signs: fever/chills, abdominal pain/severe cramps, heavy bleeding

_____ Expulsion

_____ If pregnancy occurs, notify health care provider immediately for removal (30% chance of abortion with or without removal, but infection danger if left)

_____ Consent form signed

Allergies: Yes   No

           _____ _____ Drugs

           _____ _____ Copper

           _____ _____ Iodine

Medications:

           Yes   No

           _____ _____ Ibuprofen 800 mg: Time _____

           _____ _____ Doxycycline 100 mg: Time _____

Pelvic exam

   Uterus: _____ Anteverted   _____ Midline   _____ Retroverted

           _____ Anteflexed   _____ Retroflexed

   Vaginal discharge: Vaginal _____ Yes _____ No _____ Wet smear

                  Cervical _____ Yes _____ No

Procedure

_____ Lidocaine gel to cervix

Tenaculum applied at _____ and _____

Uterus sounded to _____ cm

_____ ParaGard TCu380 A inserted using withdrawal technique with/without difficulty

416

Bleeding

     _____ None

     _____ Right side, controlled with pressure

     _____ Left side, controlled with pressure

Client tolerated the procedure: _____ Well _____ Poorly _____ Other

     Comment:

Threads cut to approximately _____ cm in length

Counseling

1. _____ Check strings after every menses (Other: _____)
2. Call if:

     _____ Fever/chills, abdominal pain/severe cramps, bad-smelling discharge

     _____ Heavy bleeding

     _____ Signs or symptoms of pregnancy

3. _____ Ibuprofen (maximum of 2400 mg/day) for cramping and/or bleeding
4. _____ No tampons for 24 hours
5. _____ Removal date: _____
6. _____ Able to feel strings
7. _____ Return appointment: _____

Appendix S

Postpartum Client History Form

1. Please check if you are having problems with any of the following:
   _____ Bleeding
   _____ Pain
   _____ Vaginal discharge
   _____ Tiredness
   _____ Urine, gas, or bowel movement control
   _____ Burning when urinating (peeing)
   _____ Pain when having sex
2. Please check how often you find yourself (not often, pretty often, very often):
   _____ Irritable
   _____ Crying
   _____ Not able to sleep
   _____ Overwhelmed
   _____ Happy
   _____ Sad
   _____ Depressed
   _____ Exhausted
   _____ Scared
   _____ Excited
   _____ Tired
   _____ Not eating well
   _____ Content
   _____ Hard to get along with
   _____ Angry
   _____ Worried
   _____ Anxious
3. On a scale of 1 to 10, with 1 being awful and 10 being wonderful, how do you think things are going with your partner?
4. On a scale of 1 to 10, how do you think things are going with you and the baby?

5. On a scale of 1 to 10, how do you think things are going with your partner and the baby?

6. Please rate how easy you think it is to take care of your baby. Let 1 be very difficult and 10 be very easy.

7. What is most helpful to you now?

8. In what area would you like to have more help?

9. What is hardest for you now?

10. Please check the things that are most stressful for you right now.

    _____ Difficult baby
    _____ Relationship with partner
    _____ Relationship with family
    _____ Money
    _____ Housing
    _____ Child care
    _____ Breastfeeding
    _____ Returning to work
    _____ Getting pregnant
    _____ My weight
    _____ Having sex
    _____ Feelings about the labor or birth
    _____ Other things

11. When you left the hospital, how were you feeding the baby?

    _____ Breastfeeding
    _____ Bottle-feeding

    How are you feeding the baby now?

    _____ Breast
    _____ Bottle

12. If you have had sex since the baby was born, please answer the following questions.

    Have you had a new sex partner since the baby was born? _____
    Did you have any pain? _____
    Were you ready to have sex? _____
    Did you have any problems with feeling dry? _____
    Did you notice any difference having sex now compared to having sex before you got pregnant? _____
    Has your partner said anything about sex being different? _____

13. What are you using or planning to use for birth control? Why is this a good method for you?

14. What medicine have you taken since the baby was born?

15. Have you made any visits to an emergency room or clinic for something other than a regular checkup since the baby was born?

16. Are you smoking?

17. Have you drunk any alcohol since the baby was born?

18. Please list any drugs you have had since the baby was born (including marijuana).

19. Are you working or planning to work for pay?

20. Please check if you would like information about any of the following.

    _____ Parenting an infant
    _____ Parenting children of other ages
    _____ Weight-loss ideas
    _____ Drug and alcohol programs
    _____ Stop-smoking programs
    _____ Anger-control programs
    _____ Support groups for women who have been abused
    _____ Counseling
    _____ Something else

21. What questions would you like to have answered today?

Appendix T

Suggestions for Discussing Condom Use With a Man

Talk about using condoms ahead of time. This may be both difficult and awkward, but it is better than bringing up the subject in the heat of lovemaking. The best-case scenario would be a grateful partner who is delighted that someone else brought up the subject. The next-best scenario is a partner who is not quite delighted but who is ready to listen. You can emphasize:

a. You are showing respect for him by not wanting to take any chances.
b. He has a chance to show respect for you.
c. This is new sex, not second-class sex. Condoms don't have to be unpleasant—they can be fun, erotic, and playful.
d. He should think of the condom as part of lovemaking rather than an interruption or bother.

The worst-case scenario is a partner who thinks safer sex is unnecessary and says, "I'm not gonna use no condom," "I don't need a condom," or "You gotta be crazy." Imagine that you are in this situation. What could you say in response?

You might buy different kinds of condoms ahead of time or visit clinics that hand them out free. Invite a friend to go with you if you are embarrassed. Invite your partner to go with you. Set aside some time to play with them to find out which kind would work best. Be aware that condoms available without cost often do not contain nonoxynol 9 (discussed later). Here is some information that might be helpful:

Size
While condoms are very elastic (try blowing one up) and adjust to a variety of penis sizes, there are a few brands for men with smaller or larger penises. If one brand does not fit, try another.

Lubrication
Some condoms are lubricated and some are not. Lubricated condoms are thought to be less likely to break. Unfortunately, lubricated condoms often

have a strong rubber taste and are, therefore, not suitable for oral sex. Lubricated condoms may be coated with a chemical known as nonoxynol 9. It provides extra protection against the AIDS virus, but some people are allergic to it. Use a condom coated with nonoxynol 9 if you can. This ingredient is listed on the outside of the condom package when present.

Use a water-soluble lubricant such as Astro glide if you need more lubrication on the condom. If you use other lubricants such as Vaseline, baby oil, Nivea Cream, hand lotion, massage oil, or Crisco, the condom is more likely to break.

The condom's tip
Condoms come with or without a tip to hold the semen (cum). Some people who like oral sex don't like the tip. Others don't mind it. Condoms with a tip on the end are less likely to break than those without a tip. If you use a condom without a tip, leave a 1/4-inch space at the end of the condom as it goes onto the penis. This leaves space for the cum when the man ejaculates. When you put on a condom, squeeze the tip or the 1/4-inch space at the end, so that no air is left in the condom. Friction can make the bubble pop.

Thickness
The thicker the condom, the less likely it is to break. But the thicker it is, the less feeling there is. Experiment to find which one is right for you. Thin is usually good for oral sex, but remember that anal sex increases the chances that a condom will break. Thicker is better—at least it is safer.

Special Features
Condoms come in different colors, and some even glow in the dark. Some are ribbed to provide extra feeling, and some are flavored with mint or fruit, including wild strawberry, to taste good. Flavored condoms may also contain nonoxynol 9.

Storage
Condoms often come with an expiration date. Don't confuse it with the date of manufacture. High temperatures can cause the condom to break. Avoid putting condoms in the glove compartment of your car on a hot day or in direct sunlight. You may have heard you shouldn't keep them in your wallet. But a recent study showed no increase in breakage after carrying the condom in a wallet for a long time. Although they may not be ideal, wallets, shoes, and the inside of a bra can be acceptable places for a condom.

Other Helpful Information
Use latex condoms rather than sheepskin condoms. Latex condoms are cheaper, protect against the AIDS virus, and are less likely to break.

If you know you are going to have sex, loosen the wrapping on the condom as you go to bed (if you have sex in bed) to avoid fumbling at an inopportune time. Use each condom one time only. Open the condom carefully. Tearing or long fingernails can damage it. Don't test it by stretching or inflating it.

Leave a paper towel and wastebasket by your bed. Put the used condom on the paper towel when you are finished with it. Later, put it in the wastebasket. Do not flush the condom down the toilet.

Leave a damp cloth and a towel by the bed. The cloth can wipe off any lubricant if oral sex is desired and you are not using a flavored condom. Later, the damp cloth can be used to freshen up each other.

Talking about condoms can lead to a better communication about sex in general. If you are new to using condoms, some suggest waiting until you are close to coming before you put the condom on. If you do this, be sure to keep the penis away from the vagina, because the precum may contain HIV and sperm. Squeeze the air out of the tip of the condom if it is the kind with the tip. If the condom does not have a tip, squeeze about 1/4 inch of the blunt end so that there will be space for the cum.

Uncircumcised men (or their partners) should pull back the foreskin before putting on the condom.

Check the condom periodically to make sure it is on.

If you are going to have oral sex and the condom is not flavored, wipe it off with a damp washcloth after putting it on. Experiment with different brands to find the one that is least objectionable or get a kind with a flavor you find pleasant.

If you are going to have anal sex, use lots of water-based lubricant and don't let the condom dry out. It might break.

After coming, pull the penis and condom out before your partner has lost his erection. Have your partner hold on to the base of the penis as it comes out so that the condom does not come off and semen does not spill out of the condom.

Appendix U

Instructions for Taking Calcium Supplements

Calcium Supplements

1. Check the label to identify the amount of elemental calcium in each tablet. Women between the ages of 19 and 50, whether or not they are pregnant or breastfeeding, need 1000 mg of elemental calcium each day. Girls in the child-bearing years under age 19 need 1300 mg of elemental calcium each day.
2. Take your calcium supplement with meals.
3. Take your supplement in divided doses, that is, with one or two of your meals each day, because the body can only absorb a certain amount of calcium at one time.
4. Keep your supplement in more than one place so that it will be easy to find.
5. Compare the price of several products, including the house labels of supermarkets.
6. To decrease your chance of having side effects such as constipation or gas when you first start your supplement, build up calcium intake gradually. Change the kind of calcium you are using if side effects continue.
7. Don't worry about getting too much calcium. Your body gets rid of any extra calcium in urine and stool.

Nutritional Sources of Calcium

1. Don't forget food sources of calcium. Good sources are dairy products, dried beans, and green, leafy vegetables. Here are some calcium-containing foods:

Food	Calcium
1 cup fat-free yogurt	450 mg
1 cup skim milk	300 mg
½ cup firm tofu	260 mg
6 oz fortified orange juice	200 mg
1 oz cheddar cheese	200 mg
½ cup collard greens	180 mg
½ cup pinto beans	45 mg
½ cup broccoli	45 mg
1 tortilla	42 mg

2. Try boosting your calcium intake by adding nonfat dry milk to recipes that use liquid milk.
3. Buy calcium-fortified orange juice and cereal.

Index

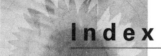

Note: Page numbers follows by *f* refer to figures; page numbers followed by *t* refer to tables; page numbers followed by *b* refer to text in boxes